Handbook of Nutrition and the Kidney

Third Edition

Handbook of Nutrition and the Kidney

Third Edition

Editors

William E. Mitch, M.D.
Garland Herndon Professor of Medicine
Emory University School of Medicine
Director, Renal Division
Emory University Hospital
Atlanta, Georgia

Saulo Klahr, M.D.
Simon Professor of Medicine
Department of Medicine
Washington University School of Medicine
Barnes-Jewish Hospital
St. Louis, Missouri

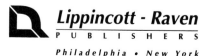

Lippincott - Raven
P U B L I S H E R S
Philadelphia • New York

Acquisitions Editor: Beth Barry
Developmental Editor: Ellen DiFrancesco
Manufacturing Manager: Dennis Teston
Production Manager: Robert Pancotti
Production Editor: Xenia Golovchenko
Cover Illustrator: Patricia Gast
Indexer: Nanette Cardon
Compositor: Lippincott–Raven Desktop Division
Printer: R R Donnelley Crawfordsville
Third edition

Printed in the United States of America

9 8 7 6 5 4 3 2 1

Library of Congress Cataloging-in-Publication Data
Handbook of nutrition and the kidney / edited by William E. Mitch, Saulo Klahr.—3rd ed.
  p. cm.
  Rev. ed. of : Nutrition and the kidney. 2nd ed. c1993.
  Includes bibliographical references and index.
  ISBN 0-7817-1534-2 (softcover)
  1. Kidneys—Diseases—Diet therapy—Handbooks, manuals, etc.
2. Kidneys—Diseases—Nutritional aspects—Handbooks, manuals, etc.
3. Kidney diseases—diet therapy—handbooks. I. Mitch, William E. II. Klahr, Saulo. III. Nutrition and the kidney.
  [DNLM: 1. Nutrition—handbooks. 2. Nutritional Requirements—handbooks. WJ 39 H2357 1998]
RC903.N87 1998
616.6'10654—dc21
DNLM/DLC
for Library of Congress   97-51461
                                                              CIP

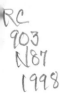

To our wives, Alexandra and Carol

Contents

Contributing Authors

J. Andrew Bertolatus, M.D.
Associate Professor of Internal Medicine, University of Iowa, College of Medicine, 200 Hawkins Drive, Iowa City, Iowa 52242

Wilfred Druml, M.D.
Medical Department III, Division of Nephrology, Vienna Medical School, Vienna General Hospital, Währinger Gürtel 18-20, A-1090 Vienna, Austria

Elizabeth Reid Gilmour, B.Sc.
Renal Dietitian, Queen Margaret Hospital, Whitefield Road, Dunfermiline, KY120SY, Scotland

Ram Gokal, M.D., F.R.C.P.
Consultant Nephrologist, Honorary Senior Lecturer, Department of Renal Medicine, Manchester Royal Infirmary, Oxford Road, Manchester M13 9WL, United Kingdom

D. Jordi Goldstein, D.Sc., R.D.
Visiting Assistant Professor of Environmental and Industrial Health, Division of Nephrology, The University of Michigan, School of Public Health, University of Michigan Medical Center, 6383 Silverbrooke West, West Bloomfield, Michigan 48322

Esther A. González, M.D.
Assistant Professor of Internal Medicine and Nephrology, Division of Nephrology, St. Louis University School of Medicine, 3635 Vista Avenue, St. Louis, Missouri 63110

Timothy H. J. Goodship, B.Sc., M.D., F.R.C.P.
Senior Lecturer in Nephrology and Consultant in Nephrology, Department of Medicine, Royal Victoria Infirmary, University of Newcastle-Upon-Tyne, Queen Victoria Road, Newcastle-Upon-Tyne NE1 4LP, United Kingdom

Raymond M. Hakim, M.D., Ph.D.
Professor of Medicine, Division of Nephrology, Vanderbilt University Medical Center, Medical Center North S-3307, Nashville, Tennessee 37232

George H. Hartley, B.Sc., S.R.D.
Renal Dieitian, Department of Nutrition and Dietetics, Freeman Hospital, High Heaton, Newcastle-Upon-Tyne NE7 7DN, United Kingdom

John Harty, M.D., F.R.C.P.
Department of Renal Medicine, Manchester Royal Infirmary, Oxford Road, Manchester M13 9WL, United Kingdom

Thomas H. Hostetter, M.D.
*Renal Division, University of Minnesota School of Medicine,
Box 736, 516 Delaware Street, SE, Minneapolis, Minnesota
55455*

Lawrence G. Hunsicker, M.D.
*Professor, Internal Medicine, Nephrology Division, University of
Iowa School of Medicine, 200 Hawkins Drive, Iowa City,
Iowa 52242-1081*

Hassan N. Ibrahim, M.D.
*Fellow of Renal Diseases and Hypertension, Department of
Medicine, University of Minnesota, 420 Delaware Street SE,
Minneapolis, Minnesota 55455*

T. Alp Ikizler, M.D.
*Assistant Professor of Medicine, Department of Medicine,
Division of Nephrology, Vanderbilt University School of
Medicine, 1161 21st Ave. S. and Garland, Nashville,
Tennessee 37232-2372*

Bertram L. Kasiske, M.D.
*Professor of Medicine, Division of Nephrology, University of
Minnesota, Hennepin County Medical Center, 701 Park
Avenue, Minneapolis, Minnesota 55415*

George A. Kaysen, M.D., Ph.D.
*Professor of Medicine; Chief, Division of Nephrology; Vice Chair
Research, Department of Internal Medicine, Division of
Nephrology, University of California, Davis, Davis, California
95616*

Saulo Klahr, M.D.
*John and Adaline Simon Professor of Medicine, Department
of Medicine, Washington University School of Medicine,
Barnes-Jewish Hospital, 216 South Kings Highway Boulevard,
St. Louis, Missouri 63110*

Bradley J. Maroni, M.D.
*Associate Professor, Department of Medicine, Emory University
School of Medicine, 1639 Pierce Drive, Atlanta, Georgia 30322*

Kevin J. Martin, M.D.
*Division of Nephrology, Department of Medicine, St. Louis
University Medical Center, 3635 Vista Avenue, St. Louis,
Missouri 63110*

William E. Mitch, M.D.
*Garland Herndon Professor of Medicine, Renal Division,
Department of Medicine, Emory University School of
Medicine, 1639 Pierce Drive, Atlanta, Georgia 30322*

Karl A. Nath, M.D.
*Professor of Medicine, Department of Medicine, University of
Minnesota and Mayo Clinic, 420 Delaware Street SE,
Minneapolis, Minnesota 55455*

Sandra Newbill Powers, B.S., R.D.
Assistant in Medicine, Division of Nephrology, Department of Medicine, Vanderbilt University School of Medicine, 215 Arts Building, Nashville, Tennessee 37232

Vernon R. Young, Ph.D., D.Sc.
Professor of Nutritional Biochemistry, School of Science, Massachusetts Institute of Technology, 77 Massachusetts Avenue, Cambridge, Massachusetts 02139

Preface

With this Third Edition, *Nutrition and the Kidney* becomes the *Handbook of Nutrition and the Kidney*, and we inaugurate some important changes: a new title; a new format for the book and the individual chapters; and a lower price, all intended to make the *Handbook* more readily available and easily accessible to the physicians, dietitians, nurses, and other professionals that provide care to patients with renal disease.

Because the requirements for protein, minerals, and other elements change significantly during advancing renal failure, the role of nutrition in treating patients with kidney disease cannot be underestimated. Since information about nutritional principles and methods of improving the nutritional conditions are of paramount importance in managing these patients, we wanted to make this material easier to find and apply for our readers. The chapters in this Third Edition have been completely revised and updated, and were written by nephrologists, dietitians, and experts in nutrition. Our goal now, as before, has been to integrate scientific foundations and clinical wisdom in providing a rational approach to the nutritional needs of patients with acute and chronic renal failure, for patients undergoing dialysis (both hemodialysis and peritoneal dialysis) or renal transplantation, for diabetic patients with nephropathy, and for those patients with the nephrotic syndrome.

We are grateful to all of the authors for their thoughtful and excellent contributions to the *Handbook*. We also acknowledge and thank Ellen DiFrancesco at Lippincott–Raven Publishers for her help and advice.

Handbook of Nutrition and the Kidney

Third Edition

Nutritional Requirements of Normal Adults

Vernon R. Young

THE NUTRIENTS

There are six general classes of nutrients: carbohydrates, fats, proteins, vitamins, minerals, and water. Those nutrients that are essential components of the diet are listed in Table 1-1. Without these elements, the individual cannot function. Without a sufficient dietary source of energy, a person can neither grow nor maintain his or her own tissues and, after a period of unsuccessful metabolic adaptation, will die. In addition to acting as a dietary energy source, food proteins provide the amino acids that are used as building blocks for the body proteins. Thus, proteins and their constituent amino acids are essential to life and fulfill a variety of physiologic roles, including their functions in the growth and maintenance of new tissue and in the regulation of internal water and acid–base balance, and as components of enzymes, antibodies, hormones, and peptide growth factors. In the course of carrying out their physiologic and functional roles, proteins and amino acids in the body turn over, and part of their nitrogen and carbon is lost through the excretory pathways, including the carbon dioxide in expired air and the urea and ammonia in urine. To maintain an adequate protein and amino acid status in the body, these losses must be balanced by a dietary supply of 1) a utilizable source of nitrogen to maintain function; and 2) the indispensable amino acids and, under specific states, the "conditionally indispensable" amino acids, to replace those lost during the course of daily metabolic transactions, deposited during growth and the repletion of tissue, or excreted with milk during lactation.

The term "conditionally indispensable" should be considered in more detail. The initial classification, proposed in 1954, of the dietary significance of the common 20 amino acids present in body proteins was to place them into one of two categories ("essential" or "nonessential"), depending on whether they were required in the diet for the maintenance of nitrogen balance in healthy adults. The essential amino acids at that time were valine, leucine, isoleucine, threonine, methionine, phenylalanine, lysine, and tryptophan. The nonessential amino acids were glycine, alanine, serine, cystine, tyrosine, aspartic acid, glutamic acid, proline, hydroxyproline, histidine, citrulline, and arginine. This is no longer satisfactory because histidine has since been shown to be an essential (indispensable) amino acid, and glycine, cystine, tyrosine, proline, and arginine, together with glutamine and taurine, are now more appropriately classified as being "conditionally indispensable." This means there are either specific dietary or host conditions under which function is best maintained or improved when these amino acids are part of the nutrient intake.

Fats, or lipids, are concentrated sources of dietary energy, and they act as carriers of the fat-soluble vitamins. The sensory properties of fats make a diet flavorful, varied, and rich, and they are

Table 1-1. The essential nutrients in human nutrition

Amino Acids	Vitamins	Elements
L-Threonine	Thiamine	Oxygen
L-Valine	Niacin	Water
L-Isoleucine	Riboflavin	Sodium
L-Leucine	Pyridoxine	Potassium
L-Lysine	Folic acid	Calcium
L-Tryptophan	Vitamin B_{12}	Magnesium
L-Methionine-cyst(e)ine	Ascorbic acid	Chloride
L-Phenylalanine-tyrosine	Biotin	Phosphorus
L-Histidine	Pantothenic acid	Iron
Taurine	Vitamin A	Copper
	Vitamin D	Zinc
Essential fatty acids	Vitamin E	Chromium
n-6 Family	Vitamin K	Manganese
n-3 Family		Selenium
		Molybdenum
		Iodine
		Fluoride

important in determining the palatability of the diet. In body tissues, they play essential roles in many enzyme reactions, in the positioning and function of cellular proteins, and in the maintenance of membrane structure and function. Dietary fats are also the source of the essential fatty acids, which are intimately involved in membrane structure and serve as precursors of the eicosanoids, with their diverse, local hormone-type actions involving gastric secretion, smooth muscle metabolism, and nervous system activity. The eicosanoids are a large family of oxygenated C_{20} fatty acids, consisting of three clans: the prostanoids (prostaglandins and thromboxanes), the leukotrienes, and the epoxides. Until recently, the unsaturated fatty acid linoleic acid (18:2), an n-6 fatty acid commonly found in vegetable oils and many other foods, was regarded as the primary essential fatty acid, together with its derivative n-6 fatty acids, of which arachidonic acid (20:4) is the most important. However, it now appears that two classes, or families, of fatty acids are essential for health (Fig. 1-1). Besides the n-6 fatty acids, a second class of essential unsaturated fatty acids includes the n-3 fatty acids, α-linolenic acid (18:3) and its longer-chain, more unsaturated, derivative docosahexanoic acid (22:6). The n-3 fatty acids are found in a wide variety of foods, including some liquid vegetable oils and green leafy vegetables, and their higher derivatives are found in shellfish, fish, and sea mammals. Finally, the n-9 fatty acid oleic acid (18:1) is the only significant dietary monosaturated fatty acid; it is not an essential dietary constituent, and at modest intakes appears to be "neutral" in terms of changing plasma cholesterol concentrations.

The requirement for n-6 fatty acids has been suggested to be from about 2% to 6% of total energy, and this probably should

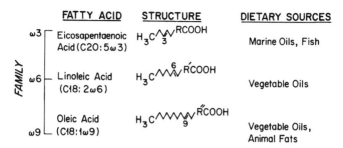

Fig. 1-1. The three families of unsaturated fatty acids and the structure of the terminal end of the fatty acid chain in each series.

include both linoleic and arachidonic acids. The dietary requirement for n-3 fatty acids in adults has not been established; in infancy it has been proposed that the requirement is from 0.5% to 1% of total energy, with a ratio of the n-6 to n-3 fatty acid intake in the range of about 4 : 10.

Clearly, fats and their constituent fatty acids provide more than just energy. Some are essential for maintaining normal metabolism and health. Conversely, excessive intakes of fats, such as saturated fats and cholesterol, can be involved in the etiology of cardiovascular disease and possibly in various types of cancer. Further, they appear to play a role in the etiology of human obesity.

A brief comment should be made concerning the isomeric form of unsaturated fatty acids, in plants and vegetables oils, which typically have the *cis* configuration (two hydrogen atoms on the same side of the double bond). There is a measurable level of *trans*-fatty acid (hydrogen atoms in the opposite direction) in commercial edible fats, which appears particularly during the hydrogenation process that changes liquid, edible oils into solid fats; the average intake of *trans*-fatty acids in the United States is about 7.6 g/day. There is some evidence that the *cis* and *trans* forms have different effects on lipid metabolism, especially with *high* levels of *trans*-fatty acids that raise serum cholesterol.

Carbohydrates account for about 45% of per capita energy intake in the United States. The nutritionally important carbohydrates may be divided into three major classes: simple sugars (monosaccharides), such as glucose and fructose; disaccharides, such as sucrose (table sugar, consisting of glucose and fructose) and lactose (milk sugar, consisting of glucose and galactose); and polysaccharides, including starch, glycogen (animal starch), celluloses, and hemicelluloses. The latter two polysaccharides contribute to the fiber component of the diet. Although they are not digested or used to a major extent by humans in the area of energy balance and requirements, there is considerable interest in the role these compounds play in the maintenance of normal gastrointestinal function, metabolism, and overall health. Dietary fiber may influence nutrient catabolism by 1) modulating absorption, 2) accelerating sterol metabolism, 3) increasing cecal bacterial mass and fermentation, and 4) changing intestinal transit time and stool weight. The various components of dietary fibers affect these different events in a specific manner, depending on their chemical form and physical structure.

The vitamins comprise another class of nutrients; 13 have been established as essential dietary constituents for humans. These are organic compounds necessary for normal growth, maintenance of health, and reproduction. Some vitamins such as thiamine, pyridoxine, and riboflavin act as organic catalysts, or coenzymes, and a lack of or low dietary intakes of these vitamins reduces the activities of enzymes responsible for promoting the conversion of food components into forms that can be used effectively by cells.

New functions, forms, and mechanisms of action of the vitamins are important. For example, retinol (vitamin A) is required for growth, vision, and reproduction, and it is now known that it carries out its function, at least in part, by binding to a nuclear receptor and enhancing transcription of specific genes. The specialized functions of retinol depend on specific retinoid derivatives. For example, II-*cis*-retinol constitutes the chromophore of the visual pigment rhodopsin, whereas 14-hydroxy-4,14-retro-retinol appears to mediate growth of lymphocytes and fibroblasts. There is a historic link between collagen synthesis and ascorbic acid, but vitamin C is also an antioxidant, maintaining iron and copper ions in some enzymes in their required reduced form and neutralizing harmful oxidants and free radicals, and it influences many enzymes and physiologic processes, a listing of which is given in Table 1-2.

Most vitamins are converted into an active form after they have been absorbed. Interactions occur between vitamins and other nutrients, affecting their bioavailability, such as ascorbic acid increasing iron bioavailability; protein intake increasing calcium

Table 1-2. Physiologic and metabolic effects of a low ascorbic acid intake

Detoxification of histamine

Phagocytic functions of leukocytes

Metabolism of drugs

Formation of nitrosamine

Tubulin function

Expression of acetylcholine receptor

Leukotriene biosynthesis

Lipid metabolism

Tetrahydrofolate reduction

Immunity

Cancer

Diabetic complications

Cataract formation

Periodontal disease

Rheumatoid arthritis

Infections

From: Padhr H. Vitamin C: newer insights into its biochemical functions. *Nutr Rev* 1991;49:65, with permission.

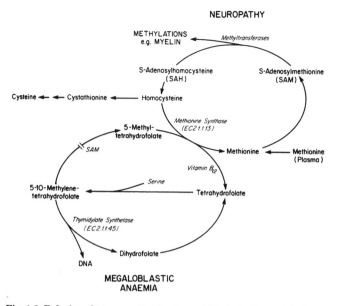

Fig. 1-2. Relations between vitamin B$_{12}$ and folate in the metabolism of one-carbon units, involving serine and DNA biosynthesis or methyl group use for synthesis of myelin and other brain structures. (From: Scott JM. Folate–vitamin B$_{12}$ interrelationships in the central nervous system. *Proc Nutr Soc* 1992;51:219, with permission.)

retention; and energy intake increasing the efficiency of protein (amino acid) utilization. As suggested in Fig. 1-2, vitamin B$_{12}$ deficiency is manifested clinically as anemia and neuropathy because of interference with the functioning of folate cofactors. These vitamins and vitamin B$_6$ are intimately involved in the metabolism of the amino acid homocysteine; it has been speculated that low concentrations of one or more of these vitamins might increase the risk of homocysteine toxicity, neuropathologies, and cognitive disturbances. Additional examples of various types of interactions between vitamins are listed in Table 1-3, indicating that changes in absorption, transport, metabolism, and excretion could potentially affect the requirement of one vitamin by another.

The minerals, or inorganic elements, are the last class of essential nutrients. The so-called macroinorganic elements—sodium, potassium, chlorine, calcium, magnesium, and phosphorus—are all present in the body in significant quantities, approximating a total of 3 kg in the adult body. The microelements, or trace minerals, total only 30 g in the body and are required in small amounts in the diet, usually less than 30 mg/day. As in the case of vitamins, interactions occur between minerals. An example of a mineral–mineral interaction is that occurring between iron and zinc: a high iron intake often reduces the efficiency of zinc absorption. For these reasons, the total amount of a mineral or of a certain vitamin in a food may not be the critical information for the nutritionist; it is more important

Table 1-3. Examples of types of vitamin–vitamin interactions

One vitamin needed for optimum absorption of another
   Vitamin B_6/vitamin B_{12}
   Folate/thiamine
A high level of one vitamin may interfere with absorption or
  metabolism of another
   Vitamin E/vitamin K
   Vitamin B_6/niacin
   Thiamine/riboflavin
One vitamin needed for metabolism of another
   Riboflavin/vitamin B_6 and niacin
One vitamin can protect against excess catabolism or urinary
  losses of another
   Vitamin C/vitamin B_6
One vitamin can protect against oxidative destruction of another
   Vitamin E/vitamin A
   Vitamin C/vitamin E
A high level of one vitamin can obscure the diagnosis of deficiency
  of another
   Folate/vitamin B_{12}

From: Machlin LJ, Langseth L. Vitamin–vitamin interactions. In: Bodwell C, Erdman JW Jr, eds. *Nutrient interactions.* New York: Marcel Dekker, 1988: 287–311. By courtesy of Marcel Dekker, Inc.

to know what *fraction* of the total is available for absorption and for meeting the physiologic needs of the host.

The major mineral elements—sodium, potassium, calcium, magnesium, and chloride—fulfill electrochemical functions. Calcium, potassium, magnesium, copper, and zinc serve as catalysts in enzyme systems, and some minerals contribute to body structure (e.g., calcium, phosphorus, and fluorine in bone and tooth formation). Other essential mineral elements include iodine for the formation of thyroid hormones, and iron as a constituent of heme, necessary for the formation of hemoglobin, which transports oxygen to body tissues and organs.

An intriguing example of mineral interactions is that iodothyronine deiodinase, which is needed for the conversion of thyroxine to triiodothyronine, the active form of the hormone, is a selenium-containing protein. In fact, selenium plays a key role in thyroid hormone metabolism; widespread iodine deficiency disorders, ranging from cretinism to goiter, are frequently associated with low selenium in the soil and potentially marginal or inadequate selenium intakes. Thus, the clinical features of selenium deficiency may not be wholly attributable to the diminished activity of the selenium-requiring enzyme glutathione peroxidase; abnormal thyroid metabolism may also be important.

THE QUANTITATIVE NEEDS FOR NUTRIENTS

The Approach

The sequence of events that leads to the appearance of symptoms of a clinical deficiency state begins with an inadequate supply of a nutrient to the body tissues (Fig. 1-3). This may result

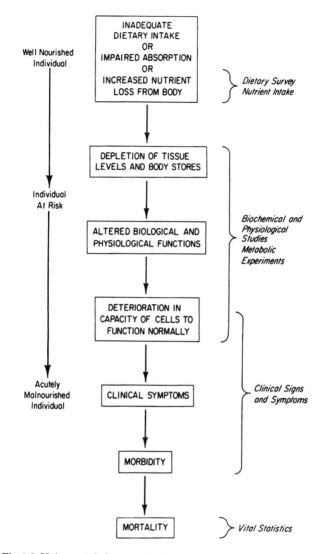

Fig. 1-3. Major metabolic steps in the sequence of events leading to the precipitation of nutrition deficiency disease and associated observations. (Adapted from Beaton GH, Patwardhan VN. Physiological and practical considerations of nutrient function and requirements. In: Beaton GH, Bengoa JM, eds. *Nutrition in preventive medicine*. World Health Organization monograph series No. 62. Geneva: World Health Organization; 1976:445–481.)

from a primary dietary deficiency or from factors that reduce the absorption, availability, or need relative to the intake of the required nutrient. One approach used for determining nutrient requirements is to assess how much of a nutrient is consumed by people in populations free of symptoms or signs associated with an inadequate intake of the nutrient. This information is then compared with nutrient intakes by people in populations in which the specific nutritional deficiency occurs.

In this way it is possible to determine an approximate range of intakes below which the disease appears and above which it is absent. This approach does not allow exact estimates of requirements because it is difficult to determine precisely how much people are consuming. Moreover, the diagnosis of subclinical deficiency is often uncertain. Nevertheless, the procedure helps to forecast the minimum levels of nutrient intake likely to maintain health in normal humans.

If the dietary intake of a nutrient, or its availability in body tissues, continues to be low and inadequate, the content of the nutrient in body tissues and fluids falls, often paralleled by a diminished rate of its excretion or conversion to end products. If the dietary insufficiency continues, biochemical and physiologic lesions develop. These might be changes in enzyme activities, changes in rates of formation of blood proteins, or a diminished capacity to use energy-yielding nutrients, reflected in changes in levels of cell and blood compounds that arise during the course of their metabolism. Those responses can be considered as characteristic of the subclinical phase of a nutritional disease, and they are followed, eventually, by the appearance of clinical signs and symptoms of nutrient deficiency.

This developmental pattern (see Fig. 1-3) provides the basis for many metabolic studies in humans to determine the quantitative needs for specific nutrients. In general, volunteers are given controlled diets in which the level of the test nutrient is altered during various dietary periods. The minimum level of intake necessary to prevent depletion of the nutrient from the body, to maintain a specific biochemical function, to prevent the development of unique signs or symptoms, or to support other criteria such as maintenance of body composition in the adult, is then determined. This approach is precise, but investigations with humans are laborious, time consuming, and expensive. Hence, it is possible to study only a relatively small number of volunteers in most experiments.

Many studies of the nutrient requirements of humans have used the metabolic balance technique. Some nutrients, or products of their metabolism, are excreted daily in urine and feces, and lost through sweat and hair. If the experimental diet is deficient in a nutrient, the amount excreted will exceed the intake. Determination of the body nutrient balance by measuring the amount in food and excreta reveals that the body is being depleted. When the intake meets the amount required by the body, the amount excreted will be equal to that in the diet and the subject is said to be in balance or equilibrium. This approach has been used for measuring the requirements for protein and amino acids (by measurement of nitrogen losses), calcium, zinc, and magnesium, but cannot be used to determine vitamin requirements or those of nutrients that are oxidized and whose carbon portion is eliminated in the expired air.

Although the metabolic balance method has proved to be useful, it has its limitations. For example, the determinations and interpretation of the significance of a particular nitrogen balance value can present a problem. First, an equilibrium, or zero, balance can be achieved over a range of protein intakes even though the rate of protein turnover in cells and organs might differ as protein intake varies. The question is whether within this range of protein (nitrogen) intake a given rate of protein turnover is better than another. This cannot be answered adequately. Second, when nitrogen intake is above the apparent minimum requirement levels, the nitrogen balance in adults has been unrealistically positive over long periods of time. Furthermore, at relatively low nitrogen intakes that might be deemed adequate to maintain nitrogen equilibrium, abnormalities in some biochemical parameters emerge when the intake is continued over an extended period of time. Therefore, nitrogen balance data do not *necessarily* provide adequate information about the status of body protein nutriture, nor do they offer sufficient evidence for establishing values for adult human protein or amino acid requirements. This problem applies also to establishing the requirements for such nutrients as calcium and zinc.

Another potential problem with using the balance technique to estimate human nutrient requirements is that the experimental studies usually involve relatively short-term experimental diet periods. This raises the question as to whether more prolonged periods would result in different estimates of nutrient balance for a given intake level.

In view of the limitations in the metabolic balance technique and interpretation of the balance data, it is important that alternative methods be developed and applied for purposes of establishing nutrient needs. A potentially valuable approach involves studying the dynamic response of body protein and amino acid metabolism in relation to alterations in the intake of indispensable amino acids. Studies in growing and adult rats have shown that when the dietary level of a specific indispensable amino acid is gradually decreased, there are significant alterations in amino acid metabolism that appear to be linked to the host's physiologic requirement. Therefore, our group has carried out a series of investigations involving nonradioactive, stable isotope tracer techniques in order to determine how kinetic parameters of whole-body amino acid and protein metabolism in adult humans respond to changes in the dietary level of an indispensable amino acid. The findings raise major doubts about the validity of currently accepted estimates of the requirements of adults for indispensable amino acid derived from metabolic nitrogen data. The validity of nutrient requirement values will depend on the nature and adequacy of the methodology used to establish them, and there remains a pressing need to develop new and alternative methods for the evaluation of nutrient requirements.

Before turning to a short account of current estimates of the requirements for specific nutrients in normal adults, it can be stated that the physiologic requirement for an essential nutrient is that minimum dietary intake on a dose-response curve which predicts a particular criterion of nutritional adequacy, such as a given blood or tissue level, indicator of enzyme activity and/or gain, and level of body nutrient balance or an agreed upon body composition.

The requirement value may not be the same when determined using different criteria, and so some expert committees have now focused on the consideration of "requirement for what?" Committees of the United Nations, dealing with requirements for vitamins and trace elements, have described basal requirements to be sufficient to maintain all demonstrable functions of the nutrient and normative requirements, which cover intake levels sufficient to maintain tissue stores or adaptive capacities judged to be desirable (see Fig. 1-4, for an example using iron).

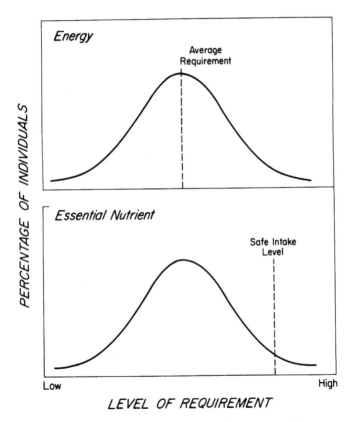

Fig. 1-4. Comparison of average requirement for energy and the recommended daily allowance (RDA) for an essential nutrient. The "safe level of intake" for protein is equivalent to the RDA. (From: Food and Agriculture Organization/World Health Organization/United Nations University (FAO/WHO/UNU). *Energy and protein requirements: report of a joint FAO/WHO/UNU expert consultation.* Technical report series no. 724. Geneva: World Health Organization; 1985:15, with permission.)

It should be appreciated that there is not necessarily a single requirement value but it will depend, in part, on the measures taken to assess nutrient intake adequacy and the interpretations made of the data. This is an important issue since, to some extent, the varying estimates of nutrient requirements among different expert groups and authorities may be due to the different judgments used to arrive at a physiologic requirement level. In the future, the description (or operational definition) of nutrient requirements may give greater uniformity to the nutrient requirement values proposed by different authorities.

Recommended Dietary Allowances

The physiologic requirement, as defined above, for a nutrient varies among apparently similar individuals. Hence, recommended dietary allowances (RDAs) have been designed as a practical value intended to cover the nutritional needs of nearly all healthy persons within a particular population. The term reference nutrient intake (RNI) has been used by a United Kingdom expert panel to replace RDAs, which really are not so much recommendations as they are reference values. Irrespective of the actual term applied, the variation in nutrient needs among individuals is important to know in order to develop appropriate dietary standards. In healthy populations of adults, this variation is assumed to be normally distributed and the mean requirement plus 2 standard deviations (SD) above the mean value is designated as the RDA. This level of intake should be sufficient to cover the requirements of about 97.5% of the population (Fig. 1-5).

Provided the intake of a nutrient is at a level equal to or moderately greater than the RDA, there is little chance that the diet would supply an inadequate amount. Although there is a range above the requirement level within which no detrimental effects occur, at some higher point the untoward effects of an excessive

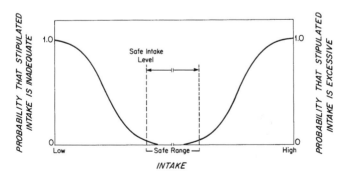

Fig. 1-5. Probability that a particular intake of an essential nutrient is inadequate or excessive for a randomly selected adult. This illustrates the concept of the same range of intake. (From: Food and Agriculture Organization/World Health Organization/United Nations University (FAO/WHO/UNU). *Energy and protein requirements: report of a joint FAO/WHO/UNU expert consultation.* Technical report series no. 724. Geneva: World Health Organization; 1985:18, with permission.)

intake may begin to emerge. The relations between two probability curves, one for meeting requirements and the other related to adverse effects, are shown in Figs. 1-4 and 1-5. These curves are separated by a *safe range of intake* that will be associated with low probabilities of either inadequacy or excess for almost all individuals. Undoubtedly, this safe range of intake could shift with the health status; an obvious example being to reduce the range for protein and phosphorus intakes in patients with renal disease.

The approach to establishing recommended or reference intakes for energy requirements differs from that of the essential nutrients, because the RDA for energy is based on the average requirements for a specific population. Diets providing intakes of energy either well above or well below the person's true requirements would result in a deterioration of health. Energy allowances for adults engaged in light to moderate activities, including pregnant and lactating women, are given in Table 1-4.

Insufficient information is available to make reliable recommendations for some of the known essential nutrients. Accordingly, these estimated safe and adequate daily dietary intakes are given in Tables 1-4 and 1-5. Several elements and compounds known to be required in the diets of some animal and microbial species are not given in either Tables 1-5 or 1-6. These include choline, which may have an RDA assigned in the future, plus taurine, carnitine, myo-inositol, and the trace elements arsenic, nickel, silicon, boron, cadmium, lead, lithium, tin, and vanadium. For adults, a safe minimum intake of sodium has been proposed to be 500 mg/day, which is less than that supplied by usual diets. It has been recommended that daily intakes of sodium chloride be limited to 6 g (2.4 g sodium) or less. The minimum requirement for potassium is considered to be 1600 to 2000 mg (40 to 50 mEq) per day, and the minimum chloride intake parallels that for sodium, on a milliequivalent basis (about 750 mg/day).

The recommended allowances are amounts considered sufficient for the maintenance of health in nearly all adults. The recommendations are not intended to be sufficient for therapeutic purposes, but to cover the additional requirements that may occur during and after recovery from infection or under conditions of malabsorption, trauma, metabolic disease, or other significant stress.

Factors Affecting Nutrient Requirements

Not everyone of the same age, body build, and sex has the same nutrient requirements. These differences may be due, in part, to variations in genetic background. Various environmental, physiologic, psychological, and pathologic influences affect the variability in physiologic requirements for nutrients among individuals (Table 1-7). For example, the growing infant or child requires higher nutrient intakes per unit of body weight than does the adult. Besides energy, for which the daily requirement declines with age because of reduced physical activity, it appears that the nutrient needs of healthy aged subjects do not differ significantly from those of young adults. Nevertheless, a characteristic of aging is an increased incidence of disease and morbidity,

Table 1-4. Recommended energy intakes for adults older than 15 years of age, with median heights and weights, according to the U.S. Food and Nutrition Board

Category	Age (yr) or Condition	Weight		Height		REE* (kcal/d)	Average Energy Allowance (kcal)†		
		kg	lb	cm	in.		Multiples of REE	Per kg	Per Day‡
Men	15–18	66	145	176	69	1760	1.67	45	3000
	19–24	72	160	177	70	1780	1.67	40	2900
	25–50	79	174	176	70	1800	1.60	37	2900
	51+	77	170	173	68	1530	1.50	30	2300
Women	15–18	55	120	163	64	1370	1.60	40	2200
	19–24	58	128	164	65	1350	1.60	38	2200
	25–50	63	138	163	64	1380	1.55	36	2200
	51+	65	143	160	63	1280	1.50	30	1900
Pregnant	1st trimester								+0
	2nd trimester								+300
	3rd trimester								+300
Lactating	1st 6 mo								+500
	2nd 6 mo								+500

REE, resting energy expenditure.
*Calculation based on Food and Agriculture Organization equations, then rounded.
†In the range of light to moderate activity, the coefficient of variation is ±20%.
‡Figure is rounded.
Adapted with permission from *Recommended dietary allowances: 10th edition.* p. 33. Copyright 1989 by the National Academy of Sciences. Published by the National Academy Press, Washington, DC.

Table 1-5. U.S. Food and Nutrition Board, National Academy of Sciences–National Research Council recommended dietary allowances* (revised 1989) for adults 15 years of age and older

Category	Age (yr) or Condition	Weight† kg	Weight† lb	Height† cm	Height† in.	Protein (g)	Fat-Soluble Vitamins Vita-min A (µg RE)‡	Vita-min D (µg)§	Vita-min E (mg α-TE)‖	Vita-min K (µg)	Water-Soluble Vitamins Vita-min C (mg)	Thia-mine (mg)	Ribo-flavin (mg)	Niacin (mg NE)¶	Vita-min B6 (mg)	Fol-ate (µg)	Vita-min B12 (µg)	Minerals Cal-cium (mg)	Phos-phorus (mg)	Mag-nesium (mg)	Iron (mg)	Zinc (mg)	Iodine (µg)	Sele-nium (µg)
Men	15-18	66	145	176	69	59	1000	10	10	65	60	1.5	1.8	20	2.0	200	2.0	1200	1200	400	12	15	150	50
	19-24	72	160	177	70	58	1000	10	10	70	60	1.5	1.7	19	2.0	200	2.0	1200	1200	350	10	15	150	70
	25-50	79	174	176	70	63	1000	5	10	80	60	1.5	1.7	19	2.0	200	2.0	800	800	350	10	15	150	70
	51+	77	170	173	68	63	1000	5	10	80	60	1.2	1.4	15	2.0	200	2.0	800	800	350	10	15	150	70
Women	15-18	55	120	163	64	44	800	10	8	55	60	1.1	1.3	15	1.5	180	2.0	1200	1200	300	15	12	150	50
	19-24	58	128	164	65	48	800	10	8	60	60	1.1	1.3	15	1.6	180	2.0	1200	1200	280	15	12	150	55
	25-50	63	138	163	64	50	800	5	8	65	60	1.1	1.3	15	1.6	180	2.0	800	800	280	15	12	150	55
	51+	65	143	160	63	50	800	5	8	65	60	1.0	1.2	13	1.6	180	2.0	800	800	280	10	12	150	55
Pregnant						60	800	10	10	65	70	1.5	1.6	17	2.2	400	2.2	1200	1200	320	30	15	175	65
Lactating	1st 6 mo					65	1300	10	12	65	95	1.6	1.8	20	2.1	280	2.6	1200	1200	355	15	19	200	75
	2nd 6 mo					62	1200	10	11	65	90	1.6	1.7	20	2.1	260	2.6	1200	1200	340	15	16	200	75

*The allowances, expressed as average daily intakes over time, are intended to provide for individual variations among most normal people as they live in the United States under usual environmental stresses. Diets should be based on a variety of common foods to provide other nutrients for which human requirements have been less well defined.

†Weights and heights of reference adults are actual medians for the U.S. population of the designated age.

‡Retinol equivalents; 1 retinol equivalent = 1 µg retinol or 6 µg β-carotene.

§As cholecalciferol; 10 µg cholecalciferol = 400 I.U. of vitamin D.

‖α-Tocopherol equivalents; 1 mg D-α-tocopherol = 1 α-TE.

¶1 NE (niacin equivalent) is equal to 1 mg of niacin or 60 mg of dietary tryptophan.

Adapted with permission from *Recommended dietary allowances: 10th edition.* Appendix. Copyright 1989 by the National Academy of Sciences. Published by the National Academy Press, Washington, DC.

Table 1-6. Estimated safe and adequate daily dietary intakes of selected vitamins and minerals for healthy adults, based on U.S. Food and Nutrition Board

Nutrient	Daily Amount
Biotin (µg)	30–100
Pantothenic acid (mg)	4–7
Copper (mg)	1.5–3.0
Manganese (mg)	2.0–5.0
Fluoride (mg)	1.5–4.0
Chromium (µg)	50–200
Molybdenum (µg)	75–250

Adapted with permission from *Recommended dietary allowances: 10th edition.* p. 284. Copyright 1989 by the National Academy of Sciences. Published by the National Academy Press, Washington, DC.

which is likely to be far more important than age per se in determining practical differences between the nutrient requirements of younger adults and elderly people.

Numerous dietary factors determine the required intake of a particular nutrient. For example, all forms of dietary iron are not equally available and the type of diet and composition of individual meals influence the availability of the iron consumed.

Table 1-7. Agent, host, and environmental factors that influence nutrient requirements and nutritional status

Agent (dietary) factors

Chemical form of nutrient

Energy intake

Food processing and preparation (may increase or decrease dietary needs)

Effect of other dietary constituents

Host factors

Age

Sex

Genetic makeup

Pathologic states
  Drugs
  Infection
  Physical trauma
  Chronic disease, cancer

Environmental factors

Physical (unsuitable housing, inadequate heating)

Biologic (poor sanitary conditions)

Socioeconomic (poverty, dietary habits and food choices, physical activity)

Acute or chronic gastrointestinal infections may interfere with the absorption of nutrients. The net result is a depletion of body nutrients followed by an increase in the physiologic requirement for nutrients during the recovery phase, to promote recovery and to compensate for the earlier losses.

Finally, various drugs can affect nutrient requirements by decreasing nutrient absorption or by altering the utilization of nutrients. For example, a reduced appetite is a frequent consequence of drug therapy, and this exaggerates the effects of drug treatment on the person's nutritional status, particularly if the diet is already marginally adequate. In addition to the inadequacy of the diet of alcoholics, ethanol interferes with the absorption or utilization of various nutrients, raising nutrient needs above those required by healthy people.

ENERGY UTILIZATION AND REQUIREMENTS

Components of the Energy Requirement

A person's energy requirement might be described with reference to the energy balance equation (Table 1-8). It is worthwhile to emphasize the major components of the energy requirement; these include *obligatory* thermogenesis, consisting of the basal metabolic rate (BMR) and the thermic effect of food, and *facultative* thermogenesis. The latter component comprises the energy transformations associated with physical activity and diet-induced thermogenesis (i.e., the more variable component of energy expenditure). With reference to the energy needs in adults, there are two important questions: 1) how large are various components of the daily energy expenditure?, and 2) do they change during the progression of the adult years, and if so, why?

An approximate "composition" of the daily energy expenditure in a relatively sedentary adult is shown in Fig. 1-6, indicating that the BMR accounts for about 60% or more of the daily energy flux. Various factors, including familial and genetic influences, nutritional, metabolic, and disease conditions, as well as gender and body composition, determine the BMR. The BMR is reduced

Table 1-8. The energy balance equation

Energy stored = energy intake – energy expenditure

Energy Intake	Energy Expenditure (Thermogenesis)
Metabolic food energy	Obligatory thermogenesis
	Basal metabolic rate (BMR)
	Thermic effect of food
	Facultative thermogenesis
	Physical activity
	Nonshivering thermogenesis
	Diet-induced thermogenesis

From: Young VR. Energy requirements in the elderly. *Nutr Rev* 1992;50:95, with permission.

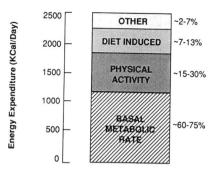

Fig. 1-6. An approximate distribution of the major components of daily energy expenditure in a sedentary adult. (From Young VR. Energy requirements in the elderly. *Nutr Rev* 1992;50:95, with permission.)

in the elderly, largely, if not entirely, because of the age-related decrease in lean body mass, especially in muscle mass.

The other component of obligatory thermogenesis is that of the thermic effect of food due to the energy transformations required for the ingestion, digestion, absorption, processing, and storage of the energy-yielding nutrients. The energy costs of the thermic effect of food vary according to the immediate metabolic fate of these nutrients, whereas the facultative component of dietary thermogenesis results from metabolic cycle activity and activation of the sympathetic nervous system.

Actual Energy Requirements

The energy requirement has been defined by Food and Agriculture Organization/World Health Organization/United Nations University (FAO/WHO/UNU), as follows:

The energy requirement of an individual is the level of energy intake from food that will balance energy expenditure when the individual has a body size and composition, and level of physical activity, consistent with long-term good health; and that will allow for the maintenance of economically necessary and socially desirable physical activity. In children and pregnant or lactating women the energy requirement includes the energy needs associated with the deposition of tissue or the secretion of milk at rates consistent with good health.

The approach followed by FAO/WHO/UNU to set or define this level of energy intake was to estimate the energy costs of various factors, expressed in relation to multiples of the BMR. These factors are 1) the BMR; 2) growth, in the case of the young; 3) physical activity, which is divided into "occupational" and "discretionary" activities; and 4) the thermic effect of food.

The maintenance component was taken to be about 1.4 times BMR for both men and women; when the other components were expressed as a function of BMR, the average daily energy requirement of an adult might be approximated as 1.55 to 1.75 times BMR (see Table 1-4). A more thorough estimation of the average energy needs of a group of healthy retired men, for example, is shown in Table 1-9. As a general guide, it appears that the average energy requirement in adults is about 1.5 times the resting energy expenditure (see Table 1-4).

Source of Energy-Yielding Nutrients

It is important to determine whether the mixture of dietary energy sources is of metabolic, pathophysiologic, or nutritional significance. This is an important issue because positive epidemiologic associations have been observed between fat intake and body composition, suggesting that the composition of the diet is a factor determining body energy balance, composition, and obesity.

Macronutrient as well as energy balance can be achieved for the following reasons: 1) dietary carbohydrate and fat have unequal effects on energy substrate metabolism and energy balance; 2) the conversion of carbohydrate to fat is not an important pathway of carbohydrate disposal in the person who is close to energy balance or when glycogen stores are depleted; 3) dietary carbohydrate promotes carbohydrate oxidation and reduces lipid oxidation, whereas dietary fat does not enhance fat oxidation or influence carbohydrate oxidation; and 4) imbalances between intake and oxidation are more likely to occur for fat than for carbohydrate because carbohydrate balance is under a stricter metabolic control than is body fat balance. From these observations, it may be concluded that 1) carbohydrate and fat balances are under different regulation; 2) appreciable storage of glycogen occurs before a significant de novo lipogenesis occurs from dietary carbohydrate; and 3) adjustment of fat oxidation to altered dietary fat occurs only after a significant expansion of adipose tissue. Excess body fat increases plasma fatty acid concentrations and promotes fat oxidation.

Table 1-9. Average energy requirement of healthy, retired elderly men (average age, 75 years; weight, 60 kg; height, 1.6 m; BMI, 23.5; estimated BMR, 54 kcal [225 kJ]/hr)

	Hr	Kcal	kJ
In bed at $1.0 \times$ BMR	8	430	1810
Occupational activities	0	0	0
Discretionary activities			
Socially desirable ($3.3 \times$ BMR)	2	355	1490
Household tasks ($2.7 \times$ BMR)	1	145	610
Cardiovascular and muscular maintenance ($4 \times$ BMR)	$1/3$	70	300
For residual time, energy needs 12 at $1.4 \times$ BMR	$2/3$	960	4020
Total (= $1.5 \times$ BMR)		1960	8200

BMI, body mass index; BMR, basal metabolic rate.
From Food and Agriculture Organization/World Health Organization/United Nations University (FAO/WHO/UNU). *Energy and protein requirements: report of a joint FAO/WHO/UNU expert consultation.* Technical report series no. 724. Geneva: World Health Organization; 1985:77; with permission.

It follows that a voluntary restriction of fat might well be desirable simply from an energy balance and requirement standpoint, regardless of the adverse effects of a high fat intake and the risks of cardiovascular and cerebrovascular disease. Appropriate consideration must be given to the *source* of the energy intake, as well as *total* energy expenditure, in determining the energy requirement and for making recommendations about energy intakes. There is no broad consensus on the "ideal" or "appropriate" mixture of the net energy from carbohydrate and lipid sources.

PROTEIN AND AMINO ACID REQUIREMENTS

The joint FAO/WHO/UNU Expert Consultation defined the protein requirement as follows:

The protein requirement of an individual is defined as the lowest level of dietary protein intake that will balance the losses of nitrogen from the body in persons maintaining energy balance at modest levels of physical activity. In children and pregnant or lactating women, the protein requirement is taken to include the needs associated with the deposition of tissues or the secretion of milk at rates consistent with good health.

Most estimates of human protein and amino acid requirements have been obtained directly, or indirectly, from measurements of nitrogen balance. The 1985 report of the FAO/WHO/UNU Expert Consultation provides an extensive discussion of the approaches used to estimate the mean requirements for protein in various age and physiologic groups. A brief summary of protein requirements of adults, including those for elderly people and women, is illustrated in Table 1-10.

The practical recommendations emerging from estimations of requirements is for a "safe protein intake" (equivalent to the

Table 1-10. Protein requirements in adults, elderly, and women: summary of essentials of the approach taken by FAO/WHO/UNU

1. Young men: Short-term N balance (mean 0.63 g/kg)
   Long-term N balance (~0.58 g/kg)
   Mean: ~0.6 g; CV 12.5%
   Hence, safe level = 0.6 + 25% = 0.75 g/kg/d
2. Young women: Concluded to be the same as for men
3. Elderly: Not lower than 0.75 g/kg/d
4. Pregnancy: Based on average 925-g protein increment + 30%, with 0.70 efficiency factor; therefore, 1.2 g, 6.1 g, and 10.7 g additional protein during 1st, 2nd, 3rd trimesters, respectively
5. Lactation: From protein secreted; + 0.7 efficiency factor + CV 12.5% (birth weight); + 16 g daily (0–6 mo); + 12 g daily (6–12 mo)

N, nitrogen; CV, coefficient of variation.
From Young VR. Protein and amino acid requirements in humans: metabolic basis and current recommendations. *Scand J Nutr* 1992;36:47, with permission.

RDA) that includes a factor accounting for the variation in protein requirements among apparently similar people. The interindividual variability in protein requirements in adults amounts to a coefficient of variation of 12.5%. Hence, a value of 25% (2 SD) above the *mean*, minimum physiologic requirement for the adult, of 0.6 g protein/kg/day, would meet the needs of all but 2.5% of people within the adult population. The mean minimum requirement should be increased to 0.75 g/kg/day to give a safe protein intake for healthy adults. Apparently, most people would require less than this to maintain an adequate state of protein nutrition; it follows that some adult subjects might require as little as 0.45 g high-quality protein/kg/day. This approach for including variability is similarly applied to the other age groups, but in the case of infants an adjustment is also made for the interindividual and intraindividual variations in growth rate.

Table 1-11 gives estimates for the amino acid requirements in various age groups. There is a marked decrease in indispensable amino acid needs, when expressed per unit of body weight, between infancy and adulthood. There also is a lower requirement for indispensable amino acids, expressed per unit of the total need for protein, in the adult compared with the infant or preschool child.

A pattern of amino acid requirements for the adult is compared in Table 1-12 with that proposed for the preschool child by the joint FAO/WHO/UNU Expert Consultation. It may be seen that these two patterns are quite similar, but the amino acid requirements for the adult are increased, on average, by a factor of 2.5.

**Table 1-11. 1985 FAO/WHO/UNU estimates of
amino acid requirements at different ages (mg/kg/d)**

Amino Acid	Infants (3–4 mo)	Children (2 yr)	School Boys (10–12 yr)	Adults
Histidine	28	?	?	8–12
Isoleucine	70	31	28	10
Leucine	161	73	44	14
Lysine	103	64	44	12
Methionine and cystine	58	27	22	13
Phenylalanine and tyrosine	125	69	22	14
Threonine	87	37	28	7
Tryptophan	17	12.5	3.3	3.5
Valine	93	38	25	10
Total (-Histidine)	714	352	216	84
Total per g protein	434	320	222	111

From Food and Agriculture Organization/World Health Organization/United Nations University (FAO/WHO/UNU). *Energy and protein requirements: report of a joint FAO/WHO/UNU expert consultation.* Technical report series no. 724. Geneva: World Health Organization; 1985:65; with permission.

Table 1-12. New, tentative amino acid requirement estimates for the human adult and the corresponding amino acid requirement pattern, compared with that for the preschool child

| Amino Acid | Adults | | 1985 FAO/WHO/ UNU Preschool Child Amino Acid Pattern (mg/g protein) |
	Tentative Requirement (mg/kg/d)	Amino Acid Pattern (mg/g protein)	
Isoleucine	23	35	28
Leucine	40	65	66
Lysine	30	50	58
Total SAA	13	25	25
Total aromatic	39	65	63
Threonine	15	25	34
Valine	20	35	35
Tryptophan	6	10	11

SAA, sulfur-containing amino acid.
Based on Young VR. Protein and amino acid requirements in humans: metabolic basis and current recommendations. *Scand J Nutr* 1992;36:47; and Food and Agriculture Organization/World Health Organization/United Nations University (FAO/WHO/UNU). *Energy and protein requirements: report of a joint FAO/WHO/UNU expert consultation.* Technical report series no. 724. Geneva: World Health Organization; 1985.

These new figures emphasize the issue of dietary protein quality and the amino acid requirement, or *scoring*, pattern to be used for the purposes of assessing food protein quality. The amino acid score, corrected for digestibility, uses the amino acid requirement pattern for the 2- to 5-year-old child, as proposed in 1985 by FAO/WHO/UNU.

INTERPRETATION AND APPLICATION OF REQUIREMENT ESTIMATES

With respect to diagnostic applications, a probability approach has been proposed for assessing the nutritional significance of observed intakes. In this procedure, the distribution of individual requirements (e.g., protein requirement) is expressed as a cumulative distribution, portraying the probability that any given intake level will be inadequate for a randomly selected person within the population (Fig. 1-7). For application of this probability approach to a population group (Fig. 1-8), the risk of inadequacy is estimated by multiplying the probability of inadequacy by the frequency of occurrence with each interval of intake and then summing across all intervals to give the expected number of affected people. This method yields an estimate of the prevalence of inadequate intakes, but it does not identify people whose intake is inadequate.

In reference to prescriptive applications, it was noted earlier that the RDA or safe level of intake is the level that meets or

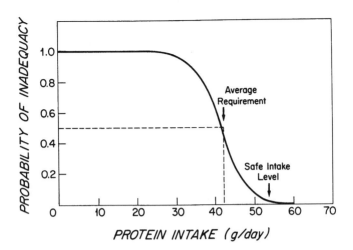

Fig. 1-7. Probability, or risk, of inadequacy of protein intake for an adult man weighing 70 kg, based on a cumulative distribution of protein requirements in this population group. (From Beaton GH. Human nutrient requirement estimates: derivation, interpretation and application in evolutionary perspective. *Food, Nutrition and Agriculture* 1992;213:3, with permission.)

exceeds the physiologic requirement for most people. Hence, for a given person this level can be "prescribed" (see Fig. 1-6) with the likelihood that there would be a very low risk of not meeting the person's actual needs.

The rule of thumb, where there is a symmetric distribution pattern in requirements, is that the group mean intake should be about 2 SDs of *intake* above the mean requirement. For example, in terms of protein requirements in adult men, the mean requirement has been estimated to be 0.6 g protein/kg body weight/day, the coefficient of variation of the requirement is 12.5%, and the variability of usual protein intake in North American men has a coefficient of variation of about 25%. Hence, the lowest acceptable group mean intake would be (2 × 0.25 × mean intake) above the average requirement of 0.6 g, or about 1.2 g/kg/day. An important point to note is that a mean intake that would be consistent with a low risk of nutritional inadequacy in this example should be higher than the RDA or safe protein intake level.

DIETARY GOALS AND GUIDELINES

With the growing epidemiologic evidence relating diet and its constituents to chronic diseases such as cardiovascular disease, cancers at certain organ sites, osteoporosis, diabetes, hypertension, and obesity, there is concern about eating enough to maintain the specific and unique physiologic functions of that nutrient. Most reports concerned with nutrient requirements have evaluated the needs for the essential fatty acids but have not

SIMULATED DISTRIBUTION OF PROTEIN INTAKES

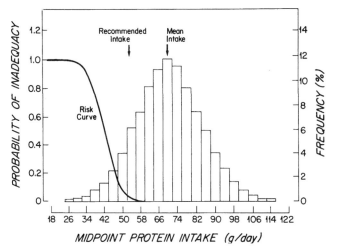

Fig. 1-8. Probability assessment of inadequacy of nutrient (e.g., protein) intake applied to a hypothetical example of the distribution of protein intake in adult men (expected inadequate intake of about 2%). (From Beaton GH. Human nutrient requirement estimates: derivation, interpretation and application in evolutionary perspective. *Food, Nutrition and Agriculture* 1992;213:3, with permission.)

considered total lipid levels or the amount and type of dietary carbohydrates. For example, β-carotene (precursor of vitamin A), ascorbic acid, and vitamin E can reduce the levels of free radicals, the highly reactive molecules that attack macromolecules, such as DNA or proteins, leading to a deterioration of cell and organ function. Use of antioxidants, possibly in combination with other strategies such as a diet rich in monounsaturated fatty acids (e.g., oleic acid), might be an attractive approach to slowing the progression of atherosclerosis. Levels of intake of specific nutrients that may be beneficial in terms of reducing the risk of certain cancers or of atherosclerosis might well be different from those established as supplying the physiologic requirements. In short, there is a difference between intakes that meet the physiologic requirements for vitamin A, and those that increase the proportion of vitamin A-rich foods in the diet. On the other hand, there should not be a contradiction between physiologic requirement estimates and levels of intake associated with meeting dietary goals in health and disease.

SELECTED READINGS

Committee on Diet and Health, Food and Nutrition Board, National Research Council. *Diet and health: implication for reducing chronic disease risk*. Washington, DC: National Academy Press; 1989.

Committee on Dietary Guidelines Implementation, Food and Nutrition Board, Institute of Medicine. *Improving America's diet and health: from recommendations to action.* Washington, DC: National Academy Press; 1991.

Department of Health. *Dietary reference values for food, energy and nutrients for the United Kingdom.* Report on health and social subjects, No. 41. London: Her Majesty's Stationery Office; 1991.

Food and Agriculture Organization/World Health Organization/United Nations University (FAO/WHO/UNU). *Energy and protein requirements: report of a joint FAO/WHO/UNU expert consultation.* Technical report series no. 724. Geneva: World Health Organization; 1985.

Flatt JP. Importance of nutrient balance in body weight regulation. *Diabetes Metab Rev* 1998;4:571.

Food and Nutrition Board, Subcommittee on Criteria for Dietary Evaluation, National Research Council. *Nutrient adequacy: assessment using food consumption surveys.* Washington, DC: National Academy Press; 1986.

Hegsted DM. Point of view: defining a nutritious diet: need for new dietary standards. *J Am Coll Nutr* 1992;11:241.

Horwitz A, MacFadyen DM, Munro HN et al, eds. *Nutrition in the elderly.* Oxford: Oxford University Press; 1989.

Kinney JM, Tucker HN, eds. *Energy metabolism: tissue determinants and cellular corollaries.* New York: Raven Press; 1992.

Kinsella JE, Lokesh B, Stone RA. Dietary n-3 polyunsaturated fatty acids and amelioration of cardiovascular disease: possible mechanisms. *Am J Clin Nutr* 1990;52:1.

Marabous N. The nutritional role of fat. *Scand J Nutr Suppl* 1992; 25:1.

Poehlman ET, Horton ES. Regulation of energy expenditure in aging humans. *Annu Rev Nutr* 1990;10:255.

Scrimshaw NS, Young VR. Requirements of human nutrition. *Sci Am* 1976;253:51.

Solomons NW. Physiological interactions of minerals. In: Bodwell C, Erdman JW, eds. *Nutrients interactions.* New York: Marcel Dekker; 1988:115–148.

Young VR. Energy requirements in the elderly. *Nutr Rev* 1992;50:95.

Young VR. Protein and amino acid requirements in humans: metabolic basis and current recommendations. *Scand J Nutr* 1992;36:47.

Young VR, Pellet PL, Bier DM. A theoretical basis for increasing estimates of the amino acid requirements in adult man, with experimental support. *Am J Clin Nutr* 1989;50:80.

Young VR, El-Khoury AE. The notion of the nutritional essentiality of amino acids revisited with a note on the indispensable amino acid requirements in adults. In: Cynober LC, ed. *Amino acid metabolism and therapy in health and nutritional disease.* Boca Raton, FL: CRC Press; 1995:191–232.

Effects of Renal Insufficiency on Nutrient Metabolism and Endocrine Function

Saulo Klahr

PRINCIPAL FUNCTIONS OF THE KIDNEY

The kidney regulates body homeostasis not only through its excretory functions but through important synthetic and degradative properties of glomerular cells and tubular epithelial cells. These properties include the synthesis of hormones, the degradation of peptides and low–molecular-weight proteins (<50 kilodaltons [kDa]), and metabolic interconversions aimed at the conservation of energy and regulation of the composition of body fluids. The kidney is not only the site of synthesis of a number of hormones (i.e., erythropoietin, 1,25-dihydroxyvitamin D_3 [1,25-dihydroxycholecalciferol], renin), but is an important catabolic site for several polypeptide hormones (e.g., insulin, glucagon, parathyroid hormone [PTH]) and glycoproteins (Table 2-1).

THE CONSEQUENCES OF RENAL INSUFFICIENCY

Accumulation of Substances Excreted by the Kidney

A decrease in glomerular filtration rate (GFR) is the hallmark of renal insufficiency. As GFR decreases, solutes that are excreted by the kidney preferentially by filtration (creatinine, urea) accumulate in body fluids and their concentration in plasma rises. Other solutes that are filtered and reabsorbed or secreted by the renal tubules may also accumulate in body fluids, including phosphates, sulfates, uric acid, and hydrogen ions. The accumulation of hydrogen ions results in the development of metabolic acidosis. Other compounds that are retained in body fluids when renal insufficiency is more advanced include phenols, guanidines, organic acids, indols, myoinositol and other polyols, polyamines, β_2-microglobulin, certain peptides, uro-

Table 2-1. Principal functions of the kidney

Excretion of metabolic waste products (urea, creatinine, uric acid)

Elimination and detoxification of drugs and toxins

Maintenance of volume and ionic composition of body fluids

Regulation of systemic blood pressure

Production of erythropoietin

Control of mineral metabolism through endocrine synthesis
  (1,25-dihydroxycholecalciferol and 24,25-dihydroxycholecalciferol)

Degradation and catabolism of peptide hormones
  (insulin, glucagon, parathyroid hormone) and low–molecular-weight proteins (β_2-microglobulin and light chains)

Regulation of metabolic processes
  (gluconeogenesis, lipid metabolism)

furemic acids, and trace elements such as aluminum, zinc, copper, and iron. β_2-Microglobulin and some trace elements can accumulate and cause dysfunction of various organs.

Decreased Flexibility in Responding to Changes in Intake

As renal function decreases, the ability of patients to respond rapidly to changes in dietary intake, particularly involving sodium, potassium, and water, is markedly restricted. Even though solute and water excretion per nephron increases as renal function falls, the fewer the number of functional nephrons, the more the range of solute or water excretion becomes restricted. Thus, the upper limit of excretion for many solutes and for water is lower, whereas the lower limit is higher in patients with renal insufficiency compared with normal subjects. As renal disease progresses, there is decreased flexibility in the capacity to respond to changes in the intakes of sodium, other solutes, and water, and this can change the volume and composition of the extracellular fluid.

Decreased Synthetic Functions of the Kidney

The loss of the kidney's synthetic functions contributes to the abnormalities seen in renal insufficiency. For example, decreased production of erythropoietin, a hormone synthesized in the kidney that plays a key role in the maturation of erythrocyte precursors in bone marrow, is a major cause of the anemia of patients with renal disease. Decreased synthesis of 1,25-dihydroxycholecalciferol (calcitriol), the active metabolite of cholecalciferol, by the diseased kidney results in decreased serum concentrations of calcitriol and decreased calcium absorption from the gastrointestinal tract. Decreased concentrations of calcitriol also contribute to the development of hyperparathyroidism and bone disease in patients with renal insufficiency.

Alterations in Degradation of Hormones and Other Peptides

The kidney is the main site of degradation of several peptides (β_2-microglobulin, light chains), proteins, and peptide hormones, including insulin, glucagon, growth hormone, and PTH (see Table 2-1). The kidney also is involved in gluconeogenesis (the synthesis of glucose from noncarbohydrate precursors) and lipid metabolism. Failure of the kidneys, therefore, leads to multiple abnormalities affecting intermediary metabolism, the concentrations of circulating hormones, and the absorption of certain nutrients. As renal failure progresses, anorexia, nausea, and vomiting may develop and compromise the intake of nutrients and energy.

RENAL METABOLISM OF PLASMA PROTEINS AND PEPTIDE HORMONES

General Considerations

The kidney is a major site for the catabolism of plasma proteins with a molecular weight <50 kDa, but not for proteins with a molecular weight >68 kDa (e.g., albumin, immunoglobulins). Because most polypeptide hormones have molecular weights <30 kDa, they are metabolized by the kidney to some extent. Renal metabolism of polypeptide hormones often involves binding of the hormone to specific receptors in the basolateral membrane of tubular cells, or glomerular filtration and tubular reabsorption. Degradation results in generation of amino acids that are returned to the circulation. Removal of peptide hormones by filtration depends on the molecular weight, shape, and charge of the molecule. For example, growth hormone, with a molecular weight of 21.5 kDa, has a filtration coefficient of 0.7, whereas insulin, with a molecular weight of 6 kDa, is freely filtered. Binding of a hormone to large proteins prevents its filtration. Other factors, including impaired renal and extrarenal degradation of a hormone or abnormal secretion, are also operative in renal disease. Most filtered peptides are reabsorbed in the proximal tubule, so that <2% of the filtered polypeptide appears in the urine. In experimental animals, nephrectomy prolongs the plasma half-life of insulin, proinsulin, glucagon, PTH, growth hormones, and the like. Consequently, the circulating levels of numerous peptide hormones are elevated in advanced renal insufficiency (Table 2-2). In most instances, successful renal transplantation rapidly returns the circulating levels of many peptide hormones to normal levels.

Insulin, Proinsulin, and C-Peptide

The major sites of insulin degradation are the kidney and the liver. In humans, <1% of the filtered insulin is excreted in the urine, and catabolism of insulin in the kidney involves both filtration–reabsorption and peritubular uptake. The kidney also catabolizes proinsulin and C-peptide. The renal extraction of all these peptides appears to be proportional to their arterial concentrations. Ligation of the renal pedicle of experimental ani-

**Table 2-2. Circulating levels of hormones
in patients with advanced renal insufficiency**

Increased	Decreased
Insulin, proinsulin, C peptide	Erythropoietin
Glucagon	1,25-dihydroxycholecalciferol
Growth hormone	Progesterone
Parathyroid hormone	Testosterone
Calcitonin	Thyroxine
Gastrin	Triiodothyronine
Endothelin	
Prolactin (particularly in women)	
Vasopressin	
Luteinizing hormone	
Follicle-stimulating hormone	
Luteinizing hormone-releasing hormone	
Secretin	
Cholecystokinin	
Vasoactive intestinal peptide	
Gastric inhibitory peptide	

mals results in a 75% rise in the levels of plasma insulin and a 300% increase in the levels of proinsulin and C-peptide. The kidney accounts for most of the catabolism of the insulin precursor proinsulin. On the other hand, the kidney accounts for only one third of the metabolic clearance rate of insulin; liver and muscle account for two thirds of the disappearance of this peptide. In patients with renal insufficiency, high plasma levels of immunoreactive insulin probably represent a greater contribution of proinsulin and C-peptide rather than the active insulin. Consequently, there may be a dissociation between the radioimmunoassay insulin level and biologically active insulin when renal function is decreased.

Glucagon

The kidney accounts for approximately one third of the metabolic clearance of glucagon. Glomerular filtration is the major route of glucagon removal. The filtered hormone is degraded in the brush border membrane of the proximal tubule and, to a lesser extent, by reabsorption and subsequent intracellular degradation of the intact hormone, so that glucagon excretion in the urine is <2% of the amount filtered. (There is some peritubular removal of glucagon.) Plasma glucagon levels are increased in patients with chronic renal insufficiency and the metabolic clearance rate of injected glucagon is markedly prolonged. Glucagon secretion in response to stimulants is exaggerated in uremic patients, but the high plasma glucagon levels in uremia are apparently due to decreased metabolic clearance rather than hypersecretion of the hormone. Immunoreactive glucagon in the circulation of patients with renal insufficiency is heterogeneous: about 20% of the total immunoreactive hormone is the biologically active, 3.5-kDa species, another 60% is a 9-kDa species with little or no biologic activity, and the remainder is a high–molecular-weight form in excess of 40 kDa. The 9-kDa species is rarely present in the plasma of normal subjects. Thus, both biologically active and inactive forms of glucagon accumulate in uremic patients. Patients with renal failure show an altered physiologic response to glucagon: they demonstrate a three- to fourfold increase in the hyperglycemic response to the hormone. Over the long term, hemodialysis corrects some of these abnormalities.

Growth Hormone and Insulin-Like Growth Factor 1

In experimental animals, the kidney accounts for approximately 40% to 70% of the metabolic clearance rate of growth hormone. Growth hormone (molecular weight, 21.5 kDa) has a somewhat restricted filtration rate of about 70% compared with insulin. It is reabsorbed extensively along the nephron, and <1% of filtered hormone is excreted in the urine. In advanced renal insufficiency, the metabolic clearance of growth hormone is markedly decreased and plasma levels of the immunoreactive hormone are increased. Abnormalities in secretion can contribute to the high growth hormone levels observed in uremic subjects. Some of the biologic effects of growth hormone are mediated by insulin-like growth factors 1 and 2 (IGF-1 and IGF-2). Because growth hormone stimulates the synthesis and release of IGFs and because circulating IGFs exert a negative effect on growth hormone secretion, these peptides form a hormonal axis.

Emerging evidence indicates that IGF-1 is involved in compensatory renal hypertrophy. Administration of IGF-1 increases GFR and kidney weight in intact animals, and after uninephrectomy, there is an increase of IGF-1 in the contralateral kidney, even though IGF-1 receptor levels are unchanged. In patients with chronic renal insufficiency, plasma levels of IGF-1 are normal, but the levels of IGF-2 are elevated. Interestingly, the biologic effects of IGF-1 and IGF-2 are blunted when assayed in the presence of uremic serum, suggesting that a uremic factor or factors interferes with the biologic activity of IGF-1 and perhaps IGF-2. However, long-term infusion of supraphysiologic amounts of growth hormone to humans increases plasma IGF-1 about threefold, causes positive nitrogen balance, and improves growth. Clinical trials focused specifically on children with renal insufficiency have shown that administration of growth hormone improves growth.

Parathyroid Hormone

Advancing renal insufficiency is usually accompanied by a rise in the circulating levels of PTH, a 9.1-kDa peptide containing 84 amino acids. This is due to increased secretion by the parathyroid glands and impaired degradation of the hormone in the liver and kidney. The greater elevation of carboxy-terminal fragments in the circulation of patients with renal insufficiency compared with amino-terminal fragments occurs because carboxy-terminal fragments depend on filtration for their catabolism, whereas amino-terminal fragments are degraded by both filtration and peritubular uptake. Intact PTH is degraded by both glomerular filtration and peritubular uptake. The metabolic fragments of PTH are derived from enzymatic breakdown of intact PTH in the liver and, to a lesser extent, in the parathyroid glands. The liver and the kidney are the principal sites of degradation, accounting for 60% and 30%, respectively, of intact PTH removal. However, the kidney appears to be the only site where the carboxy-terminal fragments of the PTH molecule are degraded. Consequently, radioimmunoassays directed against the carboxy-terminal portion of PTH reveal extremely high levels of immunoreactive PTH in the circulation of patients with renal insufficiency.

Factors that contribute to the increased levels of PTH include phosphorus retention, skeletal resistance to the effects of PTH, and decreased levels of 1,25-dihydroxycholecalciferol, culminating in hyperplasia of the parathyroid glands.

Calcitonin

Calcitonin is a peptide with a molecular weight of 3.5 kDa. The kidney accounts for about two thirds of its metabolic clearance, and calcitonin receptors are located at both peritubular sites and the brush border of tubular cells. Calcitonin is degraded at the brush border membrane of tubular cells and intracellularly in lysosomes. In renal failure, the metabolic clearance rate of calcitonin is decreased and plasma levels of the hormone are increased. The calcitonin species that accumulates in the plasma of individuals with renal insufficiency is a high–molecular-weight form that may or may not have biologic activity. Clinical consequences of elevated levels of calcitonin in patients with renal insufficiency are unknown.

Gastrin

The plasma concentration of gastrin in humans is increased after nephrectomy. The hypergastrinemia seen in patients with renal failure is due, most likely, to reduced degradation of this hormone by the kidney.

Endothelin

Endothelin 1, a potent endogenous vasoconstrictor peptide, accumulates in patients with renal insufficiency. The plasma levels are higher than in normal subjects and may contribute to hypertension in patients with renal failure.

Catecholamines

Plasma levels of norepinephrine are within normal limits in patients with mild to moderate renal insufficiency, but high levels are found in patients with advanced renal insufficiency. A threefold increase in plasma norepinephrine occurs in patients with renal insufficiency on assuming an upright position, and this response exceeds that seen in normal subjects performing the maneuver. There also is an abnormal metabolism of norepinephrine in patients with renal insufficiency because of reduced activity of tyrosine hydroxylase, the critical enzyme involved in the synthesis of norepinephrine in certain organs (e.g., heart, brain). However, the elevated levels of norepinephrine do not appear to be due to increased synthesis but rather to decreased degradation in patients with renal insufficiency.

Prolactin

Approximately 16% of prolactin is extracted during passage through the kidney. The hormone is filtered to a modest extent because its molecular weight is 23 kDa. Most of the filtered prolactin is reabsorbed by the proximal tubules (<1% appears in the urine). Very likely, the kidney contributes to the metabolic clearance of prolactin, although adequate studies in humans are lacking. Elevated plasma prolactin levels are seen in approximately 80% of women but in only 30% of men with renal insufficiency, and the increase in prolactin is not modified by the administration of dopamine or bromocriptine. There is a prolonged rise in prolactin levels after administration of thyroid-releasing factor in patients with renal insufficiency, indicating that a pituitary gland disorder plus a defect in the peripheral metabolism of the hormone are present. In fact, the metabolic clearance of prolactin is diminished to about one third in patients with renal insufficiency. Apart from galactorrhea, other biologic effects of prolactin in patients with renal insufficiency are not clearly established.

Antidiuretic Hormone (Vasopressin)

Antidiuretic hormone (ADH) is metabolized in the liver and in the kidney. The kidney accounts for about 60% of the total metabolic clearance of ADH, mainly through glomerular filtration, although there is some extraction at peritubular sites. The kidney appears to have a large capacity to remove ADH, but it is not clear whether vasopressin is filtered and reabsorbed in the proximal tubule before intracellular degradation, or whether it is degraded at the brush border membrane of proximal tubular cells. In patients with renal insufficiency, there is decreased removal of ADH, and patients undergoing long-term hemodialysis usually have high circulating levels of vasopressin.

RENAL METABOLISM OF GLYCOPROTEIN HORMONES

The kidney is a major site for the removal of several glycoprotein hormones and their metabolites, including erythropoietin, thyrotropin or thyroid-stimulating hormone (TSH), luteinizing hormone (LH), follicle-stimulating hormone (FSH), and human chorionic gonadotropin. Studies in animals suggest that the kidney accounts for 95%, 78%, and 32% of the metabolic clearance rate of LH, FSH, and erythropoietin, respectively. The renal clearance of glycoprotein hormones is relatively slow compared with that of nonglycosylated, polypeptide hormones. The filtration of glycoproteins is apparently restricted because of their larger molecular weight (usually >25 kDa). In addition, the structure of a glycoprotein may hinder its catabolism, and it is unlikely that glycoprotein hormones have peritubular receptors leading to degradation. In fact, filtered glycoproteins are reabsorbed to a lesser extent than filtered polypeptides, and a large proportion appear in the urine; the excretion of FSH is approximately 43% of the amount filtered by the kidney. A marked decrease in renal function results in reduced metabolic clearance of glycoprotein hormones, and the balance between hormone secretion and metabolism determines whether the plasma levels of glycoproteins are elevated in patients with renal insufficiency.

POTENTIAL CONSEQUENCES OF HORMONAL ALTERATIONS

Sexual dysfunction is a bothersome disorder for patients with renal insufficiency. Its cause is probably a dysfunction of the hypothalamic–pituitary–adrenal axis, characterized by elevated circulating levels of LH, FSH, prolactin, and LH-releasing hormone. These changes lead to lower levels of progesterone or testosterone in women and men, respectively. Although the pathogenesis of these abnormalities is unknown, contributory roles for PTH, anemia, and zinc deficiency have been suggested. Sexual dysfunction is manifested clinically by impotence, decreased libido, testicular atrophy, and reduced sperm count in men and amenorrhea, dysmenorrhea, and decreased libido in women. Increased levels of prolactin may cause galactorrhea, whereas high levels of LH can cause gynecomastia.

HORMONAL DEFICIENCIES IN PATIENTS WITH RENAL INSUFFICIENCY

Decreased levels of two hormones synthesized by the kidney, erythropoietin and calcitriol, contribute substantially to the metabolic abnormalities that occur in patients with renal insufficiency.

Erythropoietin

A decrease in the synthesis of erythropoietin by the diseased kidney is the most important cause of anemia in patients with renal insufficiency. Such patients have much lower erythropoietin levels than comparably anemic people with normal renal function, and therefore a hypoproliferative bone marrow leads to a hypochromic, microcytic anemia. But this is not iron deficiency, and iron overload can occur when transfusions are used to restore the hematocrit. Administration of recombinant human erythropoietin to patients with renal insufficiency corrects the anemia, increases exercise tolerance, and improves subjective indices of well-being and cognitive function. If iron deficiency occurs—gastrointestinal malabsorption of iron is present in patients with advanced renal insufficiency—parenteral administration of iron is required. When adequate iron stores are restored, erythropoietin administration corrects the anemia.

1,25-Dihydroxycholecalciferol (Calcitriol)

Vitamin D_3 is hydroxylated in the liver to 25-hydroxycholecalciferol. The enzyme 1-α hydroxylase, present in mitochondria of proximal tubular cells, catalyzes a second hydroxylation to form the active compound, 1,25-dihydroxycholecalciferol (calcitriol). Calcitriol, in turn, has several biologic effects, including increased reabsorption of calcium and phosphorus from the gastrointestinal tract. Calcitriol also facilitates PTH-induced removal of calcium from bone. The activity of the 1-α hydroxylase in the kidney is stimulated by PTH and inhibited by high levels of calcium, organic phosphates, and calcitriol in serum.

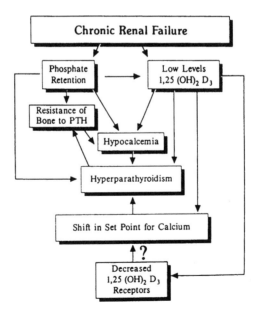

Fig. 2-1. Pathogenesis of hyperparathyroidism in renal failure.
(From Delmez JC. Renal osteodystrophy and other musculoskeletal complications of chronic renal failure. In: Greenberg A, ed. Primer on kidney diseases. New York: Academic Press; 1994:294–300, with permission.)

Besides the gut and bone, calcitriol acts directly on the parathyroid glands to reduce hypertrophy and hyperplasia of parathyroid cells in patients with renal insufficiency. The hormone reduces transcription of the prepro-PTH gene, thereby reducing the synthesis and release of PTH. Thus, the absence of calcitriol results in parathyroid hyperplasia that is not reversible because PTH production is impaired. Calcitriol deficiency also results in an upward shift of the set point for calcium-stimulated PTH release: higher serum calcium concentrations are required to achieve a standardized reduction in PTH levels. The impaired synthesis of calcitriol in renal insufficiency, most likely due to a loss of renal mass and hyperphosphatemia, may decrease intestinal calcium absorption, leading to hypocalcemia and parathyroid hyperactivity. This and other factors result in secondary hyperparathyroidism (Fig. 2-1).

ABNORMALITIES IN GLUCOCORTICOIDS AND THYROID HORMONE IN PATIENTS WITH RENAL INSUFFICIENCY

Glucocorticoids

Plasma levels of cortisol are normal or high in patients with renal insufficiency. The response of the adrenal gland to adrenocorticotropin is decreased, but the response of adrenocorticotropin to stimulatory agents such as hypoglycemia is nearly normal. Thus, the normal or high cortisol level is attributed to its reduced clearance by the diseased kidney. The net effect is that adrenal function remains normal and the expected diurnal variation remains unaltered in patients with renal insufficiency.

Thyroid Abnormalities

Abnormalities of thyroid hormones are present in patients with renal insufficiency for several reasons. Renal insufficiency affects the metabolism of thyroid hormones at different steps, including the clearance of iodide, TSH clearance, and the peripheral conversion of thyroxine (T_4) to triiodothyronine (T_3). Plasma iodide is usually high, but there are often reduced levels of total T_4, the free T_4 index, total T_3, and the free T_3 index, and normal levels of total reverse T_3. The levels of TSH are in general within normal limits, but the response to thyroid-releasing factor is blunted. The prevalence of goiter in patients with renal insufficiency is high (>33%) compared with that in the general population, but overt hypothyroidism is rare. Although many patients with renal insufficiency are subject to easy fatigability, lethargy, and cold intolerance, these changes are not accompanied by alterations in the basal metabolic rate or in the relaxation time for tendon reflexes (indicators of the biologic function of thyroid hormone).

Other Hormones

Because of decreased degradation, the levels of other hormones are high in the plasma of patients with renal insufficiency. These include gastrin, secretin, cholecystokinin, vasoactive intestinal peptide, and gastric inhibitory peptide. It is not clear whether changes in gastrointestinal physiology are due to increased levels of these hormones.

DISORDERS OF CARBOHYDRATE METABOLISM IN RENAL INSUFFICIENCY

A certain degree of glucose intolerance is present in patients with renal insufficiency. Although most patients with renal insufficiency are euglycemic when fasting, there is evidence for glucose intolerance after oral or intravenous glucose loads. The abnormal glucose metabolism of patients with renal insufficiency is characterized by fasting euglycemia, abnormal glucose tolerance, a delayed fall in blood glucose in response to insulin, hyperinsulinemia, and hyperglucagonemia (Table 2-3).

Insulin Resistance

Several studies suggest that the abnormal glucose tolerance is caused by resistance of peripheral tissues, particularly muscle, to insulin. Metabolic studies, both in vivo and in vitro, have uncovered impaired insulin-mediated glucose uptake and metabolism in these tissues. There may be a circulating factor that induces insulin resistance at the level of muscle. An increase in growth hormone in patients with renal insufficiency may also contribute to the resistance of peripheral tissues to insulin. Mechanistically, insulin binding to its receptor is apparently normal, but several studies suggest that an intracellular defect at a postreceptor step accounts for the insulin resistance. Clinically, patients with renal insufficiency can have two different responses to intravenous glucose administration: in some, the decay rate of infused glucose exceeds 1 and the circulating levels of insulin are increased, whereas in others, the decay of infused glucose is less than 1 and the plasma insulin level is either decreased or lower than predicted for the level of plasma glucose. These different responses may relate to the ability of the islets to release insulin in response to hyperglycemia.

Metabolic Acidosis

The metabolic acidosis that develops with renal insufficiency may contribute to the insulin resistance, leading to impaired glucose transport. Indeed, chronic acidosis, produced by ammonium chloride administration in normal individuals, leads to

Table 2-3. Glucose metabolism and gluconeogenic hormones in patients with renal insufficiency

1. Fasting blood glucose is usually "normal"
2. Possible spontaneous hypoglycemia
   (because of decreased gluconeogenesis, alanine deficiency)
3. Fasting hyperinsulinemia, increased plasma levels of proinsulin and peptide C
4. Increased plasma levels of immunoreactive glucagon and growth hormone
5. Decreased glucose utilization in response to insulin in peripheral tissues (mainly in muscle)
6. Impaired insulin secretion from pancreatic islets in some patients (increases in intracellular calcium in islets, as a consequence of hyperparathyroidism?)

changes in insulin-dependent glucose transport similar to those seen in patients with renal failure.

The Role of β Cells

The glucose tolerance of patients with renal insufficiency can be normal if the β cells of the pancreas secrete insulin appropriately. If this occurs, patients will have a normal fasting serum glucose, but at the expense of elevated levels of insulin in plasma.

A deficiency of calcitriol (1,25-dihydroxyvitamin D_3) may contribute to the resistance of peripheral tissues to insulin, and it is possible that calcitriol interacts with pancreatic islets to modulate the secretion of insulin. In fact, it has been reported that intravenous administration of calcitriol to dialysis patients significantly increased their secretion of insulin.

Glucose Transport in Fat Cells

Fat cells from patients with renal insufficiency also exhibit decreased glucose uptake in response to insulin compared with adipocytes obtained from normal subjects. Lipogenesis in response to insulin is also blunted, and decreased levels of insulin or resistance to its effects can decrease the activity of lipoprotein lipase, which has an important role in the removal of triglycerides.

Abnormal Insulin Release

A reduced release of insulin during the initial response to hyperglycemia has been reported, indicating a reduced sensitivity to glucose of β cells in the pancreas. PTH, apparently by enhancing the movement of calcium into the β cells, seems to impair insulin secretion from such cells. Thus, the secondary hyperparathyroidism present in patients with renal insufficiency can compromise the ability of the islets to secrete insulin appropriately and maintain normal glucose homeostasis. For two reasons, diabetic patients in whom progressive renal disease develops require decreasing doses of insulin as the disease progresses. First, they have a reduced energy intake, and second, there is a reduced degradation of insulin by the diseased kidney, leading to a decreased insulin requirement.

ENERGY NEEDS OF PATIENTS WITH RENAL INSUFFICIENCY

The energy needs of patients with chronic renal insufficiency and the calorie requirements of such patients are similar to those of normal subjects. However, energy intake in patients with renal disease tends to diminish because of the gradual onset of anorexia as the GFR decreases below 25 ml/minute. Consequently, an inadequate energy intake is common in patients with chronic renal insufficiency. This is important because anorexia also reduces protein intake and an adequate energy intake enhances the utilization of protein in patients eating low-protein diets. An intake of 150 kilojoules/kg body weight/day (35 kilocalories/kg body weight/day) is recommended for most patients with chronic renal failure, but for those older than 60 years, 130 kilojoules/kg body weight/day (30 kilocalories/kg body weight/day) may be adequate. A higher intake of energy is appropriate for patients who engage in vigorous physical activity. It is likely that reduced energy intake contributes to the malnutrition often seen in patients with renal insufficiency, but a reduction in protein intake can contribute to wasting. A low-protein diet has been prescribed for decades to patients with renal insufficiency both to ameliorate the symptoms and clinical manifestations of uremia and to attempt to slow the progression of renal disease.

PROTEIN-CALORIE MALNUTRITION

Protein-calorie malnutrition appears to play a major role in the morbidity and mortality of patients with end-stage renal failure. Several indicators of nutritional status have been used in evaluating patients with renal insufficiency (Table 2-4), including serum albumin, transferrin, cholesterol, and creatinine. Other measurements have been suggested, such as levels of prealbumin, IGF-1, amino acid profiles in plasma and muscle, and circulating levels of PTH. Finally, changes in body composition have been analyzed by measurements of anthropometry, bioelectric impedance, and total body nitrogen. Most studies of the nutritional status of patients with end-stage renal insufficiency yield a prevalence of malnutrition of 20% to 50%.

DISORDERS OF LIPID METABOLISM IN RENAL INSUFFICIENCY

Lipoproteins

Disturbances of lipoprotein metabolism are commonly present in patients with chronic renal insufficiency. In plasma, the lipoproteins function as an efficient vehicle for site-to-site transport of triglycerides and cholesterol of both endogenous and exogenous origin. The density of lipoproteins depends on the ratio between surface and core components, and five classes of

---

Table 2-4. Indicators of malnutrition in patients with renal insufficiency

Dietary intake

Spontaneous low dietary intake of protein as assessed by urea nitrogen excretion in a 24-hour urine collection (values below 0.7 g/kg/day)

Weight and anthropometric measures

Loss of weight or body weight <85% of ideal body weight

Decreased skinfold thickness, decreased midarm circumference or muscle strength

Laboratory findings

Low serum albumin levels (<3.5 g/dl)

Low serum creatinine in the presence of somewhat advanced renal insufficiency

Low serum prealbumin levels (<30 mg/dl)

Low serum transferrin levels (<200 mg/dl)

Low levels of essential amino acids in plasma or muscle

Relatively low levels of immunoreactive parathyroid hormone in patients with somewhat advanced renal insufficiency

---

lipoproteins are present in the plasma of fasting individuals: very–low-density (VLDL), intermediate-density (IDL), low-density (LDL), and high-density (HDL) lipoproteins. (Subspecies of each major lipoprotein class are also present.) Chylomicrons (large, triglyceride-rich particles of intestinal origin) are the fifth class of lipoproteins and are transiently present in plasma in the postprandial state. The protein moieties of lipoproteins, referred to as apolipoproteins (APOs), are classified by letters of the alphabet and Roman numeral suffixes. Some of these apolipoproteins, such as A-I in HDL, B-C in LDL, and B-XLVIII in chylomicrons, play a structural role. The major APOs and their function are summarized in Table 2-5.

Lipid Abnormalities

Lipid abnormalities develop in patients with chronic renal insufficiency and are not corrected by dialysis. In general, triglyceride levels are increased, HDL is reduced, and LDL, IDL, and VLDL are all increased. The mechanisms responsible for these changes have not been completely elucidated and are most likely complex. Insulin resistance and hyperparathyroidism have been implicated in the development of hypertriglyceridemia because both insulin and PTH can directly or indirectly regulate the synthesis of lipoprotein lipase. Lipoprotein lipase activity is decreased, and this may be due to inhibition by APO C-III, which accumulates in the plasma of patients with chronic renal failure. Although disorders of lipoprotein metabolism become more prevalent as renal insufficiency advances, the degree of hyperlipidemia does not necessarily correlate with the severity of renal insufficiency. Lipoprotein abnormalities may be modulated to some extent by

Table 2-5. Major human plasma apolipoproteins and their function

Protein	Molecular Weight (kDa)	Main Functions
Apo AI	28.0	LCAT activator
Apo AII	17.0	?
Apo AIV	44.5	LCAT activator
Apo B-C	550.0	Ligand for LDL receptor
Apo B-XLVIII	264.0	Structural component of chylomicrons
Apo CI	6.6	LCAT activator
Apo CII	8.9	Activator, lipoprotein lipase
Apo CIII	8.8	Inhibitor of hepatic uptake of apo E-containing particles
Apo E	34.0	Ligand for the LDL receptor; specific protein of apo (a)

Apo=apolipoprotein; LCAT=lecithin cholesterol acyltransferase; LDL=low-density lipoprotein.
Adapted from Scanu AM. Physiopathology of plasma lipoprotein metabolism. *Kidney Int* 1991;39(Suppl 31):S3–S7, with permission.

therapeutic interventions, but are only marginally affected by dialysis. Abnormalities of lipid transport and metabolism can also occur after renal transplantation. This is probably related both to the type of immunosuppressive drugs used and to persistent renal insufficiency.

Abnormalities of lipoprotein metabolism implicated in the accelerated atherogenesis seen in patients with renal insufficiency may be detectable even early in the course of the condition. Hypertriglyceridemia is the most common plasma lipid abnormality in both adults and children with renal insufficiency, although the reported prevalences differ considerably. Usually the degree of hypertriglyceridemia is moderate and plasma cholesterol levels are within the normal range, although cholesterol can be elevated, particularly in patients with more pronounced hypertriglyceridemia.

Although the exact mechanism of dyslipoproteinemia remains undefined, evidence indicates that both increased hepatic production and impaired removal of circulating triglyceride-rich LDL contribute to the defect. Triglyceride enrichment is evident not only in VLDL, but also may be detected in IDL, LDL, and HDL. There also is a redistribution of plasma cholesterol, from HDL to VLDL and IDL, even when the plasma levels of cholesterol are within normal limits. The LDL-cholesterol is usually within normal limits and the ratio of either total cholesterol or LDL-cholesterol to HDL-cholesterol is increased. The reduced levels of HDL are reflected in the reduced levels of both HDL-II and HDL-III subfractions. Patients with moderate renal insufficiency often have normal levels of plasma triglycerides and cholesterol, but more discrete changes in plasma lipids may be found, including an increase in the concentration of LDL triglyceride and a reduced concentration of HDL cholesterol. In advanced renal insufficiency, the concentration of APO A-I and A-II apolipoproteins is reduced. There are normal or slightly elevated levels of APO B and normal (or, in male patients, decreased) levels of APO E. There is usually a significantly increased concentration of APO C-III and less pronounced increases in the concentrations of APOs C-I and C-II lipoproteins. Elevated levels of APO C-III usually correlate with the level of triglycerides, but may also be found in patients with normal levels of triglycerides.

The Mechanisms of Altered Lipid Metabolism in Patients with Chronic Renal Insufficiency

The plasma concentration of lipoproteins is determined by a balance between their production and catabolism. The mechanisms underlying elevated triglycerides in patients with chronic renal insufficiency have not been completely elucidated. The predominant defect appears to be reduced lipolysis of triglyceride-rich lipoproteins, but other factors that can affect the metabolism of triglyceride-rich lipoproteins in renal insufficiency are listed in Table 2-6. Substantial evidence indicates that the transport and catabolism of triglyceride-rich lipoproteins are impaired in patients with renal insufficiency, leading to the accumulation of dyslipoproteins resulting from various degrees of catabolism, with increased concentrations of IDL and remnants of intestinal lipoproteins (chylomicron remnants). The catabolism of lipopro-

Table 2-6. Factors that may contribute to hypertriglyceridemia in patients with chronic renal insufficiency

Decreased Triglyceride Catabolism and Removal	Increased Triglyceride Production
Decreased activity of lipolytic enzymes	Increased ingestion of carbohydrates
Lipoprotein lipase	
Insulin deficiency or resistance	
Increased parathyroid hormone	
Inhibitors in uremic plasma	
Reduced apolipoprotein CII/CIII ratio	Hyperinsulinemia?
Hepatic triglyceride lipase	
Lecithin cholesterol acyltransferase	
Alterations of lipoprotein substrate	
Triglyceride-enriched LDL	
Altered apolipoprotein composition	
Increased apolipoprotein CII/E in IDL and LDL	
Modifications of lipoproteins	
Decreased receptor- and nonreceptor-mediated cellular uptake of lipoproteins	

IDL=intermediate-density lipoprotein; LDL=low-density lipoprotein.

teins rich in triglycerides is mediated mainly by lipoprotein lipase and by hepatic triglyceride lipase, which is thought to be responsible for the clearance of partially metabolized lipoproteins (possibly through the APO B and APO E receptors in the liver). Several studies have found decreased activity of lipoprotein lipase in plasma and adipose tissue of patients with renal insufficiency, and a reduced lipolytic activity after heparin administration can be detected even when the GFR is as high as 50 ml/minute, but this does not lead to an increase in plasma triglycerides. The mechanisms underlying the decrease in lipoprotein lipase activity are unknown. Insulin deficiency or insulin resistance may play a role in this process because in experimental animals, insulin administration increases the activity of lipoprotein lipase in adipose tissue. Uremic plasma may also contain a nondialyzable inhibitor of lipoprotein lipase.

Increased synthesis of triglycerides can contribute to the hypertriglyceridemia, and because there is defective catabolism, even a modest change in triglyceride synthesis (as induced by the diet) can result in significant changes in the plasma levels of triglycerides. In diabetic patients with renal failure, both increased triglyceride production due to poor metabolic control of the diabetes and reduced catabolism of triglycerides due to renal insufficiency contribute to elevated concentrations of triglyceride-rich lipoproteins. Insulin resistance may also be a factor that increases triglyceride production in renal insufficiency, although this is conjectural.

The changes in the plasma levels of lipoprotein cholesterol are thought to be secondary to the altered metabolism of triglyceride-rich lipoproteins.

PROTEIN AND AMINO ACID METABOLISM
IN PATIENTS WITH RENAL INSUFFICIENCY

There are six general classes of nutrients: carbohydrates, lipids, proteins, vitamins, minerals, and water. The first three are organic compounds that serve as sources of energy required for the biochemical and functional activities. In addition, dietary protein provides the amino acids that are needed to synthesize body proteins and support a number of physiologic processes, including growth, repair of tissues, enzymatic activity, and ion and solute transport. Protein and amino acids also function as signaling molecules and as hormones, and participate in differentiation, in immunity as antibodies, in gene expression, and so forth.

Historically, the 20 amino acids present in body proteins have been classified into two categories, essential or nonessential, depending on whether they are required in the diet for the maintenance of nitrogen balance in healthy people. The amino acids classified as essential in 1954 were leucine, isoleucine, valine, threonine, methionine, phenylalanine, lysine, and tryptophan. The nonessential amino acids were glycine, alanine, serine, cystine, tyrosine, aspartic acid, glutamic acid, proline, histidine, hydroxyproline, citrulline, and arginine. Subsequent studies have suggested this is not a satisfactory classification because histidine has been shown to be an essential amino acid, and other amino acids such as glycine, tyrosine, cystine, proline, arginine, glutamine, and taurine are now generally considered as indispensable components of the normal diet.

Patients with progressive renal insufficiency are at increased risk for the development of malnutrition. Although this can be reversed, it is a major cause of morbidity and mortality. Altered metabolism of protein and amino acids occurs in patients with chronic renal insufficiency, and as renal function decreases, nitrogenous waste products of protein metabolism accumulate, eventually resulting in symptomatic uremia. During the evolution of progressive renal insufficiency, subtle alterations occur in the concentrations of plasma proteins and in the levels of amino acids in plasma and intracellular compartments. Protein-calorie malnutrition has been found in 25% to 50% of patients entering dialysis programs in North America, and it is now established that low levels of albumin in plasma are a good predictor of morbidity and mortality in dialysis patients. Malnutrition in patients with progressive renal disease may be the result of inadequate dietary intake or increased requirements due to changes in intermediary metabolism resulting from kidney failure. In certain instances, extravascular pools of albumin may be reduced, even though the serum albumin concentration remains normal. Serum concentrations of transferrin, considered by some to be a more sensitive indicator of protein malnutrition, are low in many patients with moderate to advanced renal insufficiency, and were also found to be low in a group of patients on long-term dialysis, despite their eating sufficient protein (i.e., 1 g protein/kg body weight). Although inadequate protein or energy intake may be the major cause of malnutrition in chronic renal insufficiency, the possibility that renal failure per se disturbs one or several steps in the complex process of protein synthesis and degradation has not received sufficient study. Recent research indicates that increased catabolism of proteins may indeed occur in the muscle of patients with only moderate renal insufficiency. Metabolic alterations in patients with renal insufficiency that seem to cause net protein catabolism in muscle include higher levels of circulating glucagon and PTH, accumulation of uremic toxins, and metabolic acidosis. Metabolic acidosis produces increased proteolysis in muscle of experimental animals without altering protein synthesis. Correction of the metabolic acidosis in patients with renal insufficiency has been shown to prevent the increased proteolysis, and supplementing the diet of patients with renal insufficiency with bicarbonate can improve nitrogen balance.

Changes in Amino Acid Profiles in Renal Insufficiency

Abnormalities in plasma amino acid concentrations are present in patients with renal insufficiency. Most of these patients have a decreased ratio of essential to nonessential amino acids, a pattern that mimics that seen in malnutrition. However, the abnormalities in plasma amino acids in patients with renal insufficiency cannot be explained on the basis of malnutrition alone because they also occur when protein intake is optimal, suggesting that abnormal levels in plasma may be the result of malnutrition plus changes in amino acid metabolism brought about by the development of renal insufficiency. The plasma levels of the branched-chain amino acids, valine, leucine, and isoleucine, and their respective ketoacids, are decreased, with valine being reduced to a greater extent. The potential mechanism responsible for this decrease in branched-chain amino acids may be related to oxidation of such amino acids in skeletal muscle as a consequence of metabolic acidosis. Patients with renal insufficiency also exhibit decreases in the plasma concentration of threonine and lysine, as well as low serine levels. The latter may be due to decreased production of this amino acid from lysine in the kidney. Tyrosine levels are usually decreased, and this presumably is related to defective phenylalanine hydroxylation. The plasma levels of phenylalanine are usually normal, whereas total tryptophan is decreased in patients with uremia, despite the fact that free tryptophan levels are normal. The explanation for this is that binding of tryptophan by plasma proteins in uremic subjects is reduced. Levels of certain amino acids are increased in the plasma of patients with renal insufficiency, including glycine, citrulline, cystine, aspartate, methionine, and both 1- and 3-methylhistidine. The increase in the plasma concentration of citrulline is due to decreased conversion of this amino acid to arginine in the kidney. Interestingly, the higher citrulline level in plasma seems to correct any arginine deficit in patients with advanced renal disease. Metabolites of sulfur-containing amino acids accumulate in blood.

Intracellular Levels of Amino Acids

Measurements of intracellular levels of amino acids in patients with renal insufficiency also reveal abnormalities. Typically, intracellular muscle valine is low, but other branched-chain amino acids, leucine and isoleucine, are within normal limits. The levels of intracellular taurine are decreased despite normal plasma levels. Both cystine and methionine, two precursors of taurine synthesis, are usually increased in renal insufficiency;

thus, a low intracellular taurine level may be due to defective synthesis from these two precursors. It is possible that abnormal concentrations of amino acids in patients with renal insufficiency influence, per se, protein metabolism. Indeed, when pre-dialysis patients eating 16 to 20 g of protein per day were provided with a supplement of essential amino acids designed to modify or correct the abnormalities in amino acid levels, both nitrogen balance and the profile of intracellular amino acids improved. Decreased utilization of amino acids by the kidney can contribute to the accumulation in plasma of certain amino acids such as citrulline. The concentration of amino acids is much greater inside the cells than in plasma, however, and thus plasma levels of amino acids are not representative of intracellular amino acid levels.

VITAMINS

In patients with relatively far-advanced renal insufficiency ingesting protein-restricted diets, deficiencies of water-soluble vitamins may develop because of decreased dietary intake. Reduced concentrations of several water-soluble vitamins in serum, erythrocytes, and leukocytes have been reported, and hematologic evidence of folate deficiency was found in some patients but not in others, probably reflecting variations in dietary intake and use of vitamin supplements. In one report, patients not receiving vitamin supplements had low plasma and leukocyte concentrations of vitamin C, and a few patients had signs suggestive of mild degrees of scurvy. Plasma concentrations of other water-soluble vitamins have been reported as normal in most studies. Because the kidney is one of the routes of eliminating water-soluble vitamins and their metabolites, decreased kidney function may be a protective mechanism, especially for patients on hemodialysis, a treatment that can remove water-soluble vitamins. Vitamin deficiencies may be related to poor dietary intake, interference with vitamin absorption by other drugs, altered metabolism, and, in dialysis patients, losses of vitamins in the dialysate. The daily requirements for most vitamins in patients with renal insufficiency are not clearly defined, but there is evidence that supplements can prevent or correct vitamin deficiencies. Thus, patients with advanced renal insufficiency or those in dialysis should take supplemental folic acid and B vitamins. Vitamin replacement may need to be greater in patients undergoing high-flux dialysis.

On the other hand, supplementation with multivitamin preparations should be prescribed with caution because excessive levels of vitamins can develop in patients with advanced renal insufficiency. Vitamin C supplements should not exceed 150 to 200 mg/day because higher levels can cause the accumulation of ascorbic acid metabolites such as oxalate. Oxalate in turn can lead to complications such as calcium oxalate kidney stones and deposits of calcium oxalate in soft tissues and organs. Vitamin A is usually high in patients with advanced renal insufficiency because of an increase in the serum levels of retinol-binding protein and its decreased renal catabolism. An increase in the levels of vitamin A can cause anemia and abnormalities of lipid and calcium metabolism. Plasma levels of pyridoxal 5-phosphate are frequently low in patients with renal insufficiency. Levels of serum glutamic oxaloacetic transaminase suggest that pyridoxine deficiency is clinically relevant. Because this plasma enzyme requires pyridoxyl 5-phosphate as a cofactor, it has been suggested that a water-soluble vitamin supplement including 10 to 50 mg of pyridoxine per day and 1 to 5 mg of folate per day should be provided to avoid a deficiency state.

TRACE ELEMENTS

In patients with renal insufficiency, the metabolism of trace elements is probably deranged. The mechanisms for the alterations have not been clearly established, and the contribution of trace element deficiencies or excesses to the symptoms of advanced renal insufficiency has not been adequately studied. Highly protein-bound substances, such as copper and zinc, are lost in excessive amounts with increasing proteinuria. There are no data to support a recommendation that trace elements be given routinely to patients with chronic renal insufficiency, but there is some evidence suggesting a need for selenium, zinc, and iron. These should be given only after the adequacy of the diet in terms of calories and protein has been evaluated. The extent of zinc deficiency in advanced renal insufficiency or in patients on dialysis is debatable. Plasma levels of selenium, which has important antioxidant properties, have been reported as low, particularly in patients undergoing dialysis. However, the benefits of selenium administration in this population have not been identified. Infections or steroid therapy may artificially lower the concentration of zinc in plasma, and should be taken into account before zinc is prescribed. The accumulation of aluminum, from the administration of medicines containing it (e.g., phosphate binders), can occur. Fortunately, most dialysis centers have largely eliminated the use of aluminum as a phosphate binder in the treatment of patients with renal insufficiency. Accumulation of aluminum can cause bone disease, encephalopathy, and other clinical problems in patients with renal insufficiency.

SELECTED READINGS

Attman P-O, Samuelsson O, Alaupovic P. Lipoprotein metabolism and renal failure. *Am J Kidney Dis* 1993;21:573–592.

Ballmer PE, McNeulen MA, Hulter HW, et al. Chronic metabolic acidosis decreases albumin synthesis and induces negative nitrogen balance in humans. *J Clin Invest* 1995;95:39–45.

Castellino P, Solini A, Luzi L, et al. Glucose and amino acid metabolism in chronic renal failure: effect of insulin and amino acids. *Am J Physiol* 1992;262:F168–F176.

Fadde GZ, Haffar SM, Perna AF, et al. On the mechanism of impaired insulin secretion in chronic renal failure. *J Clin Invest* 1991;87:255–261.

Ikizler TA, Greene JH, Wingard RL, et al. Spontaneous dietary protein intake during progression of chronic renal failure. *J Am Soc Nephrol* 1995;6:1386–1391.

Ikizler TA, Hakim RM. Nutrition in end-stage renal disease. *Kidney Int* 1996;50:343–357.

Laidlaw SH, Berg RL, Kopple JD, et al. Patterns of fasting plasma amino acid levels in chronic renal insufficiency: results from the feasibility phase of the Modification of Diet in Renal Disease Study. *Am J Kidney Dis* 1994;23:504–513.

Lee P, O'Neal D, Murphy B, et al. The role of abdominal adiposity and insulin resistance in dyslipidemia of chronic renal failure. *Am J Kidney Dis* 1997;29:54–65.

Llach F. Secondary hyperparathyroidism in renal failure: the trade-off hypothesis revisited. *Am J Kidney Dis* 1995;25:663–679.

Makoff R. Vitamin supplementation in patients with renal diseases. *Dialyses-Transplantation* 1992;21:18–36.

Massry SG, Smogorzewsky MJ, Klahr S. Metabolic and endocrine dysfunctions in uremia. In: Schrier RW, Gottschalk CW, eds. *Diseases of the kidney*. 6th ed. Boston: Little, Brown; 1997: 2661–2698.

Mittman N, Avram MM. Dyslipidemia in renal disease. *Semin Nephrol* 1996;16:202–213.

Reaich D, Channon SM, Scrimgeour CM, et al. Correction of acidosis in humans with CRF decreases protein degradation and amino acid oxidation. *Am J Physiol* 1993;265:E230–E235.

Reaich D, Price SR, England BK, et al. Mechanisms causing muscle loss in chronic renal failure. *Am J Kidney Dis* 1995;26:242–247.

Richard MJ, Arnaud J, Jurkovitz C, et al. Trace elements and lipid peroxidation abnormalities in patients with chronic renal failure. *Nephron* 1991;57:10–15.

Sanaka T, Shinobe M, Ando M, et al. IGF-1 as an early indicator of malnutrition in patients with end-stage renal disease. *Nephron* 1994;67:73–81.

Schaefer F, Veldhuis D, Robertson WR, et al. Immunoreactive and bioactive luteinizing hormone in pubertal patients with chronic renal failure: the Cooperative Study of Pubertal Development in Chronic Renal Failure. *Kidney Int* 1994;45:1465–1476.

Van Renterghem D, Cornelis R, Vanholder R. Behavior of 12 trace elements in serum of uremic patients on hemofiltration. *Journal of Trace Elements and Electrolytes in Health and Disease* 1992;6: 169–174.

Williams B, Hattersley J, Layward E, et al. Metabolic acidosis and skeletal muscle adaptation to low protein diets in chronic uremia. *Kidney Int* 1991;40:779–786.

Wolfson M. Use of water soluble vitamins in patients with chronic renal failure. *Seminars in Dialysis* 1988;1:28–32.

Assessment of Nutritional Status in Renal Diseases

D. Jordi Goldstein

DEFINITION AND OBJECTIVES

Evaluation and monitoring of nutritional status is a fundamental component of providing nutrition care to patients with renal diseases. The nutritional assessment procedure includes methods to detect, diagnose, characterize, classify, and predict malnutrition. Mechanisms to monitor patient response to therapeutic intervention are also necessary parts of a comprehensive assessment protocol. Traditionally, nutritional compromise has been viewed as a secondary phenomenon that resolves spontaneously with correction of the primary disorder. Malnutrition is now recognized as a disease entity that requires diagnosis and treatment.

The global objective of nutritional assessment is to ascertain the nutritional status of a person and use the information to determine the specific intervention(s) required to maintain/obtain optimal nutrition and overall health. It has been well established that malnutrition causes substantial morbidity and mortality beyond that associated with the primary disease and can prevent patient recovery from infection, injury, and surgery. These and other adverse consequences of poor nutrition have been most comprehensively studied in hospitalized patients. The importance of routine nutritional assessment for the patient on renal replacement therapy has been scientifically documented by several studies demonstrating a direct relationship between nutritional indices and morbidity and mortality in this patient population. These observations have resulted in renewed interest in identifying specific and reliable methods to assess the nutritional status of the patient with chronic and end-stage renal disease.

METHODOLOGY

The optimal protocol to use in identifying malnutrition in a predictive, reliable, and sensitive manner for kidney patients has not been identified. This is due, in part, to a variety of metabolic, anthropometric, and biochemical abnormalities that accompany the uremic state and characterize patients receiving renal replacement therapy. The nutritional assessment procedure should detect subclinical malnutrition; diagnose frank malnutrition; identify macronutrient, micronutrient, and substrate deficiencies; ascertain the risk for the development of poor nutrition; and rate the overall nutritional status of each patient. No single measurement can accomplish all of these. Therefore, an array of indices, each representing a specific data category, are measured independently and then evaluated collectively to ascertain the nutritional status of the renal patient. Table 3-1 lists the data categories that encompass the nutritional assessment of the renal patient. Specific indices that have been used to evaluate each data category are listed in Table 3-2.

Table 3-1. Five data categories and constituents inherent to nutritional assessment

1. Clinical	2. Food and Diet Intake	3. Biochemical	4. Body Weight	5. Body Composition
Physical examination Nutrient Physical Examination (NPE)	Diet history Appetite assessment	Visceral protein stores Static protein reserves	History Actual	Adipose stores Lean body mass (skeletal muscle)
Medical history	Quantitative food intake	Other estimates of protein nutriture	Compared to standards	
Psychosocial history Demographics	Qualitative food intake Food habits and patterns	Immune competence Vitamins, minerals, and trace elements	Body mass index (BMI) Weight change over time	
Physical activity level	Fluid intake/balance	Fluid, electrolyte, and acid-base balance	Goal weight	
Current medical/ surgical issues		Lipid status		

Table 3-2. Biochemical parameters for assessing the nutritional status of the patient with renal disease

A. Visceral protein stores
Albumin
Prealbumin (thyroxin binding prealbumin)
Retinol-binding protein
Transferrin (siderophilin)
Somatomedin c (insulin-like growth factor-1)
Acute-phase proteins (ceruloplasmin, complement components,
    c-reactive protein, fibrinogen)
Fibronectin
Pseudocholinesterase
Ribonuclease
Total protein
Albumin/globulin ratio

B. Static (somatic) protein reserves
Urinary and serum creatinine
Creatinine height index
3-methylhistidine

C. Other estimates of protein reserves
Plasma amino acid profiles
Protein turnover studies
Biochemical analysis of skeletal muscle
Nitrogen balance

D. Immune competence
Total lymphocyte counts
Delayed cutaneous hypersensitivity responses: *Candida*, mumps,
    Trichophyton, streptokinase-streptodornase (sksd) and purified
    protein derivative (ppd)
Specific immunoglobulin levels
Complement proteins

E. Vitamin, mineral, trace element nutriture
Serum levels of: Water-soluble vitamins
    fat-soluble vitamins
    specific minerals and trace elements
Nutrition physical examination

F. Fluid, electrolyte, and acid-base status
Serum chemistries: Sodium, potassium, calcium, phosphorus,
    bicarbonate, chloride, glucose

G. Indirect indices of renal function and dialysis adequacy
Serum creatinine
Blood urea nitrogen

H. Anemia
Hemoglobin
Hematocrit
Mean cell corpuscular volume
Total iron-binding capacity
Serum iron
Percent transferrin saturation
Ferritin
Red blood cell count

Table 3-2 (continued)

Table 3-2. *Continued.*

Reticulocyte count
White blood cell count

I. Hyperlipidemia
Serum: Cholesterol
     Triglycerides

J. Renal osteodystrophy
Serum: Calcium
     Vitamin D
     Alkaline phosphatase

Clinical Data Categories

Physical Examination

The physical examination checks for the presence of abnormalities reflecting poor nutriture. Fat and muscle wasting can be overlooked in a muscular individual; subtle changes in hair consistency and color, skin turgor, size of the major organs and glands, and oral health are all evaluated. The objective is not to diagnose malnutrition or nutrient deficits per se, but to determine if the patient requires a more detailed evaluation.

Detection and diagnosis of specific micronutrient and macronutrient deficiencies by physical examination alone is difficult because nonspecific lesions are typically associated with multiple vitamin deficiencies. For example, a low serum folate level implies deficiency of other B-complex vitamins (i.e. niacin, thiamine, pyridoxine). This theory is being challenged by an approach called the Nutrition Physical Examination (NPE). The NPE has the capability to diagnose, treat, and document repletion of specific micronutrient and macronutrient deficiencies. Toxic states can also be identified and treated. Successful application of this process to the renal patient population is documented.

The Nutrition Physical Examination

This approach is based on the theory that the observations derived from the physical examination, when integrated with data from the medical, nursing, drug, and nutrition histories and other nutritional assessment parameters, can help the patient care team arrive at a better understanding of the patient's potential for improved health, maintained health, or prevention of complications.

The NPE divides the body into three major areas that are evaluated by physical examination for specific nutrition deficiencies. The body areas are oral and perioral structures, skin and related structures, and systems. The physical signs suggestive of a nutrient deficit for each body area are listed in Table 3-3. Evaluation of a suspect observation is done in conjunction with other data reported by medical, nursing, and health care team members. A lesion or observation determined to be nutrition specific is photographed and becomes a part of the patient's chart to describe the lesion and to document the patient's response to therapeutic intervention.

Table 3-3. Physical signs suggesting a nutrient deficit in different organs assessed by the Nutrition Physical Examination

Body Area	Signs	Deficit	Excess
		Possibilities	
Group 1 (Oral and perioral structures)			
Tongue	Aphthous-like ulcers on the dorsum or undersurface; healing leaves depapillated areas	Folic acid possibly B_{12}	
	Diminished acuteness of the sense of taste (hypogeusesthesia)	Zinc, vitamin A	
	Filiform papillary atrophy	Iron, folic acid, B_{12}, niacin, other B complex factors	
	Fissuring, edema	Niacin	
	Lobulated with atrophy	Folic acid	
	Pallor and patchy atrophy resembling geographic tongue	Biotin	
	Pebbly or granular dorsum; erythematous, purplish- red/magenta colored	Riboflavin, possibly biotin	
	Scalding sensation succeeded by reddening and hypertrophy of filiform papillae	Pyridoxine	
	Scarlet, raw, and painful with atrophy	Niacin, folic acid, possibly B_{12} and other B complex factors	
Gums	Surface partially to completely bald, smooth, and beefy red	Niacin	
	Bleeding or red and swollen, interdental gingival hypertrophy	Ascorbic acid	
	Bright red marginal discoloration of the gingiva		Vitamin A

continued

Table 3-3. *Continued.*

Body Area	Signs	Possibilities Deficit	Possibilities Excess
Group1 *Continued*			
Gums	Inflammation with generalized stomatitis and ulceration	Ascorbic acid, folic acid, and B_{12}	
Teeth	Caries	Protein-energy, fluoride, phosphorus	
	Malposition: hypoplastic line across upper primary incisors, which becomes filled with yellow-brown pigment: caries then occur and tooth may break off	Protein-energy	
	Pitting and mottling		Fluoride
Lips and Mucous Membranes	Inflammation, loss of clear differentiation at the mucocutaneous border, angular scars, cheilosis/vertical fissuring, later complicated by redness, swelling and ulceration	Riboflavin	
	Pallor	Iron	
Group 2 (Skin and related structures)			
Skin	Decubitus ulcers, delayed wound healing	Ascorbic acid, zinc, protein, possibly linoleic acid	
	Dry and rough, scaling, possibly with complaints of headache, diplopia, and dizziness	Vitamin A	
	Flaky paint dermatosis	Protein	
	Follicular hyperkeratosis (also, see hair)	Vitamin A, ascorbic acid, linoleic acid	
	Hyperpigmentation	Protein-energy, folic acid, B_{12}	

Area	Clinical sign	Nutrient
	Inflammation of mucocutaneous junctions	Niacin
	Perifollicular petechiae	Ascorbic acid, possibly vitamin A and linoleic acid
	Petechiae, unrelated to hair follicles	Vitamin K
	Pigmentation and dry scaling when exposed to sunlight/sunburn appearance with erythema, blister formation and peeling	Niacin
	Pitting edema	Protein-energy
	Reduced turgor, inelastic, "tenting"	Water, fluids
	Scaliness—becoming "crackled"	Possibly biotin
	Seborrheic inflammation accompanied by fine scaling and itching—involving face and intertriginous areas	Pyridoxine, possibly other B complex factors
	Seborrheic inflammation with erythema, thickening, dry, flaky	Linoleic acid, riboflavin
	Slate gray/hemochromatosis	Iron
	Subcutaneous ecchymoses in response to minor trauma	Vitamin K, ascorbic acid, protein-energy
	Sunburn-like erythematous eruption	Vitamin A
	Thickened and inelastic	Niacin
	Thin and inelastic	Protein-energy
	Yellow pigmentation sparing sclerae	Carotene
Eyes	Angular palpebritis	Riboflavin
	Corneal vascularization	Riboflavin, other B complex factors
	Dull, dry conjunctiva, Bitot's spots	Vitamin A
	Pallor of everted lower eyelids	Iron, folic acid
	Papilledema	Vitamin A
	Scleral icterus, mild	Pyridoxine

continued

Table 3-3. *Continued.*

		Possibilities	
Body Area	Signs	Deficit	Excess
Hair	Broken, coiled, swan-neck hairs, perifollicular hemorrhages, follicular hyperkeratosis (also, see skin)	Ascorbic acid, vitamin A	
	Easily and painlessly pluckable	Protein-energy, zinc	
	Fine, dry, brittle, stiff, lusterless and untidy, transverse depigmentation/"flag sign"	Protein-energy	Vitamin A
	Thin, sparse	Protein, biotin, zinc	
Nails	Pale, spoon-shaped (koilonychia), ridging, brittle, easily broken, thin, lusterless	Iron	
	Splinter-type hemorrhages under the nails (hemorrhages are arranged in a semi-circular lattice involving the nail beds)	Ascorbic acid	
	White-spotting	Zinc	
Group 3 (Systems and miscellaneous other) Cardiovascular Central-nervous Endocrine Gastrointestinal Immunologic Muscular-skeletal Renal Skinfolds and circumferences Other: ____		Water-soluble vitamins	

From: Kight MA. The nutrition physical examination. *CRN Quarterly;* 1987:11;10–12.

Medical History

The medical history should include any information about the patient's appetite, food intake, and ability to metabolize food. This requires past medical and surgical history, current medical diagnosis and problems, prescribed medications, drug use including alcohol, bowel habits, and weight history. Record of any major organ or gastrointestinal diseases, surgeries, or previous symptoms of malabsorption or other digestive problems, including nausea, vomiting, and diarrhea, should be noted. Impairment in fluid and electrolyte balance, hypertension/hypotension, proteinuria, and any previous symptoms of uremia that affected appetite, food intake, digestion, or nutritional status should be noted.

Psychosocial History

This evaluates the patient's mental status as well as factors regarding the economics, education level, physical home environment, food shopping and preparation capabilities, and available support systems. The goal is to create an individualized intervention that the patient or patient's support system can understand and apply. Factors that might compromise nutritional status include depression or improper food preparation and storage equipment. This component of the assessment process helps identify patients requiring social services to assist with economic needs or special services to provide regular access to food and medications.

Demographics

Information on age, marital status, gender, and ethnicity is needed to assess nutritional status. Many of the reference standards used to classify clinical indices adjust for gender and age. Knowledge of ethnicity affects the ability to individualize the diet therapy; marital status helps identify support systems.

Physical Activity

Assessment of the patient's physical capabilities is needed to maintain activities of daily living and the proper level of physical exercise for psychological and physical therapeutics.

Current Medical/Surgical Issues

Identification of nutritional implications of medical and surgical problems is imperative for the nutritional assessment procedure. For the patient with chronic, progressive disease, this requires acknowledgment of any newly diagnosed medical/surgical illnesses. The onset of hyperkalemia, for example, may suggest a catabolic state, a loss of residual renal function, or a loss of the ability to maintain potassium homeostasis. These factors, along with the information obtained from the other categories (see Table 3-1), is used for both the nutritional assessment and the formulation of nutrition interventions.

Diet and Food Intake

This category relies on subjective patient reporting to evaluate qualitative and quantitative aspects of food intake. One of the most useful outputs from this category is the calculation of nutrient intake. Other outputs include information related to past and current food intake (qualitative and quantitative), eating patterns, and specific food preferences. This information allows an approximation of the diet's adequacy. It also helps to identify nutrient factors that may be contributing to medical problems. The qualitative data are essential for the formulation of individual diet therapy, including meal plans and menus.

Diet History

The diet history is usually obtained at the initial meeting. It is an all-inclusive collection of some objective but primarily subjective information concerning the patient's food: aversions, allergies, preferences, and intake. Information on previous and current patterns assists in devising interventions to improve impaired intake, or devising an acceptable therapeutic meal plan. The most commonly used tools to obtain food intake information differ in the approach to data collection: retrospective versus prospective, and whether the information is a qualitative description of intake versus a quantitative one.

Food Record

A food record provides qualitative and approximate quantitative food intake information that is best collected prospectively. The minimal time recommended for data collection is 3 days; a reasonable maximum is 5 days. The patient should provide intake information for both weekends and weekdays so that variability can be determined. For the dialysis patient, it is strongly recommended that the food record include intake for dialysis as well as nondialysis days, in addition to the weekend versus weekday pattern. A difference in food intake between dialysis and nondialysis days has been noted in both type and amount of food selected.

The patient should be provided with instructions on how to approximate food portion sizes and servings of fluid to ensure accurate reporting. The use of food models is very helpful. The food record should include the time of day of any intake (both meals and snacks), the names of the foods eaten, the approximate amount of food ingested, the method of preparation, and special recipes or steps taken in the food preparation. The same instructions apply to fluid intake. Brand names are requested when available.

Some patients find that it is more convenient to record food intake at the end of the day. This is an inferior method because the data collection becomes retrospective and more subject to error. Calculation of the intake of total protein, protein quality, carbohydrate, fat, fatty acid classes, and other selected nutrients is best completed by a computerized nutrient analysis program.

24-Hour Food Recall

The 24-hour food recall is an interactive tool in which the clinician assists the patient in remembering qualitative and quantitative food intake via prompting. The clinician can sit with a patient during dialysis and slowly help the patient recall the previous day's intake of both food and fluid. Food models or drawings can be used to help the patient identify portion size. One 24-hour recall, however, does not provide sufficient information to ascertain total food intake.

A variation of the 24-hour recall for a dialysis patient is to meet with the patient during three consecutive treatments, or at least four sessions within a 2-week period, and obtain one 24-

hour recall at each visit. Effort should be made to obtain a recall for a weekend day, a dialysis day, and a nondialysis day. To obtain a total food intake on a dialysis day, the practitioner can ask the patient what he or she had to eat so far that day and record it. The patient or family member can finish recording for the rest of the day, or the clinician can meet with the patient at the next session help them recall what was eaten for the rest of that day. Telephoning the patient's home on a daily basis to obtain the needed information is an option but is not practical.

Food Frequency

A food frequency is a questionnaire that approximates nutrient intake by identifying the periodicity of intake of specific foods within food groups that are significant sources of a particular nutrient or nutrients (e.g., dairy products are a good source of calcium, vitamin D, and protein). A food frequency consists of listing foods according to group, such as vegetables, fruits, dairy, protein, and so forth. The patient is questioned as to how often he or she eats this food per day, per week, and per month. An approximation of the adequacy of intake of specific nutrients can be calculated from the results. Quantification of intake with a food frequency requires using techniques similar to those described for the food recall in conjunction with the frequency questionnaire.

Methodology for Office Visits

For the patient with chronic renal disease, a reasonable method to obtain diet information in one office visit is by using a food frequency checklist and obtaining a 24-hour and, if possible, 48-hour food recall. The patient should be questioned regarding differences in intake between weekdays and weekends, and between sick days and more typical days. The patient can be provided with instructions on maintaining a 3- or 5-day food record that is mailed in for evaluation. An alternative method is to mail a food record form to the patient with instructions 10 to 14 days before the scheduled visit. A telephone call to review the written instructions can be made to the patient a few days after mailing, and the completed form can be brought to the office for evaluation.

Appetite Assessment

Evaluation of the patient's appetite is an important component of the nutritional assessment procedure. This is particularly true for the renal patient with numerous medical, uremic, and treatment issues contributing to the development of a poor appetite. Impaired food intake due to a poor appetite is thought to play a role in the development of malnutrition. Despite the importance of evaluating appetite, it is often given only a subjective rating such as very poor, poor, fair, good, very good, or excellent. These informal scales have limited clinical use. An appetite and diet assessment tool (ADAT) has been developed to evaluate appetite and factors affecting dietary intake in hemodialysis patients in relation to the dose of dialysis delivered or the flux of the dialysis membrane (Fig. 3-1). The ADAT was found to be a practical tool for assessing the relationship between appetite and dietary intake in dialysis patients.

Part One: General Level of Appetite. This part has general questions about your appetite and eating habits.

1. During the past week (7 days), how would you rate your appetite?..—
   1 = very good   4 = poor
   2 = good   5 = very poor
   3 = fair

2. Have you had a change in appetite in the past week (7 days)? (0 = no, 1 = yes) ....—

3. If you answered "yes" to #2, how has your appetite changed?..—
   1 = increased
   2 = remained the same
   3 = decreased

4. Have you been sick or ill in the last 7 days? (0 = no, 1 = yes) ....—

5. During the past year (12 months), has your dry weight:..—
   1 = increased
   2 = remained the same
   3 = decreased

6. During the past week (7 days), has your dry weight: —
   1 = increased
   2 = remained the same
   3 = decreased

7. Are you satisfied with your current dry weight? (0 = no, 1 = yes) ....—

8. Who does most of your cooking?..........................—
   1 = I do   4 = home attendant
   2 = my family 5 = other
   3 = friends

9. Who does most of your food shopping?..................—
   1 = I do   4 = home attendant
   2 = my family 5 = other
   3 = friends

10. Do you have difficulty following your diet? (0 = no, 1 = yes) ....—
    If you answered "yes," which of the following describes why you are having difficulty (answer all that apply)?
    Write 0 = no, 1 = yes.

11. I do not feel like eating...................................—

12. I do not feel like preparing food.........................—

13. My diet is too expensive.................................—

14. I do not feel like the foods I am supposed to eat ....—

15. I do not understand what I am supposed to eat............—

16. I do not have control over my food choices..................—

17. Other ....—

18. Would you like to change your diet? (0 = no, 1 = yes) ....—
    If yes, how would you change it? (Please specify)

19. Do you ever go out to eat? (0 = no, 1 = yes) ....—
    If yes, where do you go? (Write 0 = no, 1 = yes for all that apply)

20. Fast food/take-out restaurant.................................—

21. Regular restaurant/cafe/diner.................................—

22. Cafeteria ....—

23. Friend's/relative's house.................................—

24. Other ....—

Fig. 3-1. An appetite and diet assessment tool for use with hemodialysis patients. From Burrowes JD, Powers SN, Cockram DB, et al.

25. If you answered yes to any above (20-24), how often during a month? ....

Which of the following do you have at home?
(0 = no, 1 = yes)

26. Stove ....

27. Refrigerator ....

28. Freezer...

29. Microwave oven ....

30. Food processor/blender ....

31. Toaster oven ....

Part Two: This part has general questions about your appetite and eating habits **on dialysis days.**

32. How would you rate your appetite on days that you have dialysis? ....

1 = very good   4 = poor
2 = good   5 = very poor
3 = fair

33. How many meals do you usually eat on days that you have dialysis? ....

34. If you eat meals, which is your biggest meal on days that you have dialysis? ....

1 = breakfast   3 = dinner
2 = lunch   4 = all are the same size

35. How many snacks do you usually eat on days that you have dialysis? ....

36. During the past week (7 days), how often did you feel hungry on days that you had dialysis? ....

1 = never   3 = often
2 = occasionally 4 = always

37. How much do you enjoy eating on days that you have dialysis?..

1 = really enjoy   4 = dislike
2 = enjoy   5. = really dislike
3 = neither enjoy or dislike

38. Do you eat while on dialysis? (0 = no, 1 = yes) ....

Part Three: This part has general questions about your appetite and eating habits on **nondialysis days.**

39. How would you rate your appetite on days that you do *not* have dialysis? ....

1 = very good   4 = poor
2 = good   5 = very poor
3 = fair

40. How many meals do you usually eat on days that you do *not* have dialysis?..

41. Which is your biggest meal on days that you do *not* have dialysis? ....

1 = breakfast   3 = dinner
2 = lunch   4 = all are the same size

42. How many snacks do you usually eat on days you do *not* have dialysis? ....

43. During the past week (7 days), how often did you feel hungry on days that you did *not* have dialysis?..............

1 = never   3 = often
2 = occasionally 4 = always

44. How much do you enjoy eating on days that you do *not* have dialysis? ....

1 = really enjoy   4 = dislike
2 = enjoy   5 = really dislike
3 = neither enjoy or dislike

Thank you for taking the time to answer these questions.

Fig. 3-1. *(continued)* Use of an appetite and diet assessment tool in the pilot phase of a hemodialysis clinical trial: Mortality and morbidity in hemodialysis study. *Jour Renal Nutrition* 1996; 229–232.

Biochemical Values

Serum biochemical values are used to assess and monitor nutritional status over time. Selected serum values pertain to visceral protein stores, static protein reserves, overall protein nutriture, immune competence, iron stores, and vitamin, mineral, and trace element status. In addition to these components, nutritional assessment involves evaluating fluid, electrolyte, and acid–base status, renal function, dialysis adequacy for the patient receiving replacement therapy, serum lipid levels, and bone health (see Table 3-2). Table 3-4 lists the normal range, the renal range, and the significance of abnormal values for the biochemical parameters used routinely to evaluate the nutritional status of the patient with renal disease.

Visceral Protein Stores

Serum levels of albumin, transferrin, prealbumin, and retinol-binding protein (RBP) are the biochemical markers most often used to assess visceral protein stores, monitor response to nutrition intervention, and identify which patients are at risk for development of complications or are responding poorly to medical/surgical treatment. The assumption—not yet proven—is that serum concentration represents hepatic protein synthetic mass and, indirectly, the functional protein mass of the internal viscera (i.e., heart, lung, kidneys, intestines).

SERUM ALBUMIN. Albumin, the most abundant plasma protein, functions to maintain plasma oncotic pressure and serves as a major carrier protein for drugs, hormones, enzymes, and trace elements. Clinically significant hypoalbuminemia occurs with different types of malnutrition besides kidney disease (i.e., protein-energy, kwashiorkor, uncomplicated), in both children and adults. In these conditions, hypoalbuminemia usually indicates other metabolic derangements as well as a poor prognosis. From these observations, serum albumin became a part of routine nutritional assessment of the hospitalized patient and, subsequently, the renal patient.

The causes of significant hypoalbuminemia associated with malnutrition are not known. Kinetic studies in animals and humans have found that when protein-energy intake is deficient, the albumin synthetic rate drops quickly, resulting in negative albumin balance. If dietary intake remains inadequate, the albumin catabolic rate decreases, reducing the rate of whole-body albumin loss. The result is a preservation of serum albumin levels despite a reduction in the rate of synthesis. The distribution also changes, with a shift from the extravascular to the intravascular space. Therefore, the relative decrease in serum albumin levels is less than the decrease in whole-body albumin levels.

Although serum albumin levels have been used extensively in clinical practice, research studies, and nutritional surveys to assess the nutritional status of the chronic and end-stage renal patient population, the reliability and sensitivity of this parameter have been questioned. The concerns are independent of the conditions that change serum albumin as a marker of visceral protein stores (Table 3-5). The utility of albumin for assessment purposes has been criticized because of its long half-life, averaging 14 to 20 days, and large body pool, 4 to 5 mg/kg, mak-

Table 3-4. Biochemical parameters commonly used to assess the nutritional status of the patient with renal disease

Laboratory Test	Reference Range	Your Lab	Renal Range	Significance of abnormal result
Serum albumin (depends on method of analysis)	3.3–5.0 g/dL Senior: 3.2–4.5 Newborn: 2.9–5.5 To age 3: 3.8–5.4 3-Adol: 3.3–5.5		Variable; desirable is >3.5 g/dl	High with dehydration, albumin infusion Low with fluid overload, chronic liver or pancreatic disease, steatorrhea, inflammatory GI disease, malnutrition, nephrotic syndrome, acute/chronic infection
Alkaline phosphatase	19–74 IU/l 12–63 Newborn: 50–275 Infant: 100–330 Child: 90–230 Adol: 100–250		WNL	High with bone disease, healing of fractures, malignancies Low with congenital hypophosphatemia, possibly in kwashiorkor, general debility, anemia (unclear mechanism), nephrotic syndrome
Blood urea nitrogen (BUN)	4–22 mg/dl Senior: 8–18 Peds: 10–20 Newborn/Infant: 8–28		60–120 mg/dl National Cooperative Dialysis Study suggests that a mid-week, predialysis BUN should range from 60–80 mg/dl	High with excessive total/low biologic value protein intake, GI bleeding, dehydration, hypercatabolism, congestive heart failure (a low cardiac output causes a decrease in GFR); transplant rejection, under dialysis Low with hepatic failure, overhydration, acute low protein intake, malabsorption, increased secretion of anabolic hormones

continued

Table 3-4. *Continued.*

Laboratory Test	Reference Range	Your Lab	Renal Range	Significance of abnormal result
Serum calcium	8.5–10.5 mg/dl		8.5–11.5 mg/dl	High with excess vitamin D/calcium, increased GI absorption, osteolytic disease, carcinoma, immobilization, aluminum bone disease, excessive vitamin A, hyperparathyroidism, dehydration, or prolonged use of tourniquet when drawing blood Low with insufficient vitamin D, in malabsorption, during bone building, postparathyroidectomy, long-term Dilantin therapy, hypoparathyroidism, low albumin
Chloride	100–106 mEq/l		WNL	High with excess salt, dehydration (concentration), some forms of metabolic acidosis, excessive treatment with medications containing chloride, primary hyperparathyroidism Low with diabetic acidosis, K^+ deficiency, metabolic alkalosis, excessive sweating, starvation, GI losses (vomiting), excessive use of diuretics, dilution; serum chloride is affected by the same conditions as serum sodium and usually moves in the same direction as sodium

Cholesterol	150–200 mg/dl Children < 200	Variable (HDL usually low in RF)	High with high cholesterol/saturated fat diet, hereditary disorders of lipid metabolism, nephrotic syndrome, glucocorticoid therapy Low in acute infection, starvation
Total CO_2	23–30 mEq/l	WNL	High in metabolic alkalosis Low in metabolic acidosis
Creatinine	0.7–1.5 mg/dl Senior: 0.6–1.2 Newborn: 0.4–1.2 0–4 yrs: 0.1–0.7 4–10 yrs: 0.2–0.9 10–16: 0.3–1.1	2–15 mg/dl 4–20 Dialysis 8–12 small pt 15–20 large pt 2.8 PreESRD	May be high with muscle damage, catabolism, myocardial infarction, muscular dystrophy, acute/chronic renal failure, use of cephalothin/cimetidine, level depends on muscle mass/muscle turnover/GFR Low with extreme muscle wasting; RF patients may have <expected values
Ferritin	12–300 µg/l (RIA) <6 mo: 25–200 6 mo–15 yr: 7–140	WNL—1500 µg/l DOQI Rec: ≥100 ng/ml	High with iron overload, many transfusions, dehydration; can be altered in inflammatory state, falsely elevated in active liver disease Low in iron deficiency
Globulin	2.3–3.5 gm/dl	WNL	High in infection, liver disease, leukemia, hyperlipidemia Low in malnutrition

continued

Table 3-4. *Continued.*

Laboratory Test	Reference Range	Your Lab	Renal Range	Significance of abnormal result
Glucose Fasting Levels)	70–100 mg/dl <50 yrs: 60–100 Senior: 55–125 Premature: 20–60 Newborn: 20–110 Child: 60–100		Variable (Usually drawn non-fasting before treatment, depends on intake)	High: diabetes, hyperthyroidism, malignancies, acute stress, emotional distress, burns, pancreatic insufficiency, diabetic acidosis, glucose intolerance, use of steroids Low with hyperinsulinemia, ETOH abuse, pancreatic tumors, liver failure, pituitary dysfunction, malnutrition, strenuous exercise
Hematocrit	39–51% 36–15% Senior: 30–54% Newborn: 40–70% Infant: 30–49% Child: 30–42% Adolescent: 34–44%		Variable (DOQI Rec: 33–36% (target for EPO, not transfusion, ≤30% is inadequate)	High in polycythemia, dehydration Low in anemias, blood loss (endogenous & dialysis), CRF, insufficient EPO
Hemoglobin	12–17 g/dl Senior: 10–17 Newborn: 14–24 Infant: 10–15 Child: 11–16		Variable (DOQI rec: 11–12 g/dl)	High in dehydration Low in overhydration, prolonged iron deficiency, anemias, blood loss, CRF

Iron	60–175 µg/dl Newborn: 100–200 4 mo–2: 40–100 Child: 85–150	>25–200 µg/dl	High in iron overload, sideroblastic anemias, estrogen or oral contraceptive therapy, hemolysis, increased for 1–2 weeks after IV iron Low in iron deficiency, reduced intake over prolonged time, EPO therapy can reduce stores, long-term blood loss, during rapid growth. Diurnal and day-to-day variations are common.
Lymphocyte count (total=% lymphocytes × WBC)	1500–4000 mm^3 (closely involved with immune response)	WNL (<1200–1500 mm^3 may be significant)	High with acute viral infections, collagen disease, hyperthyroidism, high altitude Low in malnutrition-synthesis requires adequate kcals and protein (adds power to significance of low albumin), stress, prolonged depression
Magnesium	1.4–2.3 mEq/l	WNL	High with excess intake of Mg$^+$ (in drinking water, dialysate, Mg$^+$-containing parenteral infusion or over-the-counter medications, dehydration) Low with some diuretics, diabetic ketoacidosis, hypercalcemia, ETOH abuse, diarrhea/malabsorption, pancreatitis, malnutrition, refeeding syndrome

continued

Table 3-4. *Continued.*

Laboratory Test	Reference Range	Your Lab	Renal Range	Significance of abnormal result
Mean cell corpuscular volume	81–100 fluid Preterm: 118–120 6 mo–18 mo: 70–90		WNL	High with folic acid/B_{12} deficiency, cirrhosis reticulocytosis, chronic alcoholism Low in chronic iron deficiency, anemia disease (Values in adult anemia: >120 fl—pernicious: <78 fl—microcytic; <64 fl often seen with iron deficiency anemia
Phosphorus	2.5–4.7 mg/dl Senior: 2.3–3.7 Newborn: 4–9 Infant: 4.6–6.7 Child: 4.0–6.0		4.5–6.5 mg/dl depends on medications, residual renal function, type of renal replacement therapy	High with renal insufficiency, renal bone disease. Vitamin D intoxication, diurnal rhythm-evening/afternoon as much as double morning level, Mg^+ deficiency Low with Vitamin D deficiency, decreased intake/excess P binding, malabsorption/diarrhea/vomiting, alkalosis, diabetic ketoacidosis, diuretic therapy, alcoholism, refeeding syndrome, postparathyroidectomy, osteomalacia
Potassium	3.5–5.0 mEq/l		3.5–6.0 mEq/l	High in renal insufficiency, tissue destruction, shock, acidosis, dehydration, hyperglycemia, overuse of potassium-sparing diuretics; falsely high from tourniquet compression/fist clenching before venipuncture

Test	Value	Result	Interpretation
Protein, Total	6–8.4 g dl	WNL—low	Low with diuretic therapy, ETOH abuse, vomiting/diarrhea/laxative or enema abuse, stress response, malabsorption, correction of diabetic acidosis High in dehydration, acute/chronic infectious disease, leukemia/multiple myeloma Low in malnutrition, malabsorption, cirrhosis, steatorrhea, edema, nephrotic syndrome
Reticulocyte Count	25,000 to 75,000 cells	Variable	Index of bone marrow activity—reflects early change in RBC production, response to EPO High with hemolytic anemia, significant acute bleed Low in certain anemias due to ineffective erythropoiesis (deficiency of iron, B_{12}, folic acid, B_4) or anemia of chronic disease
RBC Count (Multiply automatic counter values × 1 million for total|=)	4.4–5.7 4.0–5.3 Senior: 3.0–5.0 ($\times 10^1$/mm^3) (mil/mm^3)	WNL	High at high altitude, temporarily w/strong emotion, diurnally, cold shower, reduced plasma volume, dehydration Low with anemia, hemorrhage, infectious disease, iron deficiency

continued

Table 3-4. *Continued.*

Laboratory Test	Reference Range	Your Lab	Renal Range	Significance of abnormal result
Sodium	136–145 mEq/l		WNL Variable	High with dehydration, diabetes insipidus Low in over hydration, inappropriate ADH diuretic use, burns, starvation, adrenal insufficiency, hyperglycemia, hyperproteinemia
Transthyretin (Prealbumin or Thyroxine Binding Prealbumin)	10–40 mg/dl		Variable (Prealbumin excreted by kidneys/high in CRF)	High with administration of glucocorticoids neonate, in first few weeks of life, liver disease, malnutrition In CRF, values <30 associated with increased morbidity/mortality, values <29 associated with malnutrition.
TIBC Estimated transferrin = (.8 × TIBC) - 43	250–450 µg/dl		Varies with iron stores	High in chronic iron deficiency, pregnancy, alcoholism, acute hepatitis Low in cirrhosis, malnutrition, collagen or chrome disease/infection, iron overload
Transferrin saturation	20–55%		<10–>100% NKF-DOQI Rec: ≥20%	High in hemolytic/megaloblastic/ sideroblastic anemia, iron overload Low in absolute/relative iron deficiency

Triglycerides	40–150 mg/dl	High in liver disease, gout, pancreatitis, ETOH abuse, MI, diabetes, peritoneal dialysis, use of steroids, nephrotic syndrome
		Low in malnutrition, malabsorption
Uric acid	4.0–8.5 mg/dl 2.7–7.3 Senior: 2.9–8.8 2.4–7.2	High in gout, renal insufficiency, thiazide diuretics, starvation
	WNL to high	Low with high salicylate doses, hepatic failure
WBC count	4.5–10.6 thousand/mm^3	High in leukemia, acute infection/inflammation
	WNL	Low with in chemotherapy
Zinc	85–120 µg/dl	High in contaminated sample, hemolysis
	WNL	Low with low intake or absorption/ increased loss or needs, alcoholism, cirrhosis of the liver

CRF, chronic renal failure; DOQI, National Kidney Foundation Dialysis Outcomes Quality Initiative; EPO, erythropoietin; ESRD, end-stage renal disease; ETOH, ethanol; GFR, glomerular filtration rate; GI, gastrointestinal; RF, renal failure; TIBC, total iron-binding capacity; WBC, white blood cell; WNL, within normal limits.
*Adjust for low albumin (serum calcium−serum albumin+4).
From: McCann L, ed. *Pocket Guide to Nutrition Assessment of the Renal Patient*, 2nd ed. New York: National Kidney Foundation (1998).

**Table 3-5. Factors that independently
alter serum albumin concentrations**

A. *Disease states- change hepatic albumin synthesis or influence
albumin distribution*
Hypothyroidism
Inflammatory gastrointestinal disease
Liver disease
Malabsorption
Pancreatic disease
Protein-losing enteropathies
Nephrotic syndrome
Semistarvation (albumin shifts from extravascular
to intravascular space, resulting in an artifically
elevated serum concentration)
Sepsis and trauma (i.e., Hypermetabolism)
Steatorrhea

B. *Processes*
Inflammation
Infection

C. *Hydration status*
Dehydration results in elevated serum levels
Fluid overload results in decreased serum levels

D. *Other factors*
Body temperature
Dietary protein intake
Plasma oncotic pressure
Albumin is a negative acute-phase reactant protein:
the serum level is depressed during an acute-phase
response regardless of nutritional status
Chemotherapy
Steroids

ing albumin slow to respond to changes in visceral protein stores. It is, therefore, a late marker of malnutrition.

Studies suggest that the hypoalbuminemia observed in hemodialysis patients may be more of a response to inflammation than a consequence of malnutrition (see section on Acute-Phase Reactant Proteins).

Although recent data challenge the sensitivity of serum albumin as a marker of protein nutrition for the patient on renal replacement therapy, other data confirm serum albumin is a predictor of patient outcome. In a cross-sectional analysis of over 12,000 hemodialysis patients, Lowrie and Lew determined that serum albumin was the most powerful predictor of death compared with other indices (i.e., serum creatinine, cholesterol, and urea nitrogen). Patients who had a serum albumin <2.5 g/dl had a risk of death 20 times higher than patients with a level in the range of 4.0 to 4.5 g/dl. Patients whose serum albumin is considered to be in the normal range of 3.5 to 4.0 g/dl had double the risk of death compared with those patients whose level was in the range of 4.0 to 4.5 g/dl. Similar relationships between low serum albumin levels and risk of death have been reported for the peritoneal dialysis patient population.

Thus, in the nutritional assessment of patients undergoing renal replacement therapy, a serum albumin considered to be in a normal range places a hemodialysis patient in an *at risk* category. These data clearly confirm that the nutritional assessment process cannot rely on any one parameter, whether it be a comprehensive assessment or a preliminary nutrition screening procedure.

PREALBUMIN (THYROXINE-BINDING PREALBUMIN, TRANSTHYRETIN). Prealbumin is a carrier protein for retinol-binding protein and thus has a major role in the transport of thyroxine. Its short half-life of 2 to 3 days and its small body pool make it more sensitive than albumin to changes in protein status. This was the first visceral protein found to be low in healthy children who were eating marginal amounts of protein. In primates, prealbumin reflects overall nitrogen balance during starvation and refeeding. Decreases in serum levels occur independently of nutritional status when there is acute metabolic stress, including trauma, minor stress, and inflammation. The serum concentration has also been observed to decrease in liver disease and with iron supplementation.

The low molecular weight of prealbumin (approximately 54,980 daltons) precludes its use as a marker of nutritional status in patients with chronic renal disease who have a decreased glomerular filtration rate (GFR). Prealbumin levels have been reported to be elevated in the euvolemic patient with chronic renal failure. In hemodialysis patients, high levels have been observed and are attributed to decreased renal catabolism. A decline in the proportion of circulating free prealbumin versus that complexed with RBP may explain the diminished catabolism and, therefore, elevated levels. A concentration < 30 mg/dl (normal range, 10 to 40 mg/dl) may indicate malnutrition in the hemodialysis patient.

RETINOL-BINDING PROTEIN. This protein circulates in a 1-to-1 molar ratio with prealbumin and transports the alcohol fraction of vitamin A. Its short half-life of 10 to 12 hours and small body pool enable it to respond quickly and specifically to changes in protein status. RBP is not an appropriate marker of nutritional status for the patient with chronic or end-stage renal disease because it is catabolized in renal proximal tubular cells. With renal disease, the half-life is reported to be prolonged, and serum levels increase. Other limitations of RBP for nutritional assessment are that serum levels become low in hyperthyroidism, vitamin A deficiency, and acute catabolic states (i.e., levels change inversely with acute-phase proteins).

TRANSFERRIN (SIDEROPHILLIN). The main function of transferrin is to bind ferrous iron and to transport iron to the bone marrow. The half-life of 8 to 10 days and small body pool enable it to respond more rapidly to acute and short-term changes in protein status, compared with albumin. Studies in malnourished children as well in hospitalized patients have demonstrated a correlation between transferrin and the severity and prognosis of disease, as well as improvement in serum levels with nutrition intervention.

Before it was practical to measure transferrin levels, the total iron-binding capacity was thought to be equivalent to the amount of iron required to saturate plasma transferrin. This assumption turned out to be true only in normal and iron-deficient subjects. The most common estimate is obtained from the total iron-binding capacity (TIBC) using this formula: transferrin = $(0.8 \times \text{TIBC}) - 43$. However, this formula has not been validated as an estimate of serum transferrin in the renal patient, and a direct measure is recommended.

The utility of this protein in the nutritional assessment of the renal patient is confounded by many factors that influence the serum levels. Iron deficiency increases hepatic synthesis and plasma levels. Reduced transferrin concentrations are observed in association with uremia, protein-losing enteropathy, nephropathy, acute catabolic states, chronic infections, and iron loading. In chronic renal failure, transferrin is reliable for the evaluation of iron status. Most patients on renal replacement receive erythropoietin therapy and iron supplementation. The use of transferrin should be reserved for those patients who have a stable erythropoietin regimen with adequate iron replacement.

INSULIN-LIKE GROWTH FACTOR-1 (SOMATOMEDIN C). Insulin-like growth factor-1 (IGF-1) is a serum protein with mitogen properties and insulin-like activities; it may be a sensitive biochemical indicator of nitrogen balance. With a half-life of 2 to 6 hours, IGF-1 represents an acute-phase response. Studies of hospitalized, hypercatabolic patients indicate that IGF-1 is a better marker of nitrogen balance than other serum proteins. In humans, IGF-1 levels fall during fasting and increase with refeeding, and it has been reported to be a reliable marker of malnutrition in children. A serum concentration below 300 ng/ml indicates a poor nutritional status in hemodialysis patients.

ACUTE-PHASE REACTANT PROTEINS. This category of protein plays a role in host defense mechanisms such as the immune response and wound healing. In response to acute injury or inflammation, hepatic synthesis of acute-phase reactant proteins (APRP) increases in lieu of other visceral proteins. An inverse correlation has been reported for APRP and albumin, prealbumin, RBP, and transferrin. These latter proteins are negative APRPs because this hepatic synthesis is actually suppressed, as, for example, in response to inflammation.

Dialysis patients with hypoalbuminemia (serum albumin <3.5 g/dl) have significantly higher serum levels of APRP (β_2-macroglobulin, ferritin, and C-reactive protein) compared with hemodialysis patients with a normal serum albumin level (>4.0 g/dl). There were no other differences between the two groups, including the delivered dialysis dose or relevant nutritional indices. These and other data suggest that acute or chronic inflammation in the hemodialysis patient causes hypoalbuminemia. Inflammation causes a release of cytokines that mediate an increase in hepatic synthesis of APRP such as C-reactive protein, and a suppression of negative APRP such as albumin and other visceral proteins. With regard to patient outcome, C-reactive protein is a better predictor of death in hemodialysis patients than the serum albumin.

FIBRONECTIN. Fibronectin is a glycoprotein found in many tissues, in extracellular fluids, and on basement membranes. Plasma levels are depressed during low energy intake or with low–amino-acid or low-fat diets. Increased levels occur in wasted patients after 1 week of nutrition intervention. The serum concentration is influenced by the acute-phase response; low levels have been observed with trauma, shock, and sepsis.

PSEUDOCHOLINESTERASE AND RIBONUCLEASE. There is some evidence to suggest that both of these enzymes are sensitive markers of protein status in normal patients. The few reports that are available for pseudocholinesterase in patients with chronic renal failure have observed low serum levels in uremic patients.

Ribonuclease is an enzyme that rises in the plasma of malnourished patients who do not have renal failure. Renal failure per se can elevate plasma levels. Additional work is needed to determine if either enzyme has any useful role in the nutritional assessment of the renal patient.

TOTAL PROTEIN AND ALBUMIN/GLOBULIN RATIO. The serum total protein (TP) is not considered to be a reliable marker of visceral stores because other factors affect its concentration, including dehydration and increased globulins. An increase in globulin concentration is associated with infection, hyperlipidemia, nephrosis, and collagen disease. Malnutrition is associated with a low albumin/globulin (A : G) ratio (A : G ratio = albumin/total protein - albumin). The large number of factors that can influence TP and globulin levels in the dialysis patient (hydration issues, hyperlipidemia) prevent their inclusion for routine nutritional assessment.

Static Protein Reserves (Somatic Protein, Muscle Stores)

Measures of muscle mass are thought to be good indicators of static protein reserves because approximately 60% of total body protein is contained in muscle. Skeletal muscle is the predominant source of amino acid mobilization during periods of nutrition deficiency. Both anthropometric and biochemical markers are used to assess muscle mass. Anthropometric techniques are discussed in the section on Body Composition.

URINARY AND SERUM CREATININE. Creatinine is formed at a relatively constant rate from creatine, a compound found predominantly in muscle. Therefore, urinary creatinine is proportional to muscle creatine content, and hence to total body muscle mass. Urinary excretion of creatinine correlates with lean body mass measured by isotope dilution and ^{40}K total body counting techniques.

For the patient with renal insufficiency or deteriorating renal function, the urinary creatinine cannot be used for nutritional assessment purposes. There is no role for urinary creatinine excretion in nutritional assessment for the end-stage patient who has zero or insignificant residual renal function and accumulates creatinine.

For a chronic renal patient with a stable GFR, and for the dialysis patient, changes in serum creatinine over time (~3 months) may indicate a change in muscle mass. Verification of a change in muscle mass based on the serum creatinine must be confirmed by assessing other parameters of somatic protein stores, as well as by evaluating the patient's weight, overall food intake, and biochemical markers of visceral stores.

CREATININE HEIGHT INDEX. In normal people, creatinine production from creatine is directly related to the skeletal muscle mass. The creatinine height index (CHI) was formulated to use this relationship to assess lean body mass. The CHI is a ratio between actual urinary creatinine excretion and predicted creatinine excretion for a healthy adult who is of the same gender and age. A reduction in the CHI suggests a decrease in muscle mass.

The CHI is applicable only for renal patients who have a normal GFR, and is not useful for dialysis patients. The accuracy depends on obtaining a complete 24-hour urine collection and standard body weight charts to calculate the expected normal urinary creatinine excretion. Because of these variables, it is not possible to adjust the CHI for individual variability in muscle mass and overall body composition.

3-METHYLHISTIDINE. This amino acid is located predominately in myofibrillar protein. During muscle protein catabolism, 3-methylhistidine (3-ME) is released and excreted into the urine. A 24-hour urinary 3-ME concentration can therefore provide an estimate of muscle protein catabolism, but the method is limited by other sources of 3-ME with different protein turnover rates. In addition, dietary intake, age, gender, and metabolic stress (i.e., trauma, infection) are reported to influence 3-ME levels.

Reduced 3-ME urinary excretion in uremia has been observed. Therefore, its use should be limited to those patients who do not have an impaired GFR.

Other Estimates of Protein Nutriture

PLASMA AMINO ACID PROFILES. Specific amino acid concentrations and ratios have been used to assess protein nutrition in renal patients. This use of amino acids is derived from observations in malnourished children, in whom low levels of essential to nonessential amino acids and low concentrations of valine to glycine occur; the levels normalize with refeeding.

Abnormal serum amino acid patterns are present in patients with chronic renal disease and end-stage failure. Besides the low ratios of essential to nonessential amino acids, there are increased citrulline and cystine concentrations, and high levels of 1- and 3-methylhistidine. Decreased plasma concentrations of isoleucine, leucine, tryptophan, valine, and tyrosine may be useful in reflecting protein-calorie malnutrition in patients with advanced renal failure.

It has since been determined that only the lower essential to nonessential amino acid ratio reflects nutritional status independently. The valine to glycine ratio as well as other amino acid concentrations are affected by uremia per se. The use of plasma amino acid patterns is further limited by the fact that they reflect only very recent protein intake, and therefore cannot be used to reflect body protein status. To use amino acids as biochemical markers of protein nutrition, levels for the uremic patient eating different levels of protein must be used.

BIOCHEMICAL ANALYSIS OF SKELETAL MUSCLE. With a thin-needle biopsy, direct biochemical analysis of body tissue is possible. Alterations in the composition of human muscle that have been attributed to changes in nutritional status include electrolyte, water, and amino acid levels.

Determination of muscle DNA, RNA, and noncollagen alkali-soluble protein (ASP) can provide insight into changes of muscle protein metabolism resulting from nutritional factors. Muscle DNA changes very little in response to malnutrition and is therefore a standard reference for adults. The capacity of a cell to synthesize protein is reflected by total muscle RNA and the RNA : DNA ratio. The muscle cell size can be approximated by the ratio ASP : DNA. Human studies of starvation have demonstrated that muscle RNA content, protein content, and protein synthesis change in these conditions.

Skeletal muscle samples from chronically uremic patients treated by low-protein diet therapy or dialysis had muscle hypotrophy, reflected by increased muscle DNA concentration, and the RNA : DNA and ASP : DNA ratios were significantly lower in dialysis patients compared with control subjects. This same ratio was normal, as was muscle DNA, in a predialysis group consuming a 0.6-g protein/kg body weight/day diet. Other groups have reported similar findings with this method.

NITROGEN BALANCE STUDIES. Nitrogen balance is defined as a measure of the net change in total body protein mass. The assumption underlying the definition is that all total body nitrogen is incorporated into protein. Nitrogen comprises 16% of protein by weight, so 1 g of nitrogen = 6.25 g of protein. In nonuremic patients, a simple method of estimating nitrogen balance is by measuring urinary urea nitrogen (UUN) and dietary nitrogen intake for the same 24-hour period and completing the following calculation:

$$\frac{\text{Nitrogen}}{\text{balance}} = \frac{\text{dietary protein intake (g)}}{6.25} - [\text{UUN} + (0.031 \times \text{weight})]$$

where $0.031 \times$ weight is a constant used to account for nonurea nitrogen losses (e.g., feces, creatinine, amino acids, ammonia, uric acid). The amount of nitrogen taken in by diet versus that lost in feces and urine is compared, and nitrogen balance is determined. Normal, healthy adults are in neutral balance (nitrogen balance = 0). Nitrogen balance is positive in anabolic states such as pregnancy and growth and negative when protein catabolism exceeds anabolism. Examples include starvation, catabolic illnesses, and inadequate protein intake. Nitrogen balance is an excellent tool for determining the amount of protein required to revert a patient from a negative to a positive or neutral balance, depending on the nutrition goal.

An alternative approach for the determination of nitrogen balance has been designed for the patient with chronic or end-stage disease on dialysis therapy. Calculation of the normalized protein catabolic rate (nPCR) or urea nitrogen appearance (UNA) can be used to estimate nitrogen balance in the renal patient who is free of edema and is not in an anabolic or catabolic state. The nPCR is an adjustment that expresses the PCR in grams per kilogram body weight per day. Table 3-6 lists the formulas that can be used to calculate PCR in patients with chronic renal disease. A study example is also provided in Table 3-6.

Immune Competence

A comprehensive nutritional assessment includes tests of immune function. The total lymphocyte count and delayed cutaneous hypersensitivity responses are tests of humoral immunity and have limited use in nutritional assessment because of altered host defenses. The use of serum complement system components and serum immunoglobulins to test humoral immunity is complex because of the discrepancies concerning which pro-

Table 3-6. Formulas to calculate the protein catabolic rate in the predialysis patient

Urea clearance (ml/min)

$$C_{urea} = \frac{\text{urine urea (mg/ml)}}{\text{BUN (mg/ml)}} \times \frac{\text{urine volume (ml)}}{\text{time (min)}}$$

Urea Generation Rate (mg/min)

$$GU = C_{urea} \text{ (ml/min)} \times BUN \text{ (mg/ml)}$$

Protein Catabolic Rate (gm/day)

$$PCR = 9.35 \text{ (GU)} + 11$$

Urea generation rate (GU) calculates how much urea is accumulated in the blood (measured as blood urea nitrogen [BUN]) and how much is being excreted (measured from the urea clearance). The formula for PCR converts these measurements of urea to grams of protein/day.

Example:

Mr. W is a 42-year-old accountant: 5'5", medium frame, 60 kg; instructed on a 48-g protein diet (0.8 g/kg), 2000–2200 calories

Data:

Laboratory data	Serum urea nitrogen = 89 mg/dl (.89 mg/ml)
	Serum creatinine (Cr) = 7.4 mg/dl (.074 mg/ml)
Urine collection	Urine area = 250 mg/dl (2.5 mg/ml)
	Urine creatinine = 40 mg/dl (.4 mg/ml)
	Urine volume/24 hr = 2320 ml
	(24 hr = 1440 minutes)

1. Urea clearance
$$C_{urea} = \frac{\text{Urine urea}}{\text{BUN}} \times \frac{\text{Urine volume}}{\text{Time}}$$

$$C_{urea} = \frac{2.5 \text{ mg/ml}}{0.89 \text{ mg/ml}} \times \frac{2320 \text{ ml}}{1440 \text{ min}}$$

$$C_{urea} = 4.5 \text{ ml/min}$$

2. Urea generation rate
GU = C_{urea} × serum urea nitrogen
GU = 4.5 ml/min × .89 mg/ml
GU = 4 mg/min

3. Protein catabolic rate
PCR = 9.35 (GU) + 11
PCR = 9.35 (4) + 11
PCR = 48 g/day

Analysis of a 3-day dietary intake record:
Day 1 = 44 g protein,   2150 calories
Day 2 = 47 g protein,   2075 calories
Day 3 = 49 g protein,   2230 calories

Mean intake is 47 g protein and 2150 calories/day.
This closely matches calculated PCR of 48 g/day.
Patient is in zero nitrogen balance.

BUN, blood urea nitrogen. From: Gee C and Schroepfer C. Summary of formulas and abbreviations. In: Gee C, Schroepfer C, eds. *Urea kinetics in nutritional management of pre-end stage renal disease.* Council on Renal Nutrition, Northern California/Northern Nevada; 1993:4–5.

teins are altered in renal failure or improve with adequate nutrition.

Vitamins, Minerals, and Trace Elements

Evaluation of serum or urine levels of specific micronutrients as a component of a nutritional assessment is not routine. Table 3-7 exemplifies the influence of uremia by listing factors affecting trace element concentrations. In addition, patients with renal diseases are routinely given B-vitamins, vitamin C, vitamin E, and often vitamin D, iron, calcium, and zinc.

The NPE (see also the section on the Nutritional Physical Examination, earlier), which evaluates for the presence of nutrition-related lesions, does include assessment of micronutrient status as part of the overall nutritional assessment. Assessment using the NPE has begun to pair nutrient status with altered body composition, document nutrient-based lesions with macrophotography, demonstrate resolution of lesions and abnormal laboratory values with specific nutrient supplementation, and characterize clinical indicators associated with risk of poor outcome by statistical testing. The potential of the NPE to evaluate micronutrient and macronutrient status of the hemodialysis patient population is just beginning to be determined.

Body Weight

Initial assessment of body weight and monitoring of weight change over time is a critical component of the nutritional assessment process. Weight loss in excess of 5% to 10%, depending on the patient's overall nutritional status, or substandard weight for height, should be considered a risk factor for malnutrition. Interrelationships between weight loss over time and outcome in the renal patient population have not yet been reported.

Body mass index (weight [kg]/height [m^2]), current weight, usual weight, ideal body weight, percent usual weight, percent ideal body weight, and particularly percent weight change over a defined time period are important parameters of body weight. A database or sheet in the patient's chart that is committed to record body weight is recommended for every patient. An example of a monitoring sheet for use with the patient on renal replacement therapy that records monthly weights is shown in Fig. 3-2. Table 3-8 gives a useful formula that can be used to classify weight change over time.

Body Composition

Measures of body composition to ascertain fat stores and lean body mass are included. Other than the initial investment for skinfold calipers and an accurate tape measure, anthropometry is an inexpensive technique. The measurements obtained are compared with standards that classify the patient as normal, "at risk" for malnutrition, or having a type and degree of malnutrition. In general, measurements below the 35th to 40th percentile suggests mild depletion, below the 25th to 35th percentile moderate depletion, and below the 25th percentile, severe depletion. More sophisticated measures of body composition are available (Table 3-9).

Table 3-7. Factors affecting trace element concentration in uremia and other conditions

Inadequate intake
Absolute deficiency: protein-calorie malnutrition, anorexia, fat diets,
    low income diets, diets with alcohol providing the bulk of calories, total
    parenteral nutrition without adequate supplementation, loss of taste
    and smell
Increased requirements: rapid growth, pregnancy, lactation, tissue anabolism

Decreased availability
Interactions with other dietary constituents
Gastrointestinal dysfunction
    Inadequate digestive processes
    Secondary interactions with unabsorbed dietary constituents
    Iatrogenic
    Complexing with drugs
Drug induced alterations of gastrointestinal function

Impaired absorption
Altered binding factors
    Quantitative or qualitative
    Congenital or acquired
    Competitive uptake of other nutrients
    Inadequate functional surface
    Surgical resection
    GI mucosal disease
    Competitive uptake of other nutrients: disturbances in vitamin D
        metabolism→altered uptake, GI absorption, especially for divalent cations
Physiologically appropriate depression of absorption
Impaired mucosal "packaging"
    Inability to store
    Sequestration

Altered distribution
Defective transport
    Quantitative or qualitative changes in transport compounds
    Competitive displacement
    Altered tissue receptor sites
    Altered tissue storage compounds
    Inability to store
    Sequestration
Transient alterations in distribution: Infection, myocardial infarct, stress,
    and the like

Excessive losses
Sweat
Menstrual losses, other forms of blood loss
Urinary
    Proteinuria for protein bound elements
Fecal
    Pancreatic
    Biliary
    Gut
Upper GI losses: vomiting, nasogastric suction, enterostomies
Dialysis

Excess intake
Drugs containing trace elements (cave: homeopathy)
Increasing uptake
Altering distribution
Food and water supplies
Contamination dialysate
    Addition to tap water
    Excess presence of minerals in soil
    Environmental contamination

Table 3-7. *Continued.*

Industrial contact
Inhalation after environmental contamination
Inhalation via cigarette smoke
Parenteral fluids
Increased GI uptake
Diminished losses
Renal failure

GI, gastrointestinal. From: Vonholder R, Cornelis R, Dhondt A and Ringoir, S. Trace element metabolism in renal disease and renal failure. In: Kopple JD, Massy, SS, eds. *Nutritional management of renal disease.* Baltimore: Williams and Wilkens, 1997; 406.

Patient Name:				
Year:			**Year:**	
MONTH	ESTIMATED DRY WEIGHT (kg)	Other	ESTIMATED DRY WEIGHT (kg)	Other
JANUARY				
FEBRUARY				
MARCH				
APRIL				
MAY				
JUNE				
JULY				
AUGUST				
SEPTEMBER				
OCTOBER				
NOVEMBER				
DECEMBER				

Fig. 3-2. Estimated dry weight flow sheet.

Table 3-8. Classification of weight change over time

$$\text{Percent weight change} = \frac{(\text{usual weight} - \text{actual weight})}{(\text{usual weight})} \times 100$$

Observation period	Significant weight loss	Severe weight loss
1 week	1–2%	>2%
1 Month	5%	>5%
3 Months	7.5%	>7.5%
6 Months	10%	>10%

From: Blackburn G, Bistrian B, Maini B, et al. Nutritional and metabolic assessment of the hospitalized patient. *J Pen J Parenter Enteral Nutr* 1977;1:17.

Anthropometry

FAT STORES. Approximately half of human fat is found in the subcutaneous layer. Therefore, measurement of subcutaneous fat provides a reasonably accurate index of total body fat. The triceps skinfold thickness and subscapular skinfold are commonly used to quantify adipose tissue thickness on the limbs and trunk. Other body points that can be measured to ascertain adipose stores using skinfold thickness are biceps, abdomen, suprailiac, medial calf, and anterior thigh. Loss of fat from subcutaneous stores occurs proportionally, so repeated measures from a selected group of sites in an individual patient can provide reliable information on trends of adipose stores. In dialysis patients, it is recommended that arm measures be completed using the nonaccess arm. Otherwise, the right arm is recommended for use in measurements.

Table 3-9. Indirect methods for assessing body composition

1. Visual inspection
2. Weight-height indices
3. Determination of fat-free mass
   Body water
   Body potassium
   Body nitrogen and calcium
   Bioelectrical impedance
   Electromagnetic scanning
4. Determination of body fatness
   Densitometry
   Skinfold thickness
   Inert gas absorption
   Near infrared interactance
5. Determination of bone mineral content
   Neutron activation
   Dual energy x-ray absorptiometry

From: Lukaski H. Methodology of body composition studies. In: Watkins J, Roubenoff R, Rosenberg I, eds. *Body composition: the measure and meaning of changes with aging.* Boston: Foundation for Nutritional Advancement; 1992:13.

SKELETAL MUSCLE (SOMATIC PROTEIN MASS, STATIC PROTEIN RESERVES). Anthropometric measures of muscle mass can serve as an indirect assessment of muscle stores because approximately 60% of total body protein is located in skeletal muscle. In response to poor nutrition, skeletal muscle is the primary source of amino acids. The most commonly used anthropometric measures to assess skeletal muscle are the midarm muscle circumference (MAMC) and midarm circumference (MAC). There are several limitations to these anthropometric measures: a 10% error occurs between measurements even when performed by the same clinician, and there is a poor correlation reported between visceral stores and upper arm measurements. Therefore, anthropometric measures alone cannot be relied on to evaluate muscle and fat stores. Anthropometric measures are best used in conjunction with data from the other categories (see Table 3-1).

ADVANCED METHODS OF BODY COMPOSITION ANALYSIS. Methods available to determine fat-free mass are measures of body water, potassium, nitrogen, and calcium, and two electrical approaches, BIA (bioelectrical impedance) and electromagnetic scanning, referred to as TOBEC or EMSCAN. Techniques to estimate total body fat other than anthropometry are inert gas absorption, infrared interactance, total body carbon using neutron activation, computed tomography, magnetic resonance imaging, and dual-energy x-ray absorptiometry. These procedures are costly, require special personnel, and some carry safety issues (computed tomography). Although several of these techniques have been used for body composition analysis in renal patients, they have not been adopted for routine use. Changes in body weight are simple and easily quantified (see Table 3-8).

A recent study (n = 3000) using the BIA method observed an increased relative risk of death in hemodialysis patients with an abnormal test result.

NUTRITIONAL ASSESSMENT AND
MEDICAL MANAGEMENT ARE INTERRELATED

Biochemical values that serve as indices of nutritional status can be altered because of medical problems associated with renal disease (see Table 3-2, parts F–J), uremia, or dialysis therapy. A nutritional assessment, by virtue of the interrelationship between medicine and nutrition in renal disease, must acknowledge and integrate the medical issues to assess nutritional status as well as determine the correct nutrition intervention. Examples are described in the following sections.

Hyperkalemia

Elevated serum levels of potassium in a patient with renal insufficiency require medical evaluation for a change in renal function, urine output, prescription of medications, other medical issues or diseases (e.g., hyperglycemia, severe constipation, catabolism, metabolic acidosis). It should also be determined if the sample was hemolyzed, and dietary intake should be evaluated as a contributing factor.

Acidosis

There is good evidence that metabolic acidosis may contribute to malnutrition. Acidosis has been associated with negative nitrogen balance, reduced albumin synthesis, loss of lean muscle mass, and increased protein catabolism. The nutritional assessment process should include evaluation of the serum bicarbonate level when assessing the patient's overall nutritional status.

Blood (or Serum) Urea Nitrogen

For the adult patient on renal replacement therapy, a target, midweek blood urea nitrogen (BUN) should be in the range of 60 to 80 mg/dl. A BUN value higher than 100 mg/dl might reflect an inadequate dialysis, a catabolic state, gastrointestinal bleeding, or excessive dietary protein intake. A BUN value below 60 suggests an overly aggressive dialysis prescription, an anabolic state, or an inadequate intake of protein. This information must be integrated into the assessment process to evaluate the patient's nutritional status.

Anemia

Hematocrits < 33% in premenopausal women or <37% in adult men and postmenopausal women are indicators that anemia should be evaluated. Inclusion of the hematocrit as part of the nutritional assessment serves as a screening tool, and in conjunction with medical management, identifies the appropriate nutritional intervention.

The serum values listed in Table 3-2, parts F through J, tailor the nutritional assessment process to evaluate for altered nutrient requirements that are a consequence of the medical problems that characterize the renal patient. The values in categories F through J are the initial indices that alert the clinician that further workup is needed. When completed in this way, the nutritional assessment process can accurately identify the appropriate intervention to complement the medical management.

NUTRITIONAL ASSESSMENT PROTOCOLS

No one parameter has yet been identified that will evaluate the different variables that affect nutritional status. Therefore, the assessment procedure involves evaluating a number of different indices, each representing a body compartment or factor influencing nutritional status (see Tables 3-1 and 3-2). As a result, nutritional assessment of the renal patient has traditionally used protocols. This approach lacks scientific verification of accuracy because the protocols developed in this manner have not been formally tested for reliability and validity. Two new approaches to nutritional assessment that are undergoing formal testing in the renal patient are the NPE and the Subjective Global Assessment (SGA); the NPE is discussed in previous sections.

Subjective Global Assessment

The SGA methodology was developed in 1982 in recognition of the need to account for the many manifestations of poor nutrition, and to improve the process by including a component that could identify patients at risk for development of nutritionally mediated complications. Although this technique was originally designed to assess the nutritional status of general surgery patients, it has been validated for dialysis patients.

The SGA process requires obtaining objective information by completing a medical history and physical examination, evaluating gastrointestinal symptoms, body weight patterns, and patient functional capacity, and determining the presence of comorbid conditions that affect nutritional requirements. Evaluation of functional capacity is completed by determining if the patient has had a loss in strength or stamina due to a deterioration in nutritional status. Subjective information is also acquired such as patient-reported food intake. The patient receives a rating for each of these categories, with a rating of 1 to 2 implying severe malnutrition, 3 to 5 suggesting mild to moderate malnutrition, and 6 or 7 indicating mild malnutrition to well nourished. On completion of this evaluation, the patient is assigned to one of three groups according to his or her nutritional status: (A) well nourished, (B) mild to moderately malnourished, or (C) severely malnourished. The appropriate nutrition intervention is then formulated and implemented. An SGA rating form that has been developed specifically for use with the dialysis patient is shown as Fig. 3-3.

Limitations of the SGA include a heavy reliance on subjective clinical judgment when determining rank for each of the categories. In addition, the SGA may not identify functional impairment due to malnutrition; nor does it indicate the type and amount of nutrition that is needed for repletion. Whether the SGA becomes a gold standard for use with the renal patient population is yet to be determined.

FREQUENCY OF NUTRITIONAL ASSESSMENT

All patients with renal disease, whether newly diagnosed or new to dialysis therapy, should receive a baseline nutritional assessment. An indication of other medical problems (such as those listed in Table 3-2, parts F–J) requires further evaluation with laboratory and other testing.

A comprehensive nutritional assessment for the stable patient is recommended once each year for the predialysis patient, and twice yearly for the stable dialysis patient. Any significant medical, surgical, or metabolic events indicate that the nutritional assessment should be repeated.

Nutritional monitoring of serum proteins, weight, diet and food intake, and routine biochemistry values is recommended twice each year for the stable predialysis patient, and, ideally, once a month for the dialysis patient. A predialysis patient experiencing weight loss and reporting poor intake, with or without the presence of abnormal biochemistry values, needs to have access to formal nutrition counseling so that individual and adequate nutrition intervention can be formulated. The patient who is medically unstable and at risk for poor outcome on dialysis therapy may require weekly monitoring to note body weight and to evaluate the appropriateness of the nutrition intervention plan.

SUBJECTIVE GLOBAL ASSESSMENT RATING FORM

Patient Name/ID #:   Date:

HISTORY

Ratings: (1-2, 3-4-5, 6-7)

WEIGHT/WEIGHT CHANGE:

1. Baseline Wt: _____ (Dry weight from 6 months ago)

    Current Wt: _____ (Dry weight today)

    Actual Wt loss/past 6 mo: _____ % loss: _____ (actual loss ÷ baseline)

2. Weight change over past two weeks: _____ No change

    (Recent significant gain may _____ Increase

    negate previous loss) _____ Decrease

DIETARY INTAKE

1   No Change _____ (Adequate)

    No Change _____ (Inadequate)

2. Change: Suboptimal Intake: _____ Duration _____

    Full Liquid: _____

    Hypocaloric Liquid _____

    Starvation _____

Fig. 3-3. Subjective Global Assessment rating form. Note: The Canadian/USA study showed that a one unit increase in the seven-point scale of SGA rating was associated with a 25% decline in relative risk of death for pentoneal dialysis patients. Reproduced with permission of Linda McCann, R.N., L.D.

GASTROINTESTINAL SYMPTOMS

Symptom:*   Frequency:*   Duration:+

_____ None   _____

_____ Anorexia   _____

_____ Nausea   _____

_____ Vomiting   _____

_____ Diarrhea   _____

*Never, daily, 2-3 times/wk, 1-2 times/wk   + > 2 weeks, < 2 weeks

FUNCTIONAL CAPACITY

Description   Duration:

_____ No Dysfunction   _____

_____ Change in function   _____

_____ Difficulty with ambulation   _____

_____ Difficulty with normal activity   _____

_____ (Patient specific "normal")   _____

_____ Light activity   _____

_____ Bed/chair ridden with little   _____

_____ or no activity   _____

_____ Improvement in function   _____

Fig. 3-3. *Continued.*

DISEASE STATE/COMORBIDITIES -RELATIONSHIP TO NUTRITIONAL NEEDS

Primary Diagnosis _____

Comorbidities _____

Normal requirements _____ Increased requirements _____

Acute Metabolic Stress: _____ None _____ Low _____ Moderate _____ High

PHYSICAL EXAM

_____ Loss of subcutaneous fat (Below eye, triceps, biceps, chest) _____ Some areas _____ All areas

_____ Muscle wasting (Temple, clavicle, scapula, ribs, quadriceps, calf, knee, interosseous) _____ Some areas _____ All areas

_____ Edema (Related to undernutrition, albumin usually < 2.8 gm/dl)

_____ Ascites (Hemodialysis only -related to undernutrition)

OVERALL SGA RATING

Mild Malnutrition to Well Nourished = "6 or 7" rating in most categories or significant, continued improvement. No clear indication of normal status or severe malnutrition.

Mild-Moderately Malnourished = "3, 4, or 5" ratings.

Severely Malnourished = "1 or 2" ratings in most categories/significant physical signs of malnutrition.

Fig. 3-3. *Continued.*

SELECTED READINGS

Bergstrom J, Heimburger O, Lindholm B, et al. Elevated CRP is a strong predictor of increased mortality and low serum albumin in hemodialysis (HD) patients [abstract]. *J Am Soc Nephrol* 1995; 6:573.

Blackburn G, Bistrian B, Maini B, et al. Nutritional and metabolic assessment of the hospitalized patient. *JPEN J Parenter Enteral Nutr* 1977:1:11–22.

Burrowes JD, Powers SN, Cockram DB, et al. Use of an appetite and diet assessment tool in the pilot phase of a hemodialysis clinical trial: Mortality and Morbidity in Hemodialysis Study. *J Renal Nutr* 1996;6:229–232.

Cano N, Di Costanzo-Dufetel J, Calaf R, et al. Prealbumin–retinol-binding-protein–retinol complex in hemodialysis patients. *Am J Clin Nutr* 1988;47:664–667.

Chertow GM, Jacobs DO, Lazarus JM, et al. Phase angle predicts survival in hemodialysis patients. *J Renal Nutr* 1997;7:204:207.

Chumlea Cameron W, Go Shumei S, Vellas B. Assessment of protein-calorie nutrition. In: Kopple JD, Massry SS, eds. *Nutritional management of renal disease.* Baltimore: Williams & Wilkins; 1997: 203–228.

Churchill DN, Taylor W, Cook RJ, et al. Canadian hemodialysis morbidity study. *Am J Kidney Dis* 1992;3:214–234.

Duggan A, Huffman F. Validation of serum transthyretin (prealbumin) as a nutritional parameter in hemodialysis patients [abstract]. *J Renal Nutr* 1997;7:230.

Enia G, Sicuso C, Alati G, Zoccali C. Subjective Global Assessment of Nutrition in dialysis patients. *Nephrol Dial Transplant* 1993;8: 1094–1098.

Goldstein DJ, Frederico C. The effect of urea kinetic modeling on the nutrition management of hemodialysis patients. *J Am Diet Assoc* 1987;87:474–479.

Gee C, Schroepfer C. Summary of formulas and abbreviations. In: Gee C, Schroepfer C, eds. *Urea kinetics in nutritional management of pre-end stage renal disease.* Council on Renal Nutrition, Northern California/Northern Nevada; 1993:16.

Guarnieri G, Toigo G, Situlin R, et al. The assessment of nutritional status in chronically uremic patients. *Contrib Nephrol* 1989;72: 73–103.

Heymsfield SB, Tighe A, Wang Zi-Mian. Nutritional assessment by anthropometric and biochemical methods. In: Shils ME, Olson JA, Shike M, eds. *Modern nutrition in health and disease.* Philadelphia: Lea & Febiger; 1994:812–841.

Ikizler AT. Biochemical markers: clinical aspects. *J Renal Nutr* 1997;7:61–64.

Jacob V, LeCarpentier JE, Lalzano S, et al. IGF-1, a marker of under-nutrition in hemodialysis patients. *Am J Clin Nutr* 1990;52:39–44.

Jeejeebhoy K. Clinical and functional assessments. In: Shils ME, Olson JA, Shike M, eds. *Modern nutrition in health and disease.* Philadelphia: Lea & Febiger; 1994:805–811.

Kaysen GA, Stevenson FT, Depner T. Determinants of albumin concentration in hemodialysis patients. *Am J Kidney Dis* 1997;29: 658–668.

Kelly MP. Use of dietetic-specific nutritional diagnostic codes in clinical reasoning relevant to the nutritional management of core clinical outcome indicators in hemodialysis patients. *Adv Ren Replace Ther* 1997:4:125–135.

Kight MA. The nutrition physical examination. *CRN Quarterly* 1987: 11:9–12.

Labbe RF, Veldee MS. Nutrition in the clinical laboratory. *Clin Lab Med* 1993;13:313–327.

Lowrie EG, Lew NL. Death risk in hemodialysis patients: the predictive value of commonly measured variables and an evaluation of death rate differences between facilities. *Am J Kidney Dis* 1990;15:458–482.

Lukaski H. Methodology of body composition studies. In: Watkins J, Roubenoff R, Rosenberg I, eds. *Body composition: the measure and meaning of changes with aging*. Boston: Foundation for Nutritional Advancement; 1991:13–24.

McCann L, ed. *Pocket guide to nutritional assessment of the renal patient*. 2nd ed. New York: National Kidney Foundation; 1998.

Mitch WE. Influence of metabolic acidosis on nutrition. *Am J Kidney Dis* 1997;29:xlvi–xlviii.

Spiegel DM, Breyer JA. Serum albumin: a predictor of long-term outcome in peritoneal dialysis patients. *Am J Kidney Dis* 1994;23: 283–285.

Calcium, Phosphorus, and Vitamin D

Esther A. González and Kevin J. Martin

The regulation of calcium and phosphorus homeostasis depends on two major regulatory hormone systems, parathyroid hormone (PTH) and 1,25-dihydroxycholecalciferol (calcitriol), the active metabolite of vitamin D. Stimulation of PTH secretion results in increases in serum calcium by altering calcium mobilization from bone and increasing calcium reclamation by the kidney. PTH is also the principal regulator of renal excretion of phosphorus. By these means, PTH is responsible for the minute-to-minute regulation of mineral metabolism. Calcitriol is the principal regulator of intestinal calcium absorption. As illustrated in Fig. 4-1, these two hormone systems are themselves closely interrelated, and each regulates the production of the other in a physiologic feedback loop. Thus, PTH increases serum calcium by two mechanisms, increasing mobilization of calcium from bone and increasing renal calcium reabsorption. PTH also increases the synthesis of calcitriol by the kidney, both directly and as a consequence of increasing phosphate excretion to decrease serum phosphate. The increase in calcitriol in turn inhibits the secretion of PTH. These hormone systems undergo profound changes in the course of renal

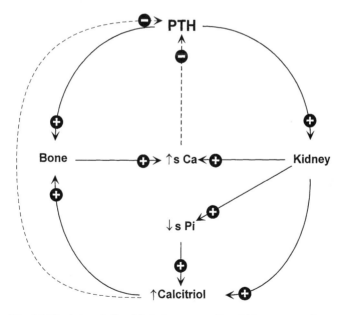

Fig. 4-1. The interrelationship between parathyroid hormone and calcitriol in the regulation of calcium and phosphorus homeostasis. sCa, serum calcium; sPi, serum inorganic phosphorus.

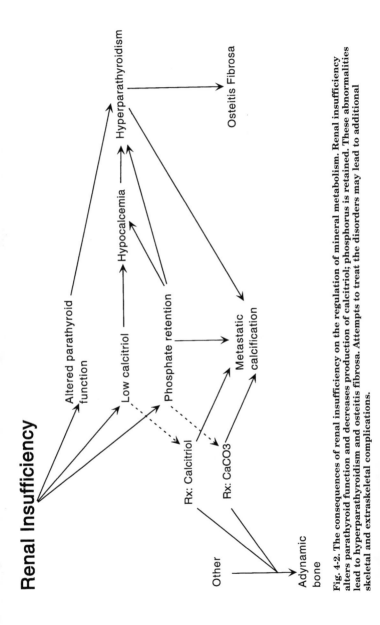

Fig. 4-2. The consequences of renal insufficiency on the regulation of mineral metabolism. Renal insufficiency alters parathyroid function and decreases production of calcitriol; phosphorus is retained. These abnormalities lead to hyperparathyroidism and osteitis fibrosa. Attempts to treat the disorders may lead to additional skeletal and extraskeletal complications.

disease because the kidney not only is the final regulator of calcium and phosphorus balance but is the principal site of calcitriol synthesis. These changes result in derangements of mineral metabolism that lead to significant morbidity in the skeletal system as well as peripheral tissues.

An example of such derangement is seen in chronic renal insufficiency as depicted in Fig. 4-2. Thus, in renal insufficiency, there are intrinsic alterations in parathyroid function that lead to abnormal calcium-regulated PTH secretion. As renal function declines, the decrease in renal mass limits the production of calcitriol, which, in turn, directly and indirectly leads to hyperparathyroidism. The decreased excretory function of the failing kidney also leads to accumulation of phosphorus, which directly and indirectly contributes to the development of hyperparathyroidism. Efforts at treating these disturbances, unless monitored closely, can cause significant morbidity.

CALCIUM

Normal Calcium Homeostasis

Calcium is the most abundant cation in the body. A 70-kg man has approximately 1.2 kg of calcium. More than 99% of the calcium is in bone and is unavailable for participation in the day-to-day regulation of calcium homeostasis. Only 1.3 g of calcium is extracellular. Exchange of calcium between bone and the extracellular fluid occurs by two mechanisms: first, the constant process of bone remodeling; and second, homeostatic mechanisms that regulate the plasma calcium concentration.

In plasma, the normal calcium concentration varies from 9 to 10.4 mg/dl. Plasma calcium is composed of three fractions (Fig. 4-3). Approximately 40% of the total serum calcium is protein bound; 75% to 90% of this fraction is bound to albumin. An additional fraction of total serum calcium is complexed to various anions (10%). The remainder is free ionized calcium (50%). The ionized calcium is the physiologically important component, and can easily be measured directly. In the absence of measurements of ionized calcium, the clinician can attempt to correct the total calcium for changes in protein concentration and changes in pH. Thus, an approximation may be obtained as follows: for every gram per deciliter that serum albumin differs from 4 g/dl, the serum calcium should be adjusted by 0.8 mg/dl. Similarly, for every 0.1 increment in pH, serum calcium should be decreased by 0.12 mg/dl. None of the many algorithms that have been formulated for this purpose is entirely accurate, and measurements of ionized calcium are recommended.

The overall scheme for calcium balance is depicted in Fig. 4-4. On a usual daily intake of approximately 1000 mg there is a net absorption of 200 mg. Approximately 200 mg enters and leaves the bone, and approximately 200 mg is excreted by the kidney to maintain balance. During growth, the need for positive calcium balance is greater, and 400 mg/day of calcium can be deposited in the growing human skeleton. The level of ionized calcium in blood is tightly controlled despite this wide range of calcium influx from the intestine and bone. Maintenance of a normal level of ionized calcium depends primarily on the parathyroid glands, which monitor plasma calcium and increase secretion of

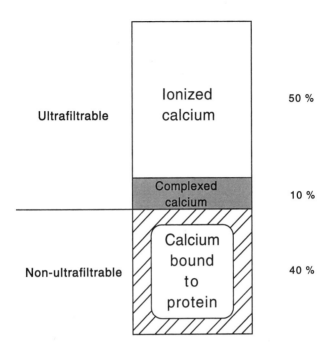

Fig. 4-3. The distribution of calcium in serum. Approximately 50% is ionized and the remainder is either bound to proteins or complexed to other anions. The ionized and complexed fractions are ultrafiltrable at the glomerulus.

PTH in response to a decrease in ionized calcium. PTH secretion results in stimulation of bone resorption, increased reabsorption of calcium by the kidney, and stimulation of calcitriol production by the kidney. These factors raise plasma calcium. The mechanism by which the parathyroid gland senses calcium has been elucidated by the cloning of a G-protein–coupled calcium receptor.

Regulation of Intestinal Calcium Absorption

Absorption of calcium across the intestinal mucosa is achieved by two processes that occur in tandem: an active transcellular transport and a passive paracellular diffusion process. The duodenum is the major site of the active transport process, whereas the passive mechanism occurs throughout the small intestine and even the colon. The absorption rate in all intestinal segments is increased by vitamin D, with the duodenum being the most responsive.

CELLULAR MECHANISMS OF ACTIVE CALCIUM TRANSPORT.   The active mechanism involves transport across the apical membrane and the cytosol and extrusion across the basolateral membrane. Initial entry involves calcium channels. In the cell, calcium is bound to a calcium-binding protein, calbindin, that

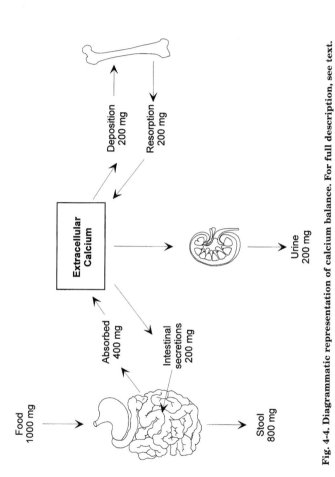

Fig. 4-4. Diagrammatic representation of calcium balance. For full description, see text.

protects the cell against a toxic increase in cytosolic calcium, and transports calcium across the cell to the basolateral membrane. An adenosine triphosphate (ATP)-dependent calcium pump in the basolateral membrane with a higher affinity for calcium than calbindin extrudes calcium from the cell. The regulation of calbindin and the plasma membrane calcium pump is vitamin D dependent. Active calcium transport becomes saturated at relatively low levels of calcium intake (<500 mg/day). When daily calcium intake exceeds 500 mg, passive paracellular absorption occurs. This mechanism is nonsaturable, but tight junction-mediated calcium transport may also be regulated by calcitriol.

THE ROLE OF VITAMIN D IN CALCIUM ABSORPTION. The major factor regulating intestinal calcium absorption is calcitriol, which acts through genomic and nongenomic mechanisms. The genomic mechanism is analogous to that of other steroid hormones; the ligand, calcitriol, binds to the vitamin D receptor (VDR), which is a member of the steroid–thyroid receptor gene superfamily of nuclear transcription factors. Calcitriol regulates the transcription of many genes, including VDR, calbindin, and the plasma membrane calcium pump. After administration of calcitriol, there is an increase in VDR, calbindin, and calcium pump synthesis, leading to increased calcium transport. There also is strong evidence for a rapid effect of calcitriol on calcium absorption (transcaltachia) that is independent of changes in gene transcription. This effect occurs, within seconds to minutes, and is too rapid to be the result of gene transcription.

OTHER FACTORS THAT AFFECT CALCIUM ABSORPTION. **Systemic Factors.** Although vitamin D is the most important systemic factor regulating calcium absorption, there are other factors. Many of these factors, such as PTH, growth hormone, estrogen, and loop diuretics, increase intestinal calcium absorption indirectly by increasing the synthesis of calcitriol. However, glucocorticoids, metabolic acidosis, and thiazide diuretics independently cause a decrease in intestinal calcium absorption.

Luminal Factors. Calcium absorption may also be influenced by substances within the intestinal lumen such as phosphate, oxalate, long-chain fatty acids, and fiber, all of which bind calcium and decrease its absorption. On the other hand, lysine, arginine, and lactose increase calcium absorption.

Calcium Handling by the Kidney

To maintain neutral balance, the kidney excretes an amount of calcium that is equal to the net intestinal calcium absorption (approximately 200 mg). The renal excretion of calcium begins with the filtration of the ultrafiltrable fraction of plasma calcium, approximately 9000 mg/day. Therefore, 8800 mg/day is reabsorbed and 200 mg/day is excreted. Approximately 70% of filtered calcium is reabsorbed in the proximal tubule, 20% in the thick ascending limb of the loop of Henle, 5% to 10% in the distal tubule, and <4% in the collecting tubule. Regulation of the amount of calcium excreted occurs mainly in the distal nephron. Transcellular transport of calcium across the renal tubular cell resembles the processes occurring in intestinal cells; as in the intestine, a large proportion occurs by the paracellular pathway.

REGULATION OF CALCIUM EXCRETION BY THE KIDNEY. Variations in calcium excretion occur in the distal tubule, where calciotropic hormones change calcium transport. In general, the process appears to be similar to calcium transport in the intestinal cell. The major factors influencing the renal handling of calcium are listed in Table 4-1.

Dietary Factors. Urinary calcium increases as urinary sodium increases; accordingly, a high dietary sodium increases calcium excretion. A high intake of calcium also increases urinary calcium excretion by increasing the filtered load if serum calcium increases, and by suppressing PTH release. A high dietary phosphate tends to decrease urine calcium excretion by decreasing the filtered load of calcium and by stimulating PTH secretion.

Hormonal Factors. The direct action of PTH is to increase calcium reabsorption by the kidney; however, an increase in serum calcium resulting from the actions of PTH on bone can override this effect, leading to hypercalciuria. The effects of calcitriol on renal calcium excretion are uncertain: a direct effect of calcitriol is to increase urinary calcium excretion independently of the changes in PTH and serum calcium.

Metabolic Disturbances. In general, acidosis is associated with an increase in urinary calcium excretion, whereas alkalosis tends to reduce urinary calcium. Hypercalcemia from any cause leads to hypercalciuria, especially if PTH secretion is suppressed. The loop diuretics increase calcium excretion by decreasing calcium reabsorption in the loop of Henle.

Genetic Factors. Defects in the calcium receptor can be associated with abnormalities such as those found in patients with familial hypocalciuric hypercalcemia.

Calcium Metabolism in Bone

Under normal circumstances, there is constant mobilization of calcium from bone and deposition of calcium in newly formed

Table 4-1. Factors involved in the renal handling of calcium

Dietary factors
Sodium
Calcium
Phosphorus

Hormonal factors
Parathyroid hormone
Calcitriol
Calcitonin

Metabolic disturbances
Acid–base
Hypercalcemia
Hypophosphatemia
Idiopathic hypercalciuria

Genetic factors
Familial hypocalciuric hypercalcemia

osteoid. This is the continuous process of normal bone remodeling occurring throughout life. During growth, calcium is deposited into the growing skeleton, but excessive bone resorption can cause skeletal loss in diseases such as hyperparathyroidism, hypercalcemia of malignancy, multiple myeloma, and osteoporosis.

Parathyroid hormone is the major regulator of bone turnover. The target cell for the effect of PTH is the osteoblast; there are indirect effects on the osteoclast. Although PTH stimulates both bone formation and bone resorption, the net effect of a sustained increase in PTH is loss of bone. Current evidence, however, indicates that intermittent elevations of PTH may actually be associated with a net increase in bone formation. Like PTH, the principal target cell for calcitriol is the osteoblast. Calcitriol is essential for normal bone growth and mineralization, but it does not appear to stimulate bone formation directly. The mechanism is complex and likely related to changes in the concentrations of extracellular calcium and phosphorus.

Bone remodeling is regulated not only by PTH and calcitriol but by insulin, growth hormone, calcitonin, insulin-like growth factor-1, glucocorticoids, sex hormones, and thyroid hormone, plus locally produced cytokines. Bone resorption may also be altered by hormone-independent mechanisms such as systemic acidosis, in which bone mineral is released from the skeleton as hydrogen ions are buffered.

Disturbances of Calcium Metabolism in Renal Disease

Renal Insufficiency

With the onset of renal insufficiency, there are several changes in mineral homeostasis that have important consequences on bone and soft tissues.

With mild to moderate renal insufficiency, intestinal calcium reabsorption is not different from normal, but with more advanced renal insufficiency, intestinal calcium absorption is reduced despite a compensatory increase in PTH secretion. The decrease in intestinal calcium absorption is likely due to lower levels of calcitriol because its production is limited by the loss of renal mass (see later).

Because intestinal calcium absorption is impaired in advanced renal failure, it is necessary to provide calcium supplements to correct the decreased efficiency of intestinal calcium absorption. In general, at least 1 g/day of supplemental calcium is required. The use of a dietary calcium supplement may have the additional benefit of limiting phosphate absorption (see later).

Symptomatic hypocalcemia is uncommon in chronic renal failure. Low levels of plasma or serum calcium are often seen in patients with hypoalbuminemia, but ionized calcium may still be normal. If hypocalcemia does occur, it acts as a profound stimulus for PTH secretion, and should be corrected with calcium supplements and other measures (see later).

Regimens that cause hypercalcemia must be avoided because hypercalcemia can hasten the progression of renal disease and cause extraskeletal calcification of blood vessels and soft tissues.

Nephrolithiasis

A detailed discussion of nephrolithiasis is beyond the scope of this chapter, but there are dietary manipulations that are essential as therapy. The most common type of kidney stone is calcium oxalate, and the most common cause of stone disease is idiopathic hypercalciuria.

DIETARY INTERVENTIONS IN HYPERCALCIURIA. Intestinal calcium absorption is elevated in many of these patients. Although hypercalciuric patients are often prescribed diets low in calcium, this is a problem because the diet increases the risk of raising urine oxalate excretion. Accordingly, severe dietary calcium restriction is not usually recommended. A dietary maneuver that is useful at least in selected patients is to add sodium cellulose phosphate to bind calcium and decrease intestinal calcium absorption. Some patients with hypercalciuria due to renal tubular acidosis require alkali supplements that increase urinary citrate excretion (an inhibitor of stone formation), which decreases the degree of hypercalciuria.

DIETARY INTERVENTIONS IN HYPEROXALURIA. Primary hyperoxaluria results from hereditary enzyme defects that raise oxalate production. Therapy is to increase the intake of fluids, citrate, and pyridoxine. In spite of these measures, renal failure from deposition of oxalate crystals often occurs.

Enteric hyperoxaluria can result from small bowel malabsorption, which allows undigested fatty acids and bile salts to reach the colon. There, the bile salts increase colonic permeability so that oxalate absorption rises. In these patients, the urine oxalate is high and urine citrate is low because of the loss of alkali from the small bowel. Therapy should be a low-oxalate, low-fat diet plus oral calcium supplements (1 to 4 g of calcium carbonate with meals) added to bind intestinal oxalate and limit its absorption. Cholestyramine may also be useful.

Milk-Alkali Syndrome

The milk-alkali syndrome is characterized by hypercalcemia, metabolic alkalosis, and renal insufficiency. It is caused by the ingestion of large quantities of calcium together with excessive alkali. It is obvious that dietary modifications are essential therapy.

PHOSPHORUS

Normal Phosphorus Homeostasis

Phosphate is a major constituent of the skeleton, and is critical for bone formation and dissolution. In addition, phosphate is essential for many synthetic actions of the cell, and is an important buffer used in the excretion of acid by the kidney. Like that of calcium, phosphate homeostasis depends on the interaction of three organ systems: the gastrointestinal tract, bone, and the kidney. Phosphate homeostasis is regulated by the two main hormones that regulate mineral metabolism, PTH and calcitriol.

Approximately 700 g of phosphorus is present in a 70-kg man, 85% of which is in the skeleton and teeth, 14% in soft tissues, and 1% the blood and extracellular fluid. The normal adult achieves neutral phosphate balance over a range of intake from 800 to 1600 mg/day. Approximately two thirds of ingested phosphorus is absorbed in the duodenum and jejunum (Fig. 4-5). Some phospho-

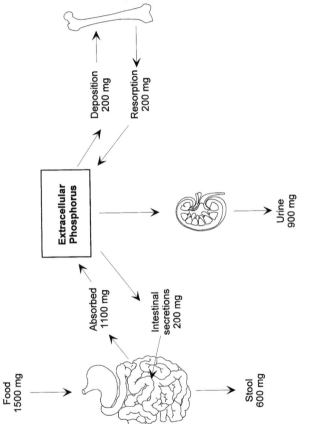

Fig. 4-5. Diagrammatic representation of phosphorus balance. For full description, see text.

rus is secreted into the intestinal lumen. Approximately 200 mg of phosphorus enters and leaves the bone each day, leaving approximately 900 mg to be excreted by the kidney.

Intestinal Absorption and Regulation of Phosphorus

Most phosphate absorption occurs in the jejunum and duodenum, primarily through a diffusional process, although a small saturable component also exists. Passive absorption is thought to be mostly by the paracellular route. The active transport process involves sodium-coupled phosphate entry by a sodium–phosphate (Na/Pi) cotransporter in the brush border membrane, for which energy is provided by Na/K ATPase.

The administration of calcitriol stimulates phosphate absorption. This effect appears to be at the level of the Na/Pi cotransporter in the brush border membrane. Changes in intestinal phosphate absorption in response to variations in dietary intake are likely mediated by changes in the levels of calcitriol, and calcitriol production in turn is regulated because a high phosphate suppresses renal 1-α-hydroxylase and hence activation of vitamin D. Regardless, the absorption of phosphorus is largely diffusional, so phosphorus in the diet is the major determinant of intestinal phosphate absorption.

There are other factors that affect intestinal phosphate absorption; a high concentration of calcium in the diet impairs phosphate uptake in the intestine. Likewise, aluminum or other divalent ions such as magnesium bind phosphates and prevent phosphate absorption.

Phosphate Handling by the Kidney

The kidney is the principal organ regulating phosphate homeostasis. Most of the circulating inorganic phosphorus is ultrafiltrable and approximately 80% is reabsorbed by the renal tubule; 60% to 70% is reabsorbed in the proximal nephron. There also is evidence for regulated phosphate reabsorption in the distal nephron.

CELLULAR MECHANISMS FOR RENAL PHOSPHATE TRANSPORT. Transepithelial phosphate transport involves uptake across the brush border membrane, translocation across the cell, and efflux across the basolateral membrane. The uptake across the brush border membrane is mediated by Na/Pi cotransporters, which are rate limiting and the major site of regulation of phosphate transport. There are also phosphate extrusion mechanisms in the basolateral membrane that appear to be primarily sodium-independent, anion exchange mechanisms.

FACTORS INFLUENCING RENAL HANDLING OF PHOSPHORUS. The major factors involved in the regulation of phosphorus excretion by the kidney are listed in Table 4-2.

Dietary and Plasma Phosphate. The kidney responds to changes in the filtered load of phosphorus by altering the urinary excretion of phosphorus. This response occurs independently of PTH, although there is also a PTH-dependent effect.

Changes in Extracellular Fluid Volume. Expansion of the extracellular fluid can increase renal phosphate excretion independently of filtered load, plasma calcium, and PTH; this response is greater if PTH is present.

Changes in Plasma Calcium. Changes in plasma calcium change the reabsorption of phosphorus by varying the glomerular filtra-

Table 4-2. Factors influencing renal handling of phosphorus

Dietary and plasma phosphate
Extracellular fluid volume
Calcium
Acid–base status
Hormones
   Parathyroid hormone
   Calcitriol
   Calcitonin
   Insulin
   Glucose
   Glucagon
   Glucocorticoids
Drugs
   Diuretics
Other factors
   ?Phosphatonin

tion rate (GFR), renal blood flow, the filtration coefficient (K_f), and PTH, as well as having direct effects on the tubule.

Acid–Base Status. In general, acidosis decreases phosphate absorption independently of PTH and plasma calcium. Alkalotic states tend to increase phosphate reabsorption. Some differences are apparent between acute and chronic acid–base disorders.

Hormones. Parathyroid hormone is the major regulator of phosphate reabsorption by the kidney. The primary site of action is the proximal convoluted and the proximal straight tubule segments. Some PTH-sensitive phosphate transport has also been demonstrated in the distal nephron. PTH exerts its effects primarily by increasing cyclic adenosine monophosphate, but activation of protein kinase C has also been implicated. Indeed, the cloned PTH/PTHrP receptor has been shown to activate both adenylate cyclase and phospholipase C.

The effects of calcitriol on phosphate handling by the kidney are somewhat controversial. In general, calcitriol reduces phosphate excretion, but the response varies with changes in serum calcium and PTH. The physiologic role of calcitonin in phosphate reabsorption is probably minor. Insulin tends to reduce phosphate excretion, whereas glucagon increases phosphate excretion. Hyperglycemia results in phosphaturia by inducing an osmotic diuresis.

Drugs and Other Factors. Acetazolamide and loop diuretics can increase phosphate excretion. Evidence suggests that an as yet uncharacterized factor, phosphatonin, may also alter the renal handling of phosphorus.

Disturbances of Phosphate Metabolism in Renal Disease

Renal Insufficiency

As renal function falls, there is a tendency for serum phosphorus to increase, reflecting the loss of the capacity to excrete phosphate. This increase in serum phosphorus results in a higher secretion rate of PTH, which acts to increase phosphate excretion and bring serum phosphorus to normal levels. The mechanisms by which phosphorus causes an increase in PTH secretion include secondary hypocalcemia, inhibition of calcitriol production, and direct effects on the parathyroid gland. This general scheme, known as the "tradeoff hypothesis," explains the development of secondary hyperparathyroidism. It was confirmed by showing that restriction of dietary phosphate in proportion to the decrement of GFR prevented the development of secondary hyperparathyroidism.

Accordingly, in the course of renal insufficiency, dietary phosphorus intake must be restricted. The phosphorus content of several foods is listed in Table 4-3. Dietary protein restriction is an essential part of dietary phosphate restriction because protein-rich foods are in general phosphate-rich foods. In practice, it is difficult to reduce dietary phosphorus intake to less than 700 mg/day. If further restriction is required, it is necessary to use strategies that bind phosphorus in the intestinal lumen to minimize phosphate absorption. Such maneuvers include supplements of calcium carbonate, calcium acetate, aluminum-containing antacids, and, more recently, nonabsorbable phosphate-binding polymers.

Other Renal Diseases

Hypophosphatemia resulting from impaired renal tubular reabsorption of phosphorus may require dietary phosphorus supplements as part of its therapy. Such conditions include hyperparathyroidism and the hypophosphatemia that follows renal transplantation. The latter condition may be due to persistent elevations of PTH or to PTH-independent mechanisms. Hypophosphatemia can also be seen as part of Fanconi syndrome and other types of renal tubular acidosis. Severe hypophosphatemia may occur in association with some mesenchymal tumors; the mechanism of this oncogenic osteomalacia is thought to be the production of a circulating phosphaturic factor, possibly phosphatonin. Similarly, the presence of a circulating phosphaturic factor has also been implicated in the pathogenesis of X-linked hypophosphatemic rickets.

VITAMIN D

Normal Vitamin D Metabolism

Figure 4-6 illustrates the normal metabolism of vitamin D. The secosteroid, vitamin D_3, is made in the skin upon the action of ultraviolet light. Native vitamin D undergoes two successive hydroxylations in the liver and kidney to form the biologically active metabolite, 1,25-dihydroxycholecalciferol, also known as calcitriol. The principal target tissues for calcitriol are the intestine, where it increases calcium absorption, and bone, where it modulates skeletal metabolism. The renal production of calcitriol is regulated mainly by PTH, calcium, and phosphorus. Calcitriol not only regulates calcium metabolism, but regulates the proliferation and differentiation of a variety of cells that are not associated with calcium metabolism.

Table 4-3. Phosphorus content of selected food items

Item	Amount	Pi (mg)
Dairy		
Milk	1 cup	278
Cheese		800
Swiss	4 oz	420
Mozzarella	4 oz	545
Cheddar	4 oz	1200
American	4 oz	212
Brie	4 oz	130
Ice cream	1 cup	1325
Yogurt	8 oz	325
Fish		
Salmon	3.5 oz	344
Fish	4 oz	400
Shrimp	3.5 oz	166
Tuna	3.5 oz	250
Crab	3.5 oz	175
Meat		
Hamburger	3.5 oz	186
Liver	3.5 oz	537
Pork	3.5 oz	300
Poultry		
Chicken	3.5 oz	190
Turkey	3.5 oz	200
Chicken livers	3.5 oz	300
Egg	1 lg	100
Vegetables		
Beans	1 cup	278
Blackeye peas	1 cup	286
Lentils	1 cup	238
Broccoli	1 cup	50
Mixed vegetables	1 cup	60
Nuts and seeds		
Peanuts	3.5 oz	466
Pumpkin seeds	3.5 oz	1144
Sunflower seeds	3.5 oz	1155
Breads and cereals		
Wheat bread	1 slice	65
Oatmeal	1 cup	130
Corn flakes	1 cup	10

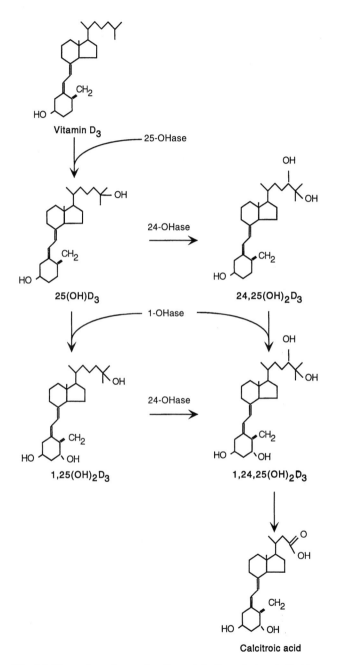

Fig. 4-6. The main pathways for the metabolism of vitamin D. 25-OHase, 25-hydroxylase; 1-OHase, 1-α-hydroxylase; 24-OHase, 24-hydroxylase.

Casual exposure to sunlight provides most of the vitamin D requirements for children and young adults, but the elderly may not have enough exposure, especially in areas without abundant sunlight. Thus, these people may be prone to the development of vitamin D deficiency. Dietary sources of vitamin D include salmon, mackerel, and fatty fish oils, including cod liver oil. Fortification of foods such as cereals, bread, and milk provides additional dietary supplements of vitamin D, and vitamin D is a component of many multivitamin preparations. It is estimated that the recommended daily allowance of vitamin D is 600 to 800 IU for adults. Vitamin D from plants, ergocalciferol, or vitamin D_2, has similar fates as vitamin D_3, and has similar biologic activities. The only structural difference between vitamins D_2 and D_3 is that the former contains a double bond between C_{22} and C_{23}, and a methyl group at C_{24}.

In plasma, vitamin D is bound to a vitamin D-binding protein and transported to the liver, where it becomes hydroxylated at the 25 position. 25-Hydroxyvitamin D_3 is the major circulating form of vitamin D. The activity of the 25-hydroxylase enzyme is not tightly regulated, and measurement of its activity is useful for the assessment of vitamin D deficiency and vitamin D intoxication. 25-Hydroxyvitamin D_3 is transported to the kidney, where it is hydroxylated in the 1-α position through the action of the enzyme, 25-hydroxyvitamin D_3 1-α-hydroxylase. Although the kidney is by far the major source of calcitriol, bone, skin, monocytes–macrophages, and the placenta also can produce calcitriol.

Calcitriol is metabolized in target tissues by several hydroxylation reactions. Both 25-hydroxyvitamin D_3 and 1,25-dihydroxyvitamin D_3 can undergo 24-hydroxylation to form 24,25-dihydroxyvitamin D_3 and 1,24,25-trihydroxyvitamin D_3, respectively. This is the first step in the degradative pathway. These metabolites are considered to have little or no biologic activity. Further metabolism results in the formation of the final metabolite, calcitroic acid.

Mechanism of Action of Calcitriol

All target tissues for calcitriol contain a nuclear VDR with a ligand-binding domain and a DNA-binding domain. Free calcitriol enters the cell and binds to the ligand-binding domain of the VDR (Fig. 4-7). The complex must form a secondary complex with another nuclear receptor, the retinoic acid X receptor. This heterodimer complex interacts with specific vitamin D response elements in DNA, leading to alterations in the transcription of the target genes, the best characterized of which are the osteocalcin, osteopontin, 24-hydroxylase, calcium-binding protein, and alkaline phosphatase genes.

Actions of Vitamin D in the Intestine

Calcitriol is the major regulator of intestinal calcium absorption. Calcitriol affects the entry of calcium through the luminal side of the plasma membrane, the movement of calcium through the cytoplasm, and the transfer of calcium across the basolateral membrane into the circulation. The mechanism by which calcitriol regulates calcium flux is not well understood; however, calcitriol has been shown to increase the production of several

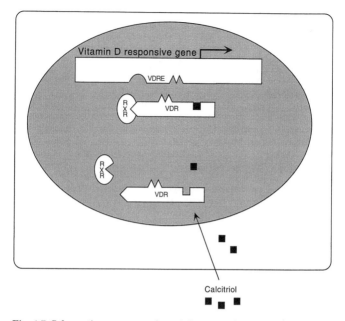

Fig. 4-7. Schematic representation of the genomic mechanism of action of calcitriol. Calcitriol binds to the vitamin D receptor (VDR), which binds to the retinoid X receptor (RXR) to form a heterodimer that then interacts with the vitamin D response element (VDRE) of specific genes.

proteins of the intestinal cell, including calcium-binding proteins, alkaline phosphatase, calcium ATPase, calmodulin, and brush border actin. Calcium-binding protein is likely to play a major role in the translocation of calcium process. As discussed, calcitriol increases intestinal calcium absorption by transcaltachia, a nongenomic mechanism. In addition, calcitriol increases intestinal phosphate absorption, but by mechanisms that are not well understood.

Actions of Vitamin D in Bone

Calcitriol plays an important role in the recruitment and differentiation of osteoclast precursors to form mature osteoclasts. Mature osteoclasts ultimately lose their ability to recognize calcitriol. Consequently, 1,25-dihydroxyvitamin D_3 influences mature osteoclasts indirectly by acting on osteoblasts. Osteoblasts contain VDRs that mediate the effects of calcitriol, causing an increase in the expression of alkaline phosphatase, osteopontin, osteocalcin, and several cytokines. The role of calcitriol in promoting the mineralization of osteoid is believed to be a consequence of actions that maintain the extracellular calcium and phosphorus concentrations in the normal range.

Alterations in Vitamin D Metabolism in Renal Insufficiency

Because the kidney is the major site of calcitriol production, it is not surprising that as renal mass decreases, there is a tendency for calcitriol production to decrease. This tendency can be offset initially by an increase in PTH secretion to increase calcitriol production directly. Ultimately, the decrease in renal mass becomes limiting and the plasma calcitriol level falls. Thus, patients with GFR <50 ml/minute have subnormal blood concentrations of calcitriol. Other factors that contribute to a low calcitriol production are acidosis and as yet unidentified substances accumulated by uremic patients. The decrease in calcitriol may be more profound in patients with interstitial renal diseases. Patients with heavy proteinuria can lose vitamin D and vitamin D-binding protein in the urine. These losses contribute to a physiologically important decrease in circulating vitamin D metabolites. The decrease in calcitriol in general results in a parallel decrease in intestinal calcium absorption in the course of renal insufficiency. Low levels of calcitriol also contribute to abnormal parathyroid gland function and may contribute to the resistance of the bones to the calcium-raising actions of PTH.

Calcitriol Supplementation in Renal Insufficiency

The mechanisms by which calcitriol deficiency contributes to the development of secondary hyperparathyroidism provide a rationale for calcitriol supplements in the course of chronic renal failure. Calcitriol and other 1-α-vitamin D sterols have been shown to be efficacious for these patients, leading to a decrease in PTH levels and histologic improvements in bone. Treatment early in the course of renal insufficiency may help prevent the development of severe parathyroid gland hyperplasia that may become refractory to therapy. Even though the rationale is strong, the routine use of vitamin D analogs in mild to moderate renal failure is not generally recommended because of a concern that these active compounds will accelerate the decline in renal function. Calcitriol can interfere with creatinine secretion, but the principal concern is that it will cause a real decline in renal function when hypercalcemia develops. In addition, hypercalcemia has the potential to aggravate metastatic calcification. We believe the risk of accelerating the loss of renal function is small, provided doses are limited to <0.5 µg/day.

An additional undesirable effect of vitamin D therapy may be that PTH is oversuppressed, resulting in the syndrome of adynamic bone disease. In advanced renal failure, vitamin D therapy can aggravate hyperphosphatemia, sharply elevating the levels of calcium–phosphorus products and the risk of extraskeletal calcification.

SELECTED READINGS

Almaden Y, Canelejo A, Hernandez A, et al. Direct effect of phosphorus on PTH secretion from whole rat parathyroid glands in vitro. *J Bone Miner Res* 1996;11:970–976.

Argiles A, Mourad G, Mion C. Oral vitamin D or calcium in the prevention of renal bone disease? *Curr Opin Nephrol Hypertens* 1996;5:329–336.

Arnold A, Brown MF, Urena P, et al. Monoclonality of parathyroid tumors in chronic renal failure and in primary parathyroid hyperplasia. *J Clin Invest* 1995;95:2047–2053.

Brown EM, Pollak M, Hebert SC. Sensing of extracellular Ca^{2+} by parathyroid and kidney cells: cloning and characterization of an extracellular Ca^{2+}-sensing receptor. *Am J Kidney Dis* 1995;25: 506–513.

Buschinsky DA. The contribution of acidosis to renal osteodystrophy. *Kidney Int* 1995;47:1816–1832.

Cai Q, Chandler JS, Wasserman RH, et al. Vitamin D and adaptation to dietary calcium and phosphorus deficiencies increase intestinal plasma membrane calcium pump gene expression. *Proc Natl Acad Sci U S A* 1993;90:1345–1349.

Cai Q, Hodgson SF, Kao PC, et al. Brief report: inhibitor of renal phosphate transport by a tumor product in a patient with oncogenic osteomalacia. *N Engl J Med* 1994;330:1645–1649.

Denda M, Finch J, Slatopolsky E. Phosphorus accelerates the development of parathyroid hyperplasia and secondary hyperparathyroidism in rats with renal failure. *Am J Kidney Dis* 1996;28: 596–602.

Econs MJ, Drezner MK. Tumor-induced osteomalacia: unveiling a new hormone. *N Engl J Med* 1994;330:1679–1681.

Farrell J, González EA, Martin KJ. The use of vitamin D in patients on dialysis. *Seminars in Dialysis* 1995;8:80–82.

Fraser DR. Vitamin D. *Lancet* 1995;345:104–107.

González EA, Martin KJ. Renal osteodystrophy: pathogenesis and management. *Nephrol Dial Transplant* 1995;10:13–21.

González EA, Martin KJ. Bone cell response in uremia. *Seminars in Dialysis* 1996;9:339–346.

Goodman WG, Coburn JW. The use of 1,25-dihydroxyvitamin D_3 in early renal failure. *Annu Rev Med* 1992;43:227–237.

Goodman WG, Ramirez JA, Belin TR, et al. Development of adynamic bone in patients with secondary hyperparathyroidism after intermittent calcitriol therapy. *Kidney Int* 1994;46:1160–1166.

Holick MF, Shao Q, Liu WW, et al. The vitamin D content of fortified milk and infant formula. *N Engl J Med* 1991;325:1178–1181.

Hruska KA, Teitelbaum S. Renal osteodystrophy. *N Engl J Med* 1995;333:166–174.

Johnson JA, Kumar R. Renal and intestinal calcium transport: roles of vitamin D and vitamin D-dependent calcium binding proteins. *Semin Nephrol* 1994;14:119–128.

Kraut JA. The role of metabolic acidosis in the pathogenesis of renal osteodystrophy. *Adv Ren Replace Ther* 1995;2:40–51.

MacDonald PN, Dowd DR, Haussler MR. New insight into the structure and functions of the vitamin D receptor. *Semin Nephrol* 1994;14:101–118.

Manolagas SC, Jilka RL. Bone marrow, cytokines, and bone remodeling. *N Engl J Med* 1995;332:305–311.

Murer H, Biber J. Molecular mechanisms in renal phosphate reabsorption. *Nephrol Dial Transplant* 1995;10:1501–1504.

Naveh-Many T, Rahamimov R, Livni N, et al. Parathyroid cell proliferation in normal and chronic renal failure rats: the effects of calcium, phosphate and vitamin D. *J Clin Invest* 1995;96:1786–1793.

Norman AW, Nemere I, Zhou LX, et al. 1,25$(OH)_2$-vitamin D_3, a steroid hormone that produces biological effects via both genomic and nongenomic pathways. *J Steroid Biochem Mol Biol* 1992;41(3-8):231–240.

Parks JH, Coe FL. Pathogenesis and treatment of calcium stones. *Semin Nephrol* 1996;6:398–411.

Portale AA, Booth BE, Halloran BP, et al. Effect of dietary phosphorus on circulating concentrations of 1,25-dihydroxyvitamin D_3 and immunoreactive parathyroid hormone in children with moderate renal insufficiency. *J Clin Invest* 1984;73:1580–1589.

Reichel H, Diebert B, Schmidt-Gayk H, et al. Calcium metabolism in early chronic renal failure: implications for the pathogenesis of hyperparathyroidism. *Nephrol Dial Transplant* 1991;6:162–169.

Ritz E, Küster S, Schmidt-Gayk H, et al. Low-dose calcitriol prevents the rise in 1,84 iPTH without affecting serum calcium and phosphate in patients with moderate renal failure (prospective placebo-controlled multicenter trial). *Nephrol Dial Transplant* 1995;10:2228–2234.

Sheikh MS, Maquire JA, Emmett M, et al. Reduction of dietary phosphorus absorption by phosphorus binders. *J Clin Invest* 1989;83:66–73.

Slatopolsky E, Weerts C, Lopez-Hilker S, et al. Calcium carbonate is an effective phosphate binder in dialysis patients. *N Engl J Med* 1986;315:157–161.

Slatopolsky E, Finch J, Denda M, et al. Phosphorus restriction prevents parathyroid gland growth: high phosphorus directly stimulates PTH secretion in vitro. *J Clin Invest* 1996;97:2534–2540.

Suki WN, Rouse D. Renal transport of calcium, magnesium, and phosphate. In: Brenner BM, ed. *The kidney*. 5th ed. Philadelphia: WB Saunders; 1996:472–515.

Sullivan W, Carpenter T, Glorieux F, et al. A prospective trial of phosphate and 1,25-dihydroxyvitamin D_3 therapy in symptomatic adults with X-linked hypophosphatemic rickets. *J Clin Endocrinol Metab* 1992;75:879–885.

Tenenhouse HS. Cellular and molecular mechanisms of renal phosphate transport. *J Bone Miner Res* 1997;12:159–164.

Tsukamoto Y, Moriya R, Nagaba Y, et al. Effect of administering calcium carbonate to treat secondary hyperparathyroidism in nondialyzed patients with chronic renal failure. *Am J Kidney Dis* 1995;25:879–886.

Yi H, Fukagawa M, Yamato H, et al. Prevention of enhanced parathyroid hormone secretion, synthesis and hyperplasia by mild dietary phosphorus restriction in early chronic renal failure in rats: possible direct role of phosphorus. *Nephron* 1995;70:242–248.

Trace Elements and Vitamins in Renal Disease

Elizabeth Reid Gilmour, George H. Hartley, and
Timothy H. J. Goodship

This chapter reviews the metabolism, concentrations, requirements, and toxicities of trace elements and vitamins in patients
with chronic renal failure before the onset of dialysis (CRF) and
during treatment with either hemodialysis or continuous ambulatory peritoneal dialysis (CAPD).

TRACE ELEMENTS

Trace elements are those elements that are present in the
body at concentrations <50 mg/kg. Nine trace elements have
been reported to be either essential or beneficial to humans, but
the biochemistry underlying the essential nature of some of
these elements has not been established.

Alteration of trace element metabolism in renal failure has
been frequently reported, but the mechanisms responsible for
these changes are poorly understood and the contribution of trace
element toxicity or deficiency to the symptoms of renal disease is
uncertain. Lack of sensitive and specific analytic techniques to
measure elements in very low concentrations contributes to our
limited knowledge of the importance of trace metals in many diseases, including renal disease. Consequently, much of the quantitative data available are inaccurate, and the absolute requirements
for trace elements in renal disease have yet to be established.
Table 5-1 gives details of the calculated daily intake of trace elements in CRF, hemodialysis, and CAPD patients compared with
the recommended dietary allowance (RDA). Table 5-2 summarizes the available data about commonly recognized alterations of
trace element metabolism in renal failure. We review some of the
toxic and nutritional aspects of trace elements in patients with
renal failure, as well as the potential clinical complications that
may arise as a result of these abnormalities. Recommendations
regarding the use of trace element supplements are suggested.

Pathophysiology

All essential elements have a regulatory pathway that maintains an optimal tissue concentration in spite of variations in
dietary supply. The amount of each element absorbed from the
diet varies because the excretion rate in urine and feces depends
on available supply in foodstuffs. Moreover, specific mechanisms
for transport of elements bound to plasma proteins are known
for some elements, and the pattern of organ or tissue uptake is
characteristic for the organ. Many enzymes in pathways of intermediary metabolism require metalloenzymes, whereas the activity of other enzymatic reactions is regulated by metal ions.
Cumulative tissue loss of specific trace elements in renal failure
has been well documented, and there are many reasons why
patients with renal failure are at increased risk for development
of trace element toxicity or deficiency. These include:

Table 5-1. Calculated daily intakes of trace elements by patients with renal failure, compared with the RDA*

	CRF	HD	CAPD	RDA
Protein (g)	40	70	100	
Potassium	Normal	Low	Normal	
Phosphorus (mg)	533	856	1163	m, 800 f, 800
Iron (mg)	5.7	9.6	13.8	m, 15 f, 15
Copper (mg)	0.7	0.9	1.3	1.5–3.0
Zinc (mg)	6.2	10.7	16.3	m, 15 f, 12

RDA, recommended dietary allowances; CRF, predialysis chronic renal failure; HD, hemodialysis; CAPD, continuous ambulatory peritoneal dialysis; m, male; f, female.
*RDAs for healthy subjects are from Subcommitee on the Tenth Edition of the RDAs. *Recommended dietary allowances*. 10th ed. Washington, DC: National Academy Press; 1989.

1. *Failure of excretion to regulate the body context*—reduced or excessive excretion leads to accumulation or depletion of trace elements.
2. *Contamination of dialysate*—toxicity may occur if the water supply or dialysis equipment is contaminated by trace elements.
3. *Loss of trace elements across the dialysis membrane.*
4. *Dietary restrictions*—Renal patients following special diets, including diets restricted in protein, are at additional risk for development of deficiency of trace elements such as zinc and selenium because foods rich in these trace elements, including meat and sea fish, are restricted. Inadequate protein and energy intake due to anorexia may also contribute to the development of a deficiency.

Iron

Anemia is an almost invariable feature of progressive renal disease. Probably the most important single cause is decreased

Table 5-2. Commonly recognized trace element abnormalities in renal failure

	CRF	HD	CAPD
Zinc	↓	↓	↓
Selenium	↓	↓	↓
Iron	↓	↓	↓
Aluminum	N–↑	N–↑	N–↑
Copper	↑	↑	↑

CRF, predialysis chronic renal failure; HD, hemodialysis; CAPD, continuous ambulatory peritoneal dialysis; N, normal.

production of erythropoietin (EPO), but uremic toxins are thought to inhibit erythropoiesis and reduce the red cell's life span. Furthermore, anemia can be aggravated by the bleeding tendency of uremia, by dialysis blood losses, and by gastrointestinal blood losses. Infection or inflammatory conditions and malignancy can inhibit a response to EPO, and aluminum accumulation or folate deficiency may lead to further worsening in the anemia of chronic dialysis patients. Additional factors that contribute to anemia include osteitis fibrosa from severe secondary hyperparathyroidism and, rarely, acute or chronic hemolysis.

Erythropoietin Therapy

Before 1985, when recombinant human EPO therapy became available, there was no satisfactory treatment for the anemia of chronic renal failure. EPO administration confers a number of advantages to the patient, such as a reduced need for blood transfusions and an increased sense of well-being.

Assessment of Iron Stores. The use of EPO requires a regular assessment of iron stores because iron depletion impairs the response to EPO, and EPO itself can cause iron deficiency.

Correction of Iron Deficiency. Because of a high incidence of iron deficiency in patients with renal failure, many clinicians routinely prescribe iron supplements to hemodialysis or CAPD patients, but controversy exists over the best method to supplement iron. Three routes of administration are available: oral, intravenous, and intramuscular. The intramuscular route is not recommended because of patient discomfort and the risk of causing a muscle hematoma. Table 5-3 lists the possible routes of iron supplementation and the preparations available.

Oral Iron Supplementation

Oral iron is the cheapest, safest, and easiest means of iron supplementation and is often the preferred route of supplementation. Ferrous sulfate, fumarate, or gluconate are the most commonly used oral iron preparations. However, the effectiveness of these preparations is reduced by poor absorption of iron from the gut, limited bioavailabilty of oral iron preparations, poor patient compliance because of the gastrointestinal side effects of the supplement, and interaction with phosphate binders. It is increasingly recognized that oral iron may not be sufficient to guarantee an adequate iron supply to the bone marrow of ure-

**Table 5-3. Routes and preparations
of available iron supplements**

Oral	Ferrous sulfate (20% elemental iron)
	Ferrous fumarate (33% elemental iron)
	Ferrous gluconate (12% elemental iron)
Intravenous	Iron dextran
	Iron sorbitol citrate
	Iron hydroxysaccharate
	Iron sodium gluconate
Intramuscular	Not commonly used

mic patients treated with EPO. A number of patients require an alternative means of supplementation.

Parenteral Iron Supplementation

The intravenous route of administration overcomes many of the problems associated with oral iron supplements. Iron dextran, iron saccharate, and iron gluconate are the most commonly used preparations, and intravenous iron can result in restoration of iron stores or even overload when intestinal barrier mechanisms are bypassed. Iron overload (as defined by a serum of ferritin > 300 ng/ml) can also occur from multiple blood transfusions. Rarely, anaphylactic reactions may occur in patients treated with iron dextran, and because iron dextran is the only intravenous formulation available in the United States, many clinicians prefer to use oral iron over intravenous iron.

Zinc

Role

Zinc is a trace element that is essential for human nutrition and is one of the most important trace elements, being an essential component of more than 200 metalloenzymes. Zinc deficiency is associated with impaired growth, delayed wound healing, impaired sexual function, neurosensory disorders, and disorders of cell-mediated immunity.

Alterations in Renal Failure

There is biochemical and clinical evidence for altered zinc metabolism in patients with renal failure. Low plasma zinc concentrations are reported in predialysis, hemodialysis, CAPD, and renal transplant patients, and in those with the nephrotic syndrome. There also have been reports of normal or elevated plasma zinc concentrations in patients with kidney failure. Uptake of zinc from the dialysate is thought to be responsible for an increased plasma zinc concentration.

Uremia. Low circulating zinc levels have been reported in patients with uremia, but it is unclear whether this results from the underlying uremia per se or from other factors such as the low zinc content of low-protein diets. It has been reported that the normalization of plasma zinc levels in dialyzed but not in undialyzed patients occurs because of a higher dietary intake by the dialysis patient; patients not receiving dialysis in this report had protein intakes of only 20 to 30 g/day.

Hemodialysis. Dialysis appears to have minimal effects on the serum zinc concentration.

CAPD. Red blood cell levels of zinc in CAPD patients are lower than in patients receiving hemodialysis or in control subjects, and it has been suggested that CAPD patients would benefit from oral zinc supplements.

Transplantation. A transient drop in zinc levels can occur in the first 2 to 4 weeks after transplantation. However, other workers have found a prolonged depression of serum zinc levels, and it has been suggested that patients with a well functioning transplanted kidney should be prescribed a zinc supplement of 15 mg/day.

Nephrotic Syndrome. Low plasma and serum zinc levels also occur in patients with nephrotic syndrome, and decreased levels of zinc in erythrocytes and hair have been found. It has been suggested that this is due to increased urinary excretion of zinc bound to proteins lost in urea. Other possible reasons include disturbed tubular transport of zinc or a decrease in intestinal absorption of zinc. It is also possible that the low plasma and serum levels reflect the loss of zinc-binding proteins such as albumin.

Symptoms in Renal Failure

Zinc deficiency has been linked to many of the symptoms of renal failure, including loss of appetite, an altered sense of taste and smell, and impaired sexual function. Several reports suggest these symptoms improve with zinc supplementation. Still, the efficacy of zinc supplementation remains controversial, because some reports do not confirm that there is improved sexual function after administration of a zinc supplement. On the other hand, there are reports of improved nerve conduction and cell-mediated immunity after zinc supplementation.

Interpretation of Zinc Levels

The measurement of either the plasma or serum zinc concentration is the most frequently used method of assessing zinc status. Although stable in normal, healthy subjects, the zinc concentration does vary in situations of stress, including renal failure. Because most plasma zinc circulates bound to albumin, a fall in the plasma zinc concentration should always be interpreted in relation to any change in the plasma albumin. Because plasma zinc is usually in the normal range unless deficiency is severe, the reliability of the measurement as an index of zinc deficiency is questionable.

Supplementation

Given the difficulties with the diagnosis of zinc deficiency and the contradictory reports of its effectiveness, routine zinc supplementation cannot be recommended.

Selenium

Role

The essentiality of selenium has been recognized only recently, but toxic effects have been known for some time. Selenium is necessary for the activity of the enzyme glutathione peroxidase. This enzyme, along with catalase, superoxidase dismutases, vitamin E, and the nonselenium-dependent glutathione transferases, acts to protect the cell against oxidative damage. Little is known about selenium homeostasis, but the kidney is thought to play an important role.

Alterations in Renal Failure

Serum selenium concentrations in patients with renal failure are low regardless of the mode of dialysis. Poor dietary protein intake or decreased gastrointestinal absorption may contribute to low levels because protein-rich foods (e.g., meat, fish) are rich in selenium. In hemodialysis patients, low blood selenium concentrations are due to losses of selenium through the dialysis membrane.

Selenium deficiency exerts diverse effects, including cardiomyopathy, ischemic heart disease, and impaired immune function. In hemodialysis patients, an association between a low plasma selenium concentration and lipid peroxidation abnormalities has been reported.

Supplementation

The usefulness of selenium supplementation in patients with renal failure remains controversial. First, selenium supplementation requires particular caution because of its potential toxicity. Second, no specific clinical abnormality present in patients with renal disease has been associated with selenium deficiency. It has been suggested that the potential association between low blood selenium concentrations and malignancy and ischemic heart disease could be important, and a few centers have recommended routine supplementation, but this is controversial.

Aluminum

Although aluminum has no known natural biologic function, it is toxic in patients with renal failure and potentially toxic in patients with normal renal function. Clinical consequences of aluminum toxicity in dialysis patients include neurologic symptoms, bone disease, myopathy, and anemia.

Common sources of aluminum in the past included dialysate fluid containing high concentrations of aluminum, which was first identified as a source of aluminum toxicity in patients with renal failure. In addition, oral aluminum hydroxide was used as a phosphate binder to control parathyroid gland function.

Mechanisms of Aluminum Intoxication

Increased bone and liver aluminum were reported in 85% of patients dying of uremia. It was suggested that accumulation of aluminum in chronic renal failure occurred because of *decreased urinary excretion* and *increased gastrointestinal absorption* of aluminum, and this was subsequently confirmed.

Studies in Europe confirmed that dialysis encephalopathy had a geographic association: centers where aluminum was present in high concentrations in the water used to prepare the dialysate had a high incidence, whereas in areas where dialysis encephalopathy was rare, the aluminum content of water was low. With the introduction of reverse osmosis treatment of dialysis water, aluminum concentrations were reduced and the incidence of encephalopathy fell.

Osteomalacia

Osteomalacia was the first bone lesion to be recognized as a component of the clinical syndrome of aluminum intoxication. Aluminum is now recognized to be important in other histologic subtypes of renal osteodystrophy; it has two predominant effects on bone—it impairs skeletal mineralization and diminishes bone cell activity. Most evidence suggests that bone aluminum concentrations <30 to 40 mg/kg have little, if any, adverse physiologic effects on bone. In patients with aluminum-related osteomalacia, concentrations usually exceed 80 mg/kg, and the histologic severity of the disease in patients with aluminum-related osteomalacia correlates with the degree of aluminum accumulation.

Current Risks

Today, aluminum toxicity most commonly results from its intestinal absorption in patients given aluminum-containing phosphate binders for prolonged periods.

Copper

Copper is essential for the activity of many enzymes, including cytochrome oxidase and zinc/copper superoxide dismutase.

Alterations in Renal Failure

Alterations in copper metabolism in patients with renal failure have been frequently reported. Hypercupremia can occur in predialysis or hemodialysis patients. Signs and symptoms of copper intoxication include hemolysis, leukocytosis, metabolic acidosis, and gastrointestinal symptoms.

Hemodialysis. In hemodialysis patients, high serum copper levels have been attributed to small amounts of copper present in cellulosic dialysis membranes because they are manufactured by the cuprammonia method; it has been shown that plasma copper is elevated despite the type of dialysis. Plasma ceruloplasmin in kidney patients does not differ from that in normal subjects, suggesting that the free copper level is high in renal failure. It is possible that renal failure impairs the hepatic metabolism of copper, but it has also been suggested that zinc deficiency results in increased copper absorption by the gut. The clinical significance of a high free copper concentration in the blood of renal failure patients is uncertain.

CAPD. In CAPD patients, plasma concentrations of copper are lower than in hemodialysis patients.

Nephrotic Syndrome. Increased urinary losses of copper and hypocupremia have been associated with the nephrotic syndrome. A close correlation exists between urinary copper excretion and urinary protein losses, indicating that copper losses are limited to loss of copper-binding proteins.

Toxicity. Acute copper poisoning has been reported in hemodialysis patients due to copper tubing used in the heating coil in contact with the dialysate. *Acute renal failure* has been reported after copper sulfate poisoning.

Ultratrace Elements

Table 5-4 summarizes the alterations of ultratrace elements and the potential clinical effects of these derangements in renal patients. The clinical significance of these changes is uncertain, but some of these elements, including strontium, tin, cadmium, and molybdenum, are potentially toxic, and their retention in patients with chronic renal failure could be clinically important.

Recommendations for Trace Element Supplementation in Renal Disease

There are no data to support a recommendation that trace elements be given routinely to patients with renal failure. There is some evidence to support the usefulness of supplementation of

Table 5-4. Summary of ultratrace element abnormalities in renal failure and their potential clinical effects

	CRF	HD	CAPD	Dialysis Induced	Clinical Features
Bromide	N	↓	↓	Yes	Disturbed sleep
Cadmium	Kidney↓ Liver↑	Kidney↓ Liver↑	N	?	
Cesium	N	N	?	?	
Chromium	N–↑	←	←	Yes	?Carcinogenic
Cobalt	N	←	←	?	?Cardiac failure, pericarditis
Lead	N–↑	N–↑	N	No	Hypertension, gastrointestinal and neurological disease
Manganese	Kidney↓ Liver↑	N	N	No	Anemia, impaired glucose tolerance
Molybdenum	Kidney↓ Liver↑	Kidney↓ Liver↑	?	?	
Nickel	→	→	?	No	Myocardial ischemia, anemia
Rubidium	→	→	→	Yes	Depression, central nervous system disturbance
Silicon	←	←	←	Yes	Respiratory and bone disease, neuropathy
Strontium	←	←	?	?	Bone disease
Tin	←	←	?	?	
Vanadium	←	←	?	No	Bone disease

CRF = predialysis chronic renal failure; HD, hemodialysis; CAPD, continuous ambulatory peritoneal dialysis; N, normal.

selenium, zinc, and *iron*, but only after the adequacy of the energy and protein content of the diet is ensured. The effects of any trace element supplements should be carefully monitored to avoid toxicity, especially with selenium, because there is a small therapeutic window (the difference between toxic and nontoxic blood levels). With respect to zinc, the presence of an infection or glucocorticoid therapy lowers the plasma zinc concentration; these problems should be excluded before prescribing a supplement. Supplementation of iron should be based on the serum ferritin concentration rather than on the levels of serum iron and transferrin, and falsely low levels occur with acute infection or chronic diseases. The administration of oral iron supplements is successful in most patients, and is preferred over parenteral iron because the intestinal mucosa regulates absorption according to the body's iron store. Iron absorption is optimized if ferrous sulfate or ferrous gluconate is taken three times a day between meals and separate from any phosphate binders, which reduce iron absorption.

VITAMINS

Vitamins are *organic compounds required in small amounts to catalyze metabolic reactions*. Because they are not adequately synthesized in the body, sufficient amounts must be provided in the diet. Vitamins are divided into fat- and water-soluble groups because of different patterns of absorption, transport, and storage. Table 5-5 gives details of the calculated daily vitamin intakes of predialysis, hemodialysis, and CAPD patients compared with the RDAs. Table 5-6 summarizes the available data on the vitamin status of these groups of patients.

Water-Soluble Vitamins

Vitamin B_1 (Thiamine)

Thiamine is activated by phosphorylation to form thiamine pyrophosphate, which is a *cofactor in oxidative decarboxylation*. Thiamine deficiency in humans causes beriberi. Dietary sources of thiamine include fresh vegetables, whole-meal cereals, fortified foods, and various meats. A diet restricted in protein or potassium also limits thiamine intake (see Table 5-3). About 10% of CRF patients prescribed a dietary protein regimen of 0.6 $g\cdot kg^{-1}\cdot day^{-1}$ will become thiamine deficient. Although it has been recommended that hemodialysis patients be routinely given supplements of thiamine, serum thiamine concentrations remain within normal limits after stopping the vitamin supplement for 1 year, and the serum thiamine concentration is normal in hemodialysis patients not receiving thiamine. On the other hand, the activity of the thiamine-dependent enzyme, transketolase, in erythrocytes is impaired in over 50% of hemodialysis patients, but this problem may be related to inhibition of the enzyme rather than a true vitamin deficiency. Daily supplementation with 30 to 45 mg of thiamine restores erythrocyte transketolase activity to normal in most patients. CAPD patients have low serum and erythrocyte thiamine concentrations and decreased erythrocyte transketolase activity. For these reasons, a routine thiamine supplement is recommended for CAPD

Table 5-5. Calculated daily intakes of vitamins by predialysis, hemodialysis, and continuous ambulatory peritoneal dialysis patients compared with recommended dietary allowances

	CRF	HD	CAPD	RDA
Protein (g)	40	70	100	
Potassium	Normal	Low	Normal	
Thiamine (mg)	1.0	1.3	1.7	m, 1.5 f, 1.1
Riboflavin (mg)	1.3	1.7	2.2	m, 1.7 f, 1.3
Pyridoxine (mg)	0.8	1.1	2.1	m, 2.0 f, 1.6
Cobalamin (μg)	2.2	3.8	5.6	m, 2.0 f, 2.0
Folic acid (μg)	79	111	279	m, 200 f, 180
Biotin (μg)	5.1	7.0	8.7	NA
Niacin (mg)	14.6	20.0	27.5	m, 19 f, 15
Pantothenic acid (mg)	2.2	3.3	4.9	NA
Ascorbic acid (mg)	36	36	157	m, 60 f, 60
Vitamin A (μg retinol equivalents)	555	965	245	m, 1000 f, 800
Vitamin E (mg α-tocopherol equivalents)	4.6	9.5	3.4	m, 10 f, 8

CRF, predialysis chronic renal failure; HD, hemodialysis; CAPD, continuous ambulatory peritoneal dialysis; RDA, recommended dietary allowance; m, male; f, female; NA, not applicable.

patients. Erythrocyte levels of thiamine in patients with the nephrotic syndrome, but without renal impairment, are normal.

Vitamin B$_2$ (Riboflavin)

Riboflavin forms flavin mononucleotide and flavin adenine dinucleotide, the cofactors necessary for oxidation–reduction reactions. Like thiamine, riboflavin is found in meat, and its intake is lowered when dietary protein is restricted (see Table 5-3). Riboflavin deficiency in humans causes corneal vascularization and dermatitis. In CRF, between 15% and 40% of patients prescribed a dietary protein intake of 0.6 g·kg^{-1}·day^{-1} become riboflavin deficient, and supplements are recommended. *There is no evidence of riboflavin deficiency in either hemodialysis or CAPD patients.* In patients with nephrotic syndrome, erythrocyte riboflavin levels are reported to be reduced or normal.

Vitamin B$_6$ (Pyridoxine)

Pyridoxine is found in meat and, again, a low-protein diet decreases pyridoxine intake. The active form of pyridoxine is

Table 5-6. Summary of vitamin status in patients with renal failure

	CRF	HD	CAPD
Thiamine	LPD↓ NPD?	N	N–↓
Riboflavin	LPD↓ NPD N–↓	↑	N
Pyridoxine	LPD↓ NPD↓	N–↓	N–↓
Cobalamin	N	N	N
Folic acid	N–↓	N–↑	N–↑
Biotin	?	↑	?
Niacin	?	N	?
Pantothenic acid	?	N	?
Ascorbic acid	↓	↑	N–↓
Vitamin A	LPD↑ NPD↑	↑	↑
Vitamin E	LPD↑ NPD N	↓	?

CRF, chronic renal failure; HD, hemodialysis; CAPD, continuous ambulatory peritoneal dialysis; LPD, low-protein diet (0.6 $g \cdot kg^{-1} \cdot d^{-1}$); NPD, normal-protein diet (1.0 $g \cdot kg^{-1} \cdot d^{-1}$); N, normal.

pyridoxal 5-phosphate, a coenzyme involved in amino acid metabolism. Pyridoxine deficiency causes symptoms similar to those of uremia. Based on measurements of either the catalytic activity of the erythrocyte enzyme, aspartate aminotransketolase, or the erythrocyte glutamic pyruvic transaminase index, as much as 50% of CRF patients are deficient. The prevalence of pyridoxine deficiency increases with time during treatment with a protein-restricted diet. Pyridoxine deficiency is also common in hemodialysis patients, and the type of hemodialysis may influence vitamin levels: compared with dialysis with cuprophane membranes, the high-flux/high-efficiency dialysis membranes increase the clearance of pyridoxal-5'-phosphate by more than 50%. This difference is associated with a significant decline in serum levels. In addition, EPO therapy can affect the levels of the vitamin by causing a fall in pyridoxine. It is recommended that pyridoxine supplementation be carefully monitored because measurement of the blood level by high-performance liquid chromatography rather than a biologic assay reveals that pyridoxal-5'-phosphate, pyridoxal, pyridoxine, and 4-pyridoxic acid have significantly elevated levels in some patients receiving supplements. Pyridoxine deficiency also occurs in CAPD patients and is corrected by supplements. In some dialysis patients, high doses (300 mg/day) have been associated with an improvement in serum cholesterol, but the clinical importance of this finding is unclear. Erythrocyte pyridoxine levels are reduced in the nephrotic syndrome and can be significantly improved by daily supplementation with 50 mg pyridoxine hydrochloride.

Vitamin B₁₂ (Cobalamin)

Meat and meat products are the major dietary sources of vitamin B_{12}, which is a necessary cofactor for many enzymes involved in isomerase and methyltransferase reactions. A deficiency state in humans is rare because of the small amounts needed, but when deficiency does occur, it causes megaloblastic anemia and neurologic problems.

There is *no evidence that the vitamin B_{12} status in CRF, hemodialysis, or CAPD is abnormal,* nor does it appear that EPO therapy affects vitamin B_{12} status. Because it is largely protein bound, losses of vitamin B_{12} during dialysis are lower than for the other water-soluble vitamins. Moreover, small amounts of vitamin B_{12} are produced by bacteria of the small bowel to augment intake.

Folic Acid

Folic acid is found in many foods, but it can be destroyed by prolonged cooking. It is needed by many enzymes involved in the transfer of one-carbon units, and folate deficiency in humans causes megaloblastic anemia. The need for a folate supplement in patients with renal disease is controversial; 10% of CRF patients have decreased folate concentrations and, like vitamin B12, folate is mainly protein bound so that dialysis losses should be small. Hemodialysis patients receiving folate supplements of 2.9 mg–7.9 mg daily have plasma and erythrocyte folate concentrations greater than the reference range in 76% and 91% of patients, respectively. Smaller doses of 1 mg twice per week are sufficient to maintain plasma levels within the optimal range for most hemodialysis patients. Folate supplements do not influence EPO requirements except when there is coexisting folate deficiency. There is no evidence to suggest folate deficiency in CAPD.

Although the folate status of dialysis patients may be normal, *supranormal levels can improve the deranged metabolism of the amino acid, homocysteine.* The hyperhomocysteinemia seen in chronic dialysis patients is believed to be an atherogenic risk factor, and may contribute to the high prevalence of cardiovascular disease in this group of patients. By acting as a methyl group donor, folate reduces serum homocysteine levels by promoting its conversion back to methionine. In predialysis, hemodialysis, and CAPD patients, it has been shown that 5 to 10 mg of folic acid daily reduces the homocysteine level by approximately 30%. After withdrawal of the supplement, homocysteine levels increase in conjunction with decreasing plasma folic acid concentrations.

Biotin, Niacin, and Pantothenic Acid

Biotin acts as a coenzyme in many of the reactions involving carboxylation of molecules. Because it is produced by intestinal microorganisms, a biotin deficiency state is rare. Niacin (nicotinic acid) is part of the two coenzymes, nicotinamide adenine dinucleotide (NAD) and NAD hydrogenase (NADH), and niacin deficiency causes pellagra, which is characterized by diarrhea, dermatitis, and dementia. Pantothenic acid is a constituent of coenzyme A and is involved in the metabolism of fatty acids, steroid hormones, cholesterol, and certain amino acids. There is *no evidence for a deficiency of biotin, niacin, or pantothenic acid in CRF, hemodialysis, or CAPD patients.* On the contrary, there is a tendency for leukocyte, erythrocyte, and plasma concentrations of those vitamins to be increased. The clinical significance of this finding is uncertain.

Vitamin C (Ascorbic Acid)

Ascorbic acid is a cosubstrate in many oxidation–reduction reactions, one of the most widely known of which is the hydroxylation of proline during the formation of collagen. Vitamin C deficiency results in scurvy. Although ascorbic acid is exclusively excreted by the kidney, its transport by residual nephrons in the damaged kidney is altered so ascorbic acid excretion is high, resulting in a low serum concentration. Ascorbic acid is easily dialyzed by either hemodialysis or CAPD. Plasma ascorbate concentrations in predialysis patients taking 5 to 1000 mg of ascorbic acid daily are subnormal in 50% of patients; ascorbic acid deficiency may also occur with a low-potassium diet because it has a low ascorbic acid content. The plasma ascorbic acid level in predialysis or hemodialysis patients who are not taking a supplement is low, and scurvy has been reported in a hemodialysis patient. Consequently, supplementation with 150 to 250 mg/day of ascorbic acid is recommended for hemodialysis patients. In CAPD patients, 15% of patients have a low serum ascorbic acid concentration and this is corrected by 100 mg ascorbic acid daily. Note that ascorbic acid supplements can have potentially harmful side effects. In hemodialysis patients, high dosage of ascorbic acid (0.5 to 1.0 g/day) results in a high serum concentration that is closely correlated with the serum oxalate concentration; even a relatively low dosage of 100 mg/day can significantly increase the serum oxalate concentrations in peritoneal dialysis patients. This is important because a high serum oxalate may contribute to the vascular disease that occurs in patients with kidney failure.

Fat-Soluble Vitamins

Vitamin A (Retinol)

Vitamin A is absorbed from the small intestine and transported in chylomicrons to the liver, where it is stored. Vitamin A is required to maintain the integrity of epithelial tissues and to form the visual pigment, rhodopsin. A high serum vitamin A level is a consistent finding in predialysis, hemodialysis, and CAPD patients. In predialysis patients, the plasma vitamin A concentration is raised in 20% of patients; there is no difference in the level between patients prescribed 0.6 and 1.0 g·kg^{-1}·day^{-1} dietary protein. However, there is a correlation between the serum creatinine and serum vitamin A concentration, indicating a causal relationship with renal failure. In fact, elevated serum concentrations of vitamin A have been found both in hemodialysis patients taking supplements and those not taking supplements; the plasma concentration is also raised in CAPD patients. Hypervitaminosis A persists in dialysis patients because neither hemodialysis nor CAPD clear the vitamin. The major factor causing a high vitamin A plasma level in kidney failure is an increase in the retinol-binding protein serum concentration. Although hypervitaminosis A is common in renal failure, toxicity is seldom seen because most of the vitamin is bound to the protein and is therefore inactive. In the nephrotic syndrome, serum vitamin A levels are high because of an increase in the serum retinol-binding protein concentration.

Vitamin E (Tocopherol)

Vitamin E acts as a scavenger for oxygen-free radicals. Because it is the major fat-soluble antioxidant, there is interest in the protective effect of vitamin E against lipid peroxidation. Dietary intake of vitamin E is independent of the quantity of protein taken. Studies of the vitamin E status in renal patients report variable findings: serum vitamin E levels in predialysis patients have been found to be decreased, normal, and elevated with an unrestricted or a low-protein diet (0.6 g·kg^{-1}·day^{-1}). In hemodialysis patients, the findings are equally contradictory; plasma vitamin E levels are reported to be increased, normal, or decreased. On the other hand, the platelet vitamin E is reported to be low and is corrected after supplementation. A significant factor that affects vitamin E status is EPO therapy, which is associated with both an increase in vitamin E levels and a decrease in erythrocyte lipid peroxidation as measured by erythrocyte malonaldehyde concentration. Thus, in addition to stimulating erythropoiesis, EPO appears to improve the antioxidant capacity of erythrocytes by increasing their vitamin E concentration. Finally, serum vitamin E levels are increased in the nephrotic syndrome, presumably because of higher levels of vitamin E binding protein produced in response to protein losses.

Recommendations for Supplementation

Whether vitamin supplements should be prescribed for patients with renal disease depends on the degree of renal insufficiency, the mode of renal replacement therapy, the dietary prescription, concurrent medication, and the patient's nutritional status. There is *no evidence that supplements of cobalamin, folic acid, biotin, niacin, pantothenic acid, vitamin A, or vitamin E are required to correct deficiencies in any group of patients. Pharmacologic doses of folate and vitamin E may, respectively, lower homocysteine levels and protect against lipid peroxidation.* Supplements of thiamine, riboflavin, pyridoxine, and vitamin C need to be prescribed when circumstances described in this chapter are present.

SELECTED READINGS

Trace Elements

Alfrey AC. In: Zurukzoglu W, Papadimitriou M, Pyrpasopoulos M, et al., eds. *Trace element alterations in uremia. Proceedings of the Eighth International Congress of Nephrology.* Basel: Karger; 1981: 1007–1013.

Alfrey AC, Hegg A, Craswell P. Metabolism and toxicity of aluminum in renal failure. *Am J Clin Nutr* 1980;33:1509–1516.

Antoniou LD, Shalhoub RJ. Zinc-induced enhancement of lymphocyte function and viability in chronic uremia. *Nephron* 1985;40:13–21.

Berlyne G, Dudek E, Adler AJ, et al. Silicon metabolism: the basic facts in renal failure. *Kidney Int* 1984;28(Suppl 17):S175–S177.

Bonomini M, Di Paolo B, De Risio F, et al. Effects of zinc supplementation in chronic haemodialysis patients. *Nephrol Dial Transplant* 1993;8:1166–1168.

Bonomini M, Forster S, De Risio F, et al. Effects of selenium supplementation on immune parameters in chronic uraemic patients on haemodialysis. *Nephrol Dial Transplant* 1995;10:1654–1661.

D'Haese PC, De Broe ME. Adequacy of dialysis: trace elements in dialysis fluids. *Nephrol Dial Transplant* 1996;11(Suppl 2):92–97.

Gallieni M, Brancaccio D, Cozzolino M, et al. Trace elements in renal failure: are they clinically important? *Nephrol Dial Transplant* 1996;11:1232–1234.

Girelli D, Olivieri O, Stanzial AM, et al. Low platelet glutathione peroxidase activity and serum selenium concentration in patients with chronic renal failure: relations to dialysis treatments, diet and cardiovascular complications. *Clin Sci* 1993;84:611–617.

Horl WH, Cavill I, Macdougall IC, et al. How to diagnose and correct iron deficiency during r-huEPO therapy: a consensus report. *Nephrol Dial Transplant* 1996;11:246–250.

Hosokawa S, Yoshida O. Role of trace elements on complications in patients undergoing chronic hemodialysis. *Int J Artif Organs* 1992; 15:5–9.

Saint-Georges MD, Bonnefont DJ, Bourely BA, et al. Correction of selenium deficiency in hemodialyzed patients. *Kidney Int* 1989;36 (Suppl 27):S274–S277.

Sondheimer JH, Mahajan SK, Rye DL, et al. Elevated plasma copper in chronic renal failure. *Am J Clin Nutr* 1988;47:896–899.

Sprenger KBG, Budnschu D, Lewis K, et al. Improvement of uremic neuropathy and hypogeusia by dialysate zinc supplementation: a double blind study. *Kidney Int* 1983;24(Suppl 16):S315–S318.

Thomson NM, Stevens BJ, Humphrey TJ, et al. Comparison of trace elements in peritoneal dialysis, hemodialysis, and uremia. *Kidney Int* 1983;23:9–14.

Vitamins

Allman MA, Pang E, Yau DF, et al. Elevated plasma vitamers of vitamin B_6 in patients with chronic renal failure on regular haemodialysis. *J Clin Nutr* 1992;46:679–683.

Arnadottir M, Brattstrom L, Simonsen O, et al. The effect of high-dose pyridoxine and folic acid supplementation on serum lipids and plasma homocysteine concentrations in dialysis patients. *Clin Nephrol* 1993;40:236–240.

Blumberg A, Hanck A, Sander G. Vitamin nutrition in patients on continuous ambulatory peritoneal dialysis (CAPD). *Clin Nephrol* 1983; 20:244–250.

Chauveau P, Chadefaux B, Coude M, et al. Long-term folic acid (but not pyridoxine) supplementation lowers elevated plasma homocysteine level in chronic renal failure. *Miner Electrolyte Metab* 1996;22:106–109.

Descombes E, Hanck AB, Fellay G. Water soluble vitamins in chronic hemodialysis patients and need for supplementation. *Kidney Int* 1993;43:1319–1328.

Janssen MJFM, van Guldener C, de Jong GMT, et al. Folic acid treatment of hyperhomocysteinemia in dialysis patients. *Miner Electrolyte Metab* 1996;22:110–114.

Kasama R, Koch T, Canals-Navas C, et al. Vitamin B6 and hemodialysis: the impact of high-flux/high-efficiency dialysis and review of the literature. *Am J Kidney Dis* 1996;27:680–686.

Kopple JD, Mercurio K, Blumenkrantz MJ, et al. Daily requirements for pyridoxine supplements in chronic renal failure. *Kidney Int* 1988;19:694–704.

Loughrey CM, Young IS, Lightbody JH, et al. Oxidative stress in haemodialysis. *Q J Med* 1994;87:679–683.

Lubrano R, Taccone-Galluci M, Piazza A, et al. Vitamin E supplementation and oxidative status of peripheral blood mononuclear cells and lymphocyte subsets in hemodialysis patients. *Nutrition* 1992;8:94–97.

Maggi E, Bellazzi R, Falaschi F, et al. Enhanced LDL oxidation in uremic patients: an additional mechanism for accelerated atherosclerosis. *Kidney Int* 1994;45:876–883.

Mydlik M, Derziova K, Guman M, et al. Vitamin B_6 requirements in chronic renal failure. *Int Urol Nephrol* 1992;24:453–457.

Nenov D, Paskalev D, Yankova T. Lipid peroxidation and vitamin E in red blood cells and plasma in hemodialysis patients under rhEPO treatment. *Artif Organs* 1995;19:436–439.

Panzetta O, Cominacini L, Garbin U, et al. Increased susceptibility of LDL to in vitro oxidation in patients on maintenance hemodialysis: effects of fish oil and vitamin E administration. *Clin Nephrol* 1995;44:303–309.

Shah GM, Ross EA, Sabo A, et al. Effects of ascorbic acid and pyridoxine supplementation on oxalate metabolism in peritoneal dialysis patients. *Am J Kidney Dis* 1992;20:42–49.

Westhuyzen J, Adams CE, Fleming SJ. Evidence for oxidative stress during in vitro dialysis. *Nephron* 1995;70:49–54.

Management of Lipid Abnormalities in the Patient with Renal Disease

Bertram L. Kasiske

Abnormalities in circulating lipoproteins are common in patients with renal disease. The pathogenesis and specific type of lipid abnormality vary according to the type of renal disease and the modality of treatment. The pattern of lipid abnormalities can be quite different in nephrotic syndrome, in renal insufficiency without nephrotic syndrome, with hemodialysis or peritoneal dialysis, and after transplantation. Consequently, the management of lipid abnormalities in each of these clinical settings is often different.

To date, there have been no studies carried out in patients with renal disease to determine whether treating hyperlipidemia reduces morbidity or mortality. However, there is little reason to believe that the risk of hyperlipidemia is any less in patients with renal disease than in the general population. In the general population, primary and secondary intervention trials have shown that treating abnormal levels of total cholesterol, low-density lipoprotein (LDL), triglycerides, and high-density lipoprotein (HDL) reduces the risk of cardiovascular disease events. In the absence of more specific data, it is reasonable to base the management of specific lipoprotein abnormalities in patients with renal disease on guidelines established for the general population.

The National Cholesterol Education Program (NCEP) guidelines recommend an individualized treatment strategy based on both the specific lipoprotein abnormalities and the overall cardiovascular disease risk profile. In general, these (or similar guidelines) can be used for patients with renal disease. No matter which guidelines are used, the threshold for beginning treatment should be reduced for patients who have established coronary heart disease (CHD). It should also be reduced for patients with risk factors, such as age ($\geq$ 45 years for men and $\geq$ 55 years for women), hypertension, diabetes, cigarette smoking, or a positive family history for premature CHD. The NCEP guidelines suggest that diet modification should be started if LDL cholesterol is $\geq$ 160 mg/dl (4.1 mmol/l) in people without CHD and less than two risk factors; $\geq$ 130 mg/dl (3.4 mmol/l) in patients without CHD but two or more risk factors; and > 100 mg/dl (2.6 mmol/l) in patients with CHD. Pharmacologic treatment should be considered if LDL cholesterol is $\geq$ 190 mg/dl (4.1 mmol/l) in people without CHD and less than two risk factors; $\geq$ 160 mg/dl (3.4 mmol/l) in patients without CHD but two or more risk factors; and > 130 mg/dl (2.6 mmol/l) in patients with CHD.

For most patients, a lipid-lowering diet, such as the American Heart Association's Step I diet, should be an integral part of therapy. The key elements of such a diet include low total fat (< 30% of total calories), low saturated fat (< 10% of total calories), and low cholesterol (< 300 mg/day) content. Even when extensive

123

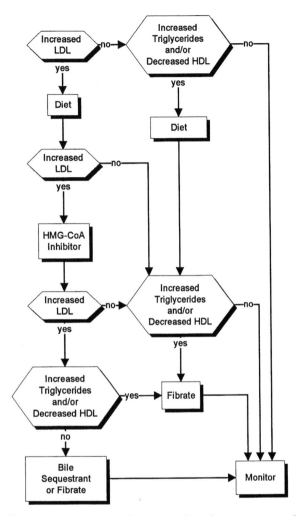

Fig. 6-1. An easy-to-remember approach to the management of hyperlipidemia in patients with renal disease. This approach gives primary consideration to increases in low-density lipoprotein (LDL) cholesterol because the evidence that reducing lipoproteins prevents coronary heart disease events is strongest for LDL cholesterol. It also emphasizes pharmacologic agents that have the greatest potential for lowering lipoproteins with the fewest adverse effects. See Table 6-1 for further details on drug dosing. Exercise and other drugs are appropriate for some patients.

dietary education cannot be provided, a patient can be instructed that the most effective part of a lipid-lowering diet is avoiding animal fat. Substituting vegetable for animal protein is also helpful and easy for patients to remember. Weight reduction in overweight people and increased physical activity should be used to reduce lipoprotein levels when appropriate. Diet and exercise are important, and they can often be used in conjunction with pharmacologic treatment when lipoprotein levels are very high and the risk of CHD is great.

Drug treatment should be targeted at specific lipoprotein abnormalities (Fig. 6-1). Because the preponderance of data from studies in the general population have established that reducing

Table 6-1. Pharmacologic therapy for hyperlipidemia

Agent	Daily dose	Dosing interval	Precautions
HMG-CoA reductase inhibitors			
Fluvastatin (Lescol)	20–40 mg	24 h	↓ Dose if taking CsA
Pravastatin (Pravacol)	10–40 mg	24 h	↓ Dose if taking CsA
Lovastatin (Mevacor)	20–80 mg	24 h	↓ Dose if taking CsA
Simvastatin (Zocor)	5–40 mg	24 h	↓ Dose if taking CsA
Atorvastatin (Lipitor)	10–80 mg	24 h	↓ Dose if taking CsA
Cerivastatin (Baycol)	0.2–3.4 mg	24 h	↓ Dose if taking CsA or if ↓ Ccr
Fibric acid derivatives			
Gemfibrozil	1200 mg	12 h	↓ Dose if ↓ Ccr
Bile acid sequestrants			
Cholestyramine powder (Questran)	4–24 g	8–24 h	Avoid if ↑ triglycerides Administer apart from CsA
Colestipol granules (Colestid)	5–30 g	8–12 h	Avoid if ↑ triglycerides Administer apart from CsA
Other agents			
Probucol* (Lorelco)	500–1000 mg	12 h	May reduce HDL
Nicotinic acid	1.5–3 g	4–6 h	Frequent adverse effects

HMG-CoA, 3-hydroxy-3-methylglutaryl coenzyme A; CsA, cyclosporine A; Ccr, creatinine clearance.
*No longer available in the United States.

LDL cholesterol reduces the risk of cardiovascular disease, it is reasonable to give priority to a strategy that reduces LDL in patients with renal disease (see Fig. 6-1). The most effective agents for reducing LDL cholesterol are the 3-hydroxy-3-methylglutaryl coenzyme A (HMG-CoA) reductase inhibitors, bile acid sequestrants, and nicotinic acid (Table 6-1). The HMG-CoA reductase inhibitors are the most effective and are associated with the fewest adverse effects. Bile acid sequestrants frequently cause adverse gastrointestinal symptoms and should not be used in patients with elevated triglycerides because they may increase triglyceride levels. Nicotinic acid is inexpensive, but is associated with a high incidence of flushing or other adverse effects that limit its usefulness. Fibric acid analogs are generally most effective agents for reducing triglycerides and increasing HDL. The rationale for using fibric acid analogs was strengthened by the results of the Helsinki Heart Study, which demonstrated that reducing triglycerides and increasing HDL by using a fibric acid analog is effective in reducing cardiovascular risk. Experimental data suggest that oxidized LDL may be important in the pathogenesis of atherosclerosis. Although probucol is an antioxidant that reduces LDL, there are no clinical trials showing that probucol reduces cardiovascular disease events. In addition, the decrease in HDL caused by probucol makes its use as first-line therapy less attractive.

NEPHROTIC SYNDROME

Abnormalities and Pathogenesis

Total Cholesterol and Low-Density Lipoprotein

Increased total cholesterol is invariably found in patients with nephrotic-range proteinuria (>3 g/24 hours). The degree of increase is in rough proportion to the degree of proteinuria and the lowering of serum albumin. Much of the increase in total cholesterol is due to increased LDL. Although the pathogenesis of hyperlipidemia in nephrotic syndrome is still not completely understood, it appears that both overproduction and decreased catabolism of lipoproteins play a role. In addition, the corticosteroids and cyclosporine A often used to treat patients with nephrotic syndrome may also contribute to elevations of total and LDL cholesterol.

Triglycerides and High-Density Lipoprotein

Although not all patients with nephrotic-range proteinuria have increased triglycerides, this abnormality is very common. Hypertriglyceridemia is most common in patients with severe proteinuria. Hypertriglyceridemia probably results from increased hepatic secretion of very–low-density lipoprotein (the predominant triglyceride-bearing lipoprotein) and from a decrease in triglyceride catabolism. Although HDL levels are often normal in patients with nephrotic syndrome, the pattern of HDL particles is usually perturbed. Specifically, the immature, proatherogenic HDL$_3$ is often increased, whereas the level of more mature HDL$_2$ is reduced. These abnormalities in HDL are not surprising because the catabolism of triglyceride-bearing lipoproteins is directly linked to the formation and maturation of HDL.

Other Lipoprotein Abnormalities

As expected, levels of apolipoprotein (apo) B, the major protein in LDL, are particularly high in nephrotic patients. However, apo C and E are also frequently increased. Interestingly, the ratio of apo C-II to apo C-III is reduced. Because apo C-II activates and C-III inhibits lipoprotein lipase, the reduced ratio of C-II to C-III could help explain the reduced catabolism of triglycerides. Several studies in patients without renal disease have shown that the level of lipoprotein(a) [Lp(a)] is an independent risk factor for myocardial infarction. In vitro data suggest that Lp(a) may be prothrombogenic. Although the mechanisms are unclear, the blood level of Lp(a) appears to be increased in patients with nephrotic syndrome.

Possible Consequences

Cardiovascular Disease

There have been no controlled intervention trials to prove or disprove the hypothesis that abnormalities of lipoproteins in nephrotic syndrome contribute to cardiovascular disease. Indeed, there have been few studies examining the true incidence of cardiovascular disease in patients with nephrotic syndrome. However, there are anecdotal reports of coronary artery disease occurring in very young children (Kallen et al., 1977). An autopsy study found a very high prevalence of coronary lesions in patients with nephrotic syndrome compared with age- and sex-matched control subjects (Curry and Roberts, 1977). However, this study included patients with diabetes and systemic lupus erythematosus, and it is unclear whether factors other than hyperlipidemia played a role in the pathogenesis of the coronary artery disease.

A retrospective study of 142 patients with nephrotic syndrome excluded diabetics, but nevertheless reported that there is a 5.5-fold increase in the risk of cardiovascular disease, and a 2.8-fold increase in the risk of cardiovascular disease death compared with control subjects (Ordóñez et al., 1993). The increased risk was independent of hypertension and cigarette smoking. However, plasma lipid levels were measured only once, so the role of hyperlipidemia in the pathogenesis of coronary artery disease in this study is unclear. Thus, there are still no conclusive data implicating hyperlipidemia in the pathogenesis of cardiovascular disease in patients with nephrotic syndrome, but there is no reason to suspect that the risk of cardiovascular disease in hyperlipidemic patients with nephrotic syndrome is any less than that in the general population.

Renal Disease Progression

Data in experimental animal models suggest that hyperlipidemia may cause or contribute to chronic renal injury. Some clinical studies have shown that lipid abnormalities correlate with the rate of renal disease progression, and epidemiologic studies suggest that in many patients, the chances for development of end-stage renal disease are roughly proportional to the degree of proteinuria, and this, in turn, tends to be correlated with the degree of hyperlipidemia. The large-scale intervention trials that are needed to determine whether hyperlipidemia contributes to renal disease progression in humans have not been carried out.

Treatment

The best treatment of any condition is to remove the underlying cause. There is no evidence that hyperlipidemia of short duration is particularly harmful, so that treatment of hyperlipidemia can probably be delayed for patients in whom therapy of the underlying renal disease is likely to induce a remission. When achieving a remission is not likely, consideration should be given to reducing the degree of proteinuria. A low-protein diet can theoretically reduce proteinuria, but low-protein diets should be used carefully in patients with nephrotic syndrome (see Chapter 9). Treatment of hypertension may also help reduce proteinuria. In particular, converting enzyme inhibitors have been shown to reduce the degree of proteinuria and to decrease lipoprotein levels in patients with nephrotic syndrome (Fig. 6-2). In patients who respond with a reduction in proteinuria, converting enzyme inhibitors can be expected to reduce both total and LDL cholesterol. Some of the capacity to reduce proteinuria with the use of a converting enzyme inhibitor may be independent of a decrease in blood pressure, so consideration may be given to their use even in normotensive patients.

When proteinuria and hyperlipidemia persist, specific treatment of the hyperlipidemic pattern should be considered. Guidelines that take into account factors raising the overall cardiovascular disease risk, such as those of the NCEP, should be considered in deciding when therapy should be initiated. Hyperlipidemia is typically so severe in patients with nephrotic syndrome that most are candidates for treatment, and the first line of therapy should be dietary restriction. This measure can produce modest reductions in total and LDL cholesterol (see Fig. 6-2), but manipulating the diet has had little consistent effect on triglycerides and HDL in nephrotic patients (see Fig. 6-2). Most diets investigated include a reduced total and saturated fat content, as well as reduced cholesterol intake. A cholesterol-free, vegetarian and soya-bean diet has been shown to be especially effective.

The influence of a dietary fish oil supplement has been investigated in nephrotic patients but there is no consistent effect of the fish oil supplement on total cholesterol, LDL, or HDL. Fish oil does appear to reduce triglycerides in patients with nephrotic syndrome and may have beneficial effects to reduce platelet aggregability and blood viscosity while increasing red blood cell deformability to reduce the tendency of nephrotic patients to form blood clots. If fish oil supplements are used, they should be administered with an antioxidant because there is a tendency for the omega-3 fatty acids in fish oil to be destroyed by oxidation.

The response to dietary manipulation alone is usually inadequate in patients with nephrotic proteinuria. Therefore, it is often appropriate to begin pharmacologic therapy at the same time as changing the diet, especially in patients with markedly abnormal lipoproteins or a high risk for coronary artery disease. Because elevations in LDL are the rule, an HMG-CoA reductase inhibitor is the drug of first choice in most patients. Of all therapies studied in patients with nephrotic syndrome, the HMG-CoA reductase inhibitors caused the greatest and most consistent reductions in total and LDL cholesterol (see Fig. 6-2). Triglycerides were also significantly reduced, and HDL was increased by HMG-CoA reductase inhibitors in patients with

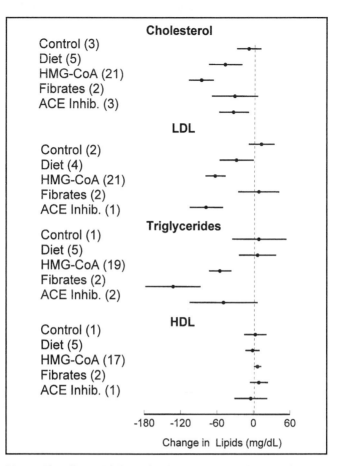

Fig. 6-2. The effects of different lipid-lowering therapies in patients with nephrotic syndrome. Shown are the mean and 95% confidence intervals (solid horizontal lines) for the change in lipid levels (mg/dl) before and during therapy. The number of studies pooled is shown in parentheses. Failure of a 95% confidence interval to cross zero indicates $P < 0.05$. Results from both controlled and uncontrolled trials are included. HMG-CoA, 3-hydroxy-3-methylglutaryl coenzyme A reductase inhibitor; ACE, angiotensin-converting enzyme. (Data from Massy ZA, Ma JZ, Louis TA, et al. Lipid-lowering therapy in patients with renal disease. *Kidney Int* 1995;48:188–198, with permission.)

nephrotic syndrome (see Fig. 6-2). The dose of HMG-CoA reductase inhibitors must be reduced in patients treated with cyclosporine A because it increases blood levels of HMG-CoA reductase inhibitors and the risk of myopathy.

Despite the predicable response to HMG-CoA reductase inhibitors, most patients will have persistent hyperlipidemia. It is a mistake for physicians and patients to become discouraged if the plasma cholesterol level remains high even though there has been a significant reduction after therapy. Data from studies in the general population suggest that each 1% reduction in cholesterol reduces the risk of cardiovascular disease by 2%. This emphasizes that even a partial response will be of great benefit to patients with very high lipid levels. Nevertheless, consideration should be given to adding a second agent along with an HMG-CoA reductase inhibitor if plasma lipoprotein levels remain substantially increased. Unfortunately, there are few studies reporting the effects of combination therapy in patients with nephrotic syndrome. Therefore, patients should be monitored closely if combination therapy is used in nephrotic patients.

Consideration can be given to adding a fibric acid analog to an HMG-CoA reductase inhibitor, especially if triglycerides are elevated. When used alone, fibric acid analogs reduce total cholesterol, but are most effective in decreasing triglycerides (see Fig. 6-2). The dose of the fibric acid analog should be lowered according to the level of renal function. The risk of myositis and rhabdomyolysis increases with combination therapy, so high doses of the fibric acid analog should be avoided, particularly if used in combination with an HMG-CoA reductase inhibitor.

In theory, a bile acid sequestrant might be useful when combined with an HMG-CoA reductase inhibitor, at least in patients who do not have elevated triglycerides. However, bile acid sequestrants only modestly reduced total and LDL cholesterol and triglycerides increased in nephrotic patients treated with sequestrants. The addition of a bile acid sequestrant failed to improve the results with an HMG-CoA reductase inhibitor substantially. Adverse effects of bile acid sequestrants, particularly gastrointestinal symptoms, frequently limit their usefulness.

Nicotinic acid should be attractive for treating hyperlipidemia because it is relatively inexpensive, but there are virtually no data regarding the safety and efficacy of nicotinic acid in nephrotic patients. There are also few data on using nicotinic acid in combination therapy, and adverse reactions to nicotinic acid are common.

Probucol is theoretically advantageous because it lowers serum cholesterol and is an antioxidant, and oxidized LDL could be important in the pathogenesis of atherosclerosis. Unfortunately, when probucol was given to nephrotic patients, there were only small reductions in total cholesterol, LDL, and triglycerides. In other patient populations, probucol tends to reduce HDL, and this response would make it less attractive for patients with the nephrotic syndrome.

RENAL INSUFFICIENCY

Abnormalities and Pathogenesis

Total Cholesterol and Low-Density Lipoprotein

Renal insufficiency per se does not appear to increase plasma LDL, but patients may have increased LDL for reasons that are unrelated to renal function. Otherwise, an increase in total cholesterol more often results from an increase in triglyceride-rich lipoproteins.

Triglycerides and High-Density Lipoprotein

Renal insufficiency can increase plasma triglycerides and decrease HDL, and higher triglyceride levels may appear when renal function falls below 30 to 40 ml/minute. This appears to be largely due to the decreased catabolism of triglyceride-rich lipoproteins, which, in turn, may be due to abnormalities in lipase activity. Indeed, the activity of lipases that catabolize triglycerides appears to be inversely proportional to the level of renal function. Because the formation of HDL is linked to the catabolism of triglyceride-bearing lipoproteins, HDL tends to decline with decreasing renal function. A decrease in lipase activity has been attributed to parathyroid hormone excess, insulin resistance, as well as abnormalities in apolipoprotein cofactors in patients with renal insufficiency. In particular, the low levels of apo C-II and high levels of apo C-III seen in patients with renal insufficiency could be the cause of reduced lipase activity.

Other Lipoprotein Abnormalities

Even patients with normal plasma levels of cholesterol and triglycerides frequently have abnormalities in apolipoproteins; apo B and apo C-III are often elevated, and apo A-I (associated with HDL) is frequently decreased. The hallmark of the dyslipidemia of renal insufficiency is a low ratio of apo A-I/apo C-III, occurring even in people with normal triglycerides. These patients can also have a high proatherogenic ratio of apo B/apo A-I. All of these apolipoprotein abnormalities are accentuated in people with increased triglycerides.

Laboratory data suggest that oxidized LDL may play a role in the pathogenesis of atherosclerosis, and this is of interest because patients with renal insufficiency often have elevated levels of oxidized LDL. In addition, the susceptibility of LDL to oxidation appears to be increased in patients with renal insufficiency. There is limited information about the levels of plasma Lp(a), a suspected risk factor for cardiovascular disease, in patients with mild or moderate renal insufficiency.

Possible Consequences

Few studies have examined the incidence of cardiovascular disease in nonnephrotic patients with renal insufficiency. Therefore, the relative contribution that lipid abnormalities may make on the pathogenesis of cardiovascular disease in this population is unknown. Decisions to treat hyperlipidemia are based on inferences made from data on the risk of hyperlipidemia in the general population; there are circumstantial data, but no proof, that lipid abnormalities may contribute to renal disease progression.

Treatment

A low-fat diet reduces total cholesterol in patients with renal insufficiency and should probably be used as first-line therapy as long as nutrition is closely monitored (Fig. 6-3).In patients with elevated triglycerides, a fibric acid analog seems a logical agent to add to the diet because they reduce total cholesterol and triglycerides, and tend to increase HDL in patients with renal insufficiency (see Fig. 6-3). The dose of fibric acid analogs should be reduced according to the degree of renal function impairment, to prevent myopathy. In the less frequently encountered patients with elevated LDL, an HMG-CoA reductase inhibitor is effective

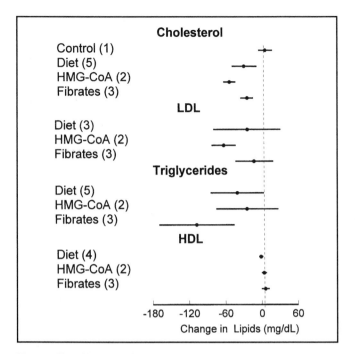

Fig. 6-3. The effects of different lipid-lowering therapies in patients with renal insufficiency. Shown are the mean and 95% confidence intervals (solid horizontal lines) for the change in lipid levels (mg/dl) before and therapy. The number of studies pooled is shown in parentheses. Failure of a 95% confidence interval to cross zero indicates $P < 0.05$. Results from both controlled and uncontrolled trials are included. HMG-CoA, 3-hydroxy-3-methylglutaryl coenzyme A reductase inhibitor. (Data from Massy ZA, Ma JZ, Louis TA, et al. Lipid-lowering therapy in patients with renal disease. *Kidney Int* 1995;48:188–198, with permission.)

in reducing total and LDL cholesterol in patients with renal insufficiency (see Fig. 6-3).

HEMODIALYSIS

Abnormalities and Pathogenesis

Total Cholesterol and Low-Density Lipoprotein

As is the case for renal insufficiency in pre–end-stage renal disease, LDL levels are usually normal or low in patients on hemodialysis.

Triglycerides and High-Density Lipoprotein

The same abnormalities in lipase activity present in patients with renal insufficiency probably contribute to the increased plasma levels of triglycerides and lower HDL of hemodialysis patients. The heparin used during dialysis may interfere with lipase activity and contribute to increased triglycerides and decrease HDL.

Other Lipoprotein Abnormalities

The same apolipoprotein abnormalities of predialysis renal insufficiency are common in patients treated with hemodialysis. There also is an enhanced susceptibility of LDL to oxidation.

Lipoprotein(a) reportedly is elevated in many hemodialysis patients. As in the general population, levels of Lp(a) are inversely proportional to the levels of genetically determined high-molecular-weight apo(a) isoforms. Although dialysis patients tend to have increased Lp(a) levels, compared with normal control subjects, dialysis patients with a greater proportion of the low–molecular-weight Lp(a) type have higher plasma Lp(a) levels than dialysis patients with high–molecular-weight isoforms.

Possible Consequences

There is no doubt that the morbidity and mortality from atherosclerosis are very high in hemodialysis patients. Most investigators believe that cardiovascular disease is the leading cause of death in the dialysis population, but the extent to which lipoprotein abnormalities contribute to the pathogenesis of atherosclerotic cardiovascular disease among hemodialysis patients is unclear. Both low and high total serum cholesterol levels have been associated with increased mortality in hemodialysis patients. The association between a low serum cholesterol level and mortality could theoretically be explained by poor nutrition or increased lipoprotein catabolism from infections, occult malignancy, or other comorbid conditions. Certainly, it cannot be inferred that treating a high serum cholesterol will increase mortality in hemodialysis patients, but the association between high serum cholesterol levels and increased mortality suggests, but does not prove, that lipid abnormalities may contribute to cardiovascular disease in the dialysis population.

Lipoprotein(a) has been reported to be an independent risk factor for coronary artery disease in hemodialysis patients (Cressman et al., 1992). Lp(a) levels have also been reported to be associated with the degree of atherosclerosis in extracranial carotid arteries of patients on hemodialysis (Kronenberg et al., 1994). Unfortunately, there are no established therapies for increased Lp(a) levels.

Treatment

A low-fat, low-cholesterol diet can be tried in hyperlipidemic hemodialysis patients, but nutritional adequacy must be closely monitored to ensure that calorie intake is adequate. Dietary therapy has been shown to improve triglyceride levels in hemodialysis patients (Fig. 6-4), and also can reduce total and LDL cholesterol when these are elevated (see Fig. 6-4). With the availability of erythropoietin therapy, at least some hemodialysis patients may be able to exercise regularly, and exercise can

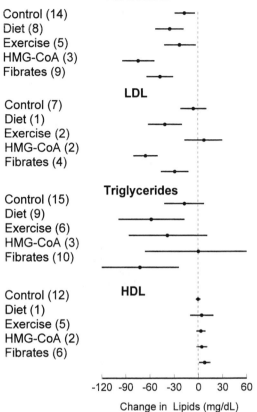

Fig. 6-4. The effects of different lipid-lowering therapies in patients on hemodialysis. Shown are the mean and 95% confidence intervals (solid horizontal lines) for the change in lipid levels (mg/dl) before and during therapy. The number of studies pooled is shown in parentheses. Failure of a 95% confidence interval to cross zero indicates $P < 0.05$. Results from both controlled and uncontrolled trials are included. HMG-CoA, 3-hydroxy-3-methylglutaryl coenzyme A reductase inhibitor. (Data from Massy ZA, Ma JZ, Louis TA, et al. Lipid-lowering therapy in patients with renal disease. *Kidney Int* 1995;48:188–198, with permission.)

improve lipid levels in these patients (see Fig. 6-4). Fish oil supplements can also improve the lipid profiles of hemodialysis patients (Fig. 6-5).

When dietary therapy fails, low-dose fibric acid analogs are a logical choice for hyperlipidemic hemodialysis patients because these patients often have high triglycerides. Fibric acid analogs effectively reduce not only triglycerides, but total and LDL cholesterol (see Fig. 6-4), and may increase HDL. The occasional patient with a high plasma LDL level may respond to an HMG-CoA reductase inhibitor (see Fig. 6-4).

The use of low–molecular-weight heparin has been reported to improve hyperlipidemia in hemodialysis patients, although the degree of improvement is not striking (see Fig. 6-5). This conclu-

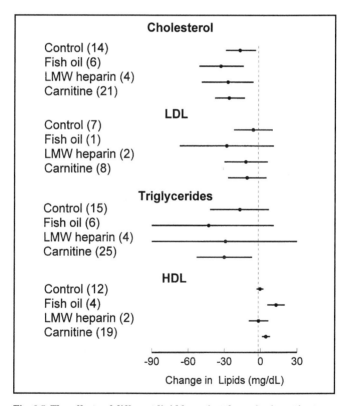

Fig. 6-5. The effects of different lipid-lowering therapies in patients on hemodialysis, a continuation of Fig. 6-4. Shown are the mean and 95% confidence intervals (solid horizontal lines) for the change in lipid levels (mg/dl) before and therapy. The number of studies pooled is shown in parentheses. Failure of a 95% confidence interval to cross zero indicates $P < 0.05$. Results from both controlled and uncontrolled trials are included. LMW, low–molecular-weight heparin. (Data from Massy ZA, Ma JZ, Louis TA, et al. Lipid-lowering therapy in patients with renal disease. *Kidney Int* 1995;48:188–198, with permission.)

sion may be confounded by the inclusion of patients receiving different types of low–molecular-weight heparin. Some trials have shown that the use of high-flux dialysis membranes may improve lipid profiles, but more controlled trials are needed to confirm these observations.

A relatively large number of studies have reported that carnitine supplements can improve plasma lipid levels in hemodialysis patients. Total cholesterol, LDL, triglycerides, and HDL seem to be favorably affected by carnitine supplements (see Fig. 6-5), although many of these trials were uncontrolled.

PERITONEAL DIALYSIS

Abnormalities and Pathogenesis

Total Cholesterol and Low-Density Lipoprotein

Unlike hemodialysis, continuous ambulatory peritoneal dialysis (CAPD) is often accompanied by increased plasma total and LDL cholesterol levels. The reason for this is unclear. Speculation has centered on the role of the increased caloric intake from the dextrose in the peritoneal dialysis solution plus the loss of proteins in the dialysate. Besides the loss of albumin, the loss of proteins that play a role in regulating lipoprotein metabolism could theoretically affect lipoprotein levels.

Triglycerides and High-Density Lipoprotein

Like hemodialysis, CAPD is associated with increased plasma triglycerides and decreased HDL levels. Presumably, the mechanisms relate to decreased renal function and are similar to those found in patients on hemodialysis.

Other Lipoprotein Abnormalities

The LDL from CAPD patients may be more susceptible to oxidation than LDL from normal subjects, and proatherogenic Lp(a) levels are increased. Although the cause of the higher Lp(a) level is unknown, it appears to correlate with the amount of protein lost into the dialysate and the allelic variation of apo(a) isoforms. As in hemodialysis patients, however, variations in the genetically determined isoform frequency do not explain the increase in plasma Lp(a) in CAPD patients.

Possible Consequences

Cardiovascular disease is the most common cause of death in CAPD patients, but there are few studies examining the relationship between hyperlipidemia and cardiovascular disease. In one retrospective, case–control study of CAPD patients, cholesterol and LDL were increased in patients with cardiovascular disease compared with patients without cardiovascular disease (Webb and Brown, 1993). Peritoneal dialysis patients with coronary artery disease appear to have a higher frequency of low–molecular-weight Lp(a) isoforms and higher Lp(a) levels compared with peritoneal dialysis patients without coronary artery disease.

Treatment

There are virtually no studies investigating the efficacy of dietary manipulation in the management of hyperlipidemia in

CAPD patients. Regardless, a change in the diet would seem to be a prudent first step, as long as overall nutrition is not compromised. If this is not sufficient, HMG-CoA reductase inhibitors are a logical second step for patients with increased LDL cholesterol because these drugs effectively reduce total and LDL cholesterol in CAPD patients (Fig. 6-6). HMG-CoA reductase inhibitors also tend to reduce triglycerides and increase HDL cholesterol levels. Fibric acid analogs appear to be the most effective drugs for reducing triglycerides in CAPD patients (see Fig. 6-6). As in any patient with decreased renal function, the doses of fibric acid analogs should be reduced to avoid myopathies.

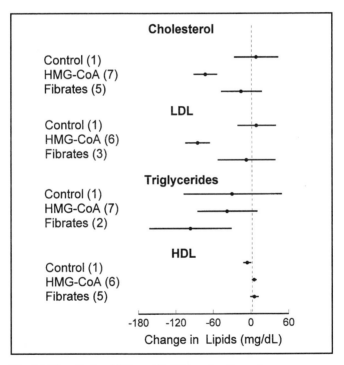

Fig. 6-6. The effects of different lipid-lowering therapies in patients on continuous ambulatory peritoneal dialysis. Shown are the mean and 95% confidence intervals (solid horizontal lines) for the change in lipid levels (mg/dl) before and therapy. The number of studies pooled is shown in parentheses. Failure of a 95% confidence interval to cross zero indicates $P < 0.05$. Results from both controlled and uncontrolled trials are included. HMG-CoA, 3-hydroxy-3-methylglutaryl coenzyme A reductase inhibitor.
(Data from Massy ZA, Ma JZ, Louis TA, et al. Lipid-lowering therapy in patients with renal disease. *Kidney Int* 1995;48:188–198, with permission.)

TRANSPLANTATION

Abnormalities and Pathogenesis

Total Cholesterol and Low-Density Lipoprotein

Total and LDL cholesterol levels are frequently high in the plasma of renal transplant recipients. The pathogenesis is probably multifactorial, but the corticosteroids and cyclosporine A can increase plasma LDL and total cholesterol levels. Patients with acute rejection episodes tend to receive higher doses of these immunosuppressive medications and usually have higher cholesterol levels. Many transplant patients also have proteinuria, and this can contribute to high plasma levels of cholesterol and LDL.

Triglycerides and High-Density Lipoprotein

Plasma triglycerides are frequently increased after renal transplantation. Besides the influences of corticosteroids and cyclosporine A, obesity and renal allograft dysfunction can contribute to the increase in triglycerides. Plasma HDL levels tend to be normal or even high after renal transplantation; this may be a result of corticosteroid therapy, because withdrawal of corticosteroids leads to reduced plasma HDL. Unfortunately, the composition and the reverse cholesterol transport function of HDL may not be normal in transplant recipients, so the normal or high plasma HDL levels after renal transplantation (or the lower plasma HDL levels after steroid withdrawal) may not be associated with the same risk profile for cardiovascular disease as similar HDL changes in the general population.

Other Lipoprotein Abnormalities

Studies have suggested that plasma LDL isolated from renal transplant recipients may be more susceptible to oxidation than that from normal control subjects. Fortunately, plasma Lp(a) levels decline after renal transplantation, and most studies suggest that it is normal in renal transplant recipients who do not have proteinuria or graft dysfunction.

Possible Consequences

Cardiovascular Disease

The incidence of cardiovascular disease is high after renal transplantation. Epidemiologic studies indicate that posttransplantation hyperlipidemia is an independent risk factor for cardiovascular disease events in the late posttransplantation period. Although this association does not prove a cause-and-effect relationship, it suggests that the risk of hyperlipidemia may be at least as great as it is in the general population with similar abnormalities in plasma lipids.

Chronic Renal Allograft Rejection

Experimental studies suggest that hyperlipidemia may contribute to the pathogenesis of the intragraft vascular disease that characterizes chronic rejection. Epidemiologic studies of rather small groups have found that elevated plasma lipid levels are correlated with the subsequent development of chronic rejection. Although these associations do not prove cause and effect, they do suggest the need for clinical trials to determine whether treating hyperlipidemia will prolong survival of the transplanted kidney.

A randomized, controlled trial found that chronic administration of an HMG-CoA reductase inhibitor reduced the incidence of acute renal allograft rejection after renal transplantation (Katznelson et al., 1996). The number of patients studied was very small, and the incidence of acute rejection in the placebo group was much higher than that usually seen today in most transplant centers. Larger, multicenter trials are underway to examine the effects of HMG-CoA reductase inhibitors on both allograft rejection and cardiovascular disease events.

Treatment

Patients should be maintained on the lowest possible doses of corticosteroids and cyclosporine A compatible with long-term allograft survival. In selected, stable patients, corticosteroids can be reduced to very low doses, and in some patients, corticosteroids have been successfully withdrawn, resulting in lower plasma levels of cholesterol and LDL. Cyclosporine A withdrawal is also associated with an improved lipoprotein profile.

Newer immunosuppressive agents, such as FK 506 and mycophenolic acid mofetil, appear to cause less hyperlipidemia compared with cyclosporine A. These agents can be used to reduce the doses of prednisone and cyclosporine A used after transplantation, and may lower plasma lipid levels. Ongoing clinical trials are exploring the possibility of substituting newer immunosuppressive agents for corticosteroids and cyclosporine, thereby reducing the risk of cardiovascular disease in the late posttransplantation period.

Dietary manipulation has been shown to be effective in reducing the total and LDL cholesterol and triglyceride elevations that are so common in the plasma after transplantation (Fig. 6-7). However, the effects of diet changes usually are modest, and a pharmacologic agent is often necessary. When hyperlipidemia is marked and the risk for cardiovascular disease is high, consideration should be given to starting the low-lipid diet and pharmacologic therapy simultaneously.

Of all agents studied, the HMG-CoA reductase inhibitors appear to be most consistently effective in treating hyperlipidemia after renal transplantation. Plasma levels of total and LDL cholesterol are substantially reduced by HMG-CoA reductase inhibitors, and triglycerides are also lower (see Fig. 6-7). Blood levels of HMG-CoA reductase inhibitors are increased by the concomitant use of cyclosporine A, so the dose of HMG-CoA reductase inhibitors should be reduced in these patients to avoid myositis and rhabdomyolysis. There is no convincing evidence that any HMG-CoA reductase inhibitor is safer than any other in renal transplant recipients.

A number of studies have examined the safety and efficacy of fibric acid analogs after renal transplantation. Not surprisingly, these drugs are particularly effective in reducing plasma triglycerides and also total cholesterol and LDL (see Fig. 6-7). The reductions in total cholesterol and LDL are not as dramatic as with HMG-CoA reductase inhibitors, and HDL is not substantially altered.

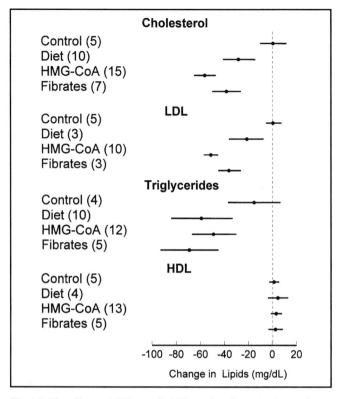

Fig. 6-7. The effects of different lipid-lowering therapies in renal transplant recipients. Shown are the mean and 95% confidence intervals (solid horizontal lines) for the change in lipid levels (mg/dl) before and therapy. The number of studies pooled is shown in parentheses. Failure of a 95% confidence interval to cross zero indicates $P < 0.05$. Results from both controlled and uncontrolled trials are included. HMG-CoA, 3-hydroxy-3-methylglutaryl coenzyme A reductase inhibitor. (Data from Massy ZA, Ma JZ, Louis TA, et al. Lipid-lowering therapy in patients with renal disease. *Kidney Int* 1995;48:188–198, with permission.)

There are few data about the use of other agents after renal transplantation. Probucol can decrease cholesterol and LDL, but also reduces HDL. The latter response has led most clinicians to avoid using this agent in renal transplant recipients. Niacin has not been extensively studied, probably because of the high incidence of adverse effects. Bile acid sequestrants have not been adequately studied in renal transplant recipients, and the theoretical concern that bile acid sequestrants will limit the bioavailability of cyclosporine A has not been substantiated in clinical trials. Many patients cannot tolerate high doses of bile acid sequestrants; lower doses of newer preparations may be more effective and better tolerated.

Information about the effectiveness of combining an HMG-CoA reductase inhibitor with a bile acid sequestrant is limited. This is an attractive option because their mechanisms of action are different, and adverse effects from the combination should be less. However, patients should be instructed to take cyclosporine A and the bile acid sequestrant at different times to minimize the chances of reduced cyclosporine A absorption. Although combining an HMG-CoA reductase inhibitor with a fibric acid analog may be effective, the risk of myositis and rhabdomyolysis will rise.

SELECTED READINGS

Cressman MD, Heyka RJ, Paganini EP, et al. Lipoprotein(a) is an independent risk factor for cardiovascular disease in hemodialysis patients. *Circulation* 1992;86:475–482.

Curry RC, Roberts WC. Status of the coronary arteries in the nephrotic syndrome: analysis of 20 necropsy patients aged 15 to 35 years to determine if coronary atherosclerosis is accelerated. *Am J Med* 1977;63:183–192.

D'Amico G, Gentile MG, Manna G, et al. Effect of vegetarian soy diet on hyperlipidaemia in nephrotic syndrome. *Lancet* 1992;339: 1131–1134.

Expert Panel on Detection Evaluation and Treatment of High Blood Cholesterol in Adults. Summary of the Second Report of the National Cholesterol Education Program (NCEP) (Adult Treatment Panel II). *JAMA* 1993;269:3015–3023.

Frick MH, Elo O, Haapa K, et al. Helsinki Heart Study: primary-prevention trial with gemfibrozil in middle-aged men with dyslipidemia: safety of treatment, changes in risk factors, and incidence of coronary heart disease. *N Engl J Med* 1987;317: 1237–1245.

Ghanem H, van den Dorpel MA, Weimar W, et al. Increased low density lipoprotein oxidation in stable kidney transplant recipients. *Kidney Int* 1996;49:488–493.

Gokal R, King J, Bogle S, et al. Outcome in patients on continuous ambulatory peritoneal dialysis and haemodialysis: 4-year analysis of a prospective multicenter study. *Lancet* 1987;2:1105–1109.

Gonwa T, Atkins C, Velez R, et al. Metabolic consequences of cyclosporine-to-azathioprine conversion in renal transplantation. *Clin Transplant* 1988;2:91–96.

Groggel GC, Cheung AK, Ellis-Benigni K, et al. Treatment of nephrotic hyperlipoproteinemia with gemfibrozil. *Kidney Int* 1989; 36:266–271.

Hirata K, Kikuchi S, Saku K, et al. Apolipoprotein(a) phenotypes and serum lipoprotein(a) levels in maintenance hemodialysis patients with/without diabetes mellitus. *Kidney Int* 1993;44:1062–1070.

Hricik DE, Bartucci MR, Mayes JT, et al. The effects of steroid withdrawal on the lipoprotein profiles of cyclosporine-treated kidney and kidney-pancreas transplant recipients. *Transplantation* 1992; 54:868–871.

Jensen RA, Lal SM, Diaz-Arias A, et al. Does cholestyramine interfere with cyclosporine absorption? A prospective study in renal transplant patients. *ASAIO J* 1995;41:M704–M706.

Josephson MA, Fellner SK, Dasgupta A. Improved lipid profiles in patients undergoing high-flux hemodialysis. *Am J Kidney Dis* 1992; 20:361–366.

Kallen RJ, Brynes RK, Aronson AJ, et al. Premature coronary ather-osclerosis in a 5-year-old with corticosteroid refractory nephrotic syndrome. *American Journal of Diseases of Children* 1977;131: 976–980.

Kasiske BL, O'Donnell MP, Kim Y, et al. Treatment of hyperlipid-emia in chronic progressive renal disease. *Curr Opin Nephrol Hypertens* 1993;2:602–608.

Katznelson S, Wilkinson AH, Kobashigawa JA, et al. The effect of pravastatin on acute rejection after kidney transplantation: a pilot study. *Transplantation* 1996;61:1469–1474.

Keogh A, Day R, Critchley L, et al. The effect of food and cholestyra-mine in the absorption of cyclosporine in cardiac transplant recip-ients. *Transplant Proc* 1988;20:27–30.

Krolewski AS, Warram JH, Christlieb AR. Hypercholesterolemia: a determinant of renal function loss and deaths in IDDM patients with nephropathy. *Kidney Int* 1994;45(Suppl 45):S125–S131.

Kronenberg F, Kathrein H, König P, et al. Apolipoprotein(a) pheno-types predict the risk for carotid atherosclerosis in patients with end-stage renal disease. *Arteriosclerosis and Thrombosis* 1994;14: 1405–1411.

Lowrie EG, Lew NL. Commonly measured laboratory variables in hemodialysis patients: relationships among them and to death risk. *Semin Nephrol* 1992;12:276–283.

Maggi E, Bellazzi R, Falaschi F, et al. Enhanced LDL oxidation in uremic patients: an additional mechanism for accelerated athero-sclerosis? *Kidney Int* 1994;45:876–883.

Maki DD, Ma JZ, Louis TA, et al. Long-term effects of antihyperten-sive agents on proteinuria and renal function. *Arch Intern Med* 1995;155:1073–1080.

Markell MS, Sumrani N, Sarn Y, et al. Prospective randomized double-blind trial of probucol vs. placebo in hypercholesterolemic renal transplant recipients [abstract]. *Transplantation* 1993;4:948.

Massy ZA, Ma JZ, Louis TA, et al. Lipid-lowering therapy in patients with renal disease. *Kidney Int* 1995;48:188–198.

Ordóñez JD, Hiatt RA, Killebrew EJ, Fireman BH. The increased risk of coronary heart disease associated with nephrotic syndrome. *Kidney Int* 1993;44:638–642.

Ravid M, Neumann L, Lishner M. Plasma lipids and the progression of nephropathy in diabetes mellitus type II: effect of ACE inhibitors. *Kidney Int* 1995;47:907–910.

Samuelsson O, Aurell M, Knight-Gibson C, et al. Apolipoprotein-B-containing lipoproteins and the progression of renal insufficiency. *Nephron* 1993;63:279–285.

Samuelsson O, Attman P-O, Knight-Gibson C, et al. Lipoprotein abnormalities without hyperlipidaemia in moderate renal insuffi-ciency. *Nephrol Dial Transplant* 1994;9:1580–1585.

Seres DS, Strain GW, Hashim SA, et al. Improvement of plasma lipoprotein profiles during high-flux dialysis. *J Am Soc Nephrol* 1993;3:1409–1415.

Spitalewitz S, Porush JG, Cattran D, Wright N. Treatment of hyper-lipidemia in the nephrotic syndrome: the effects of pravastatin therapy. *Am J Kidney Dis* 1993;22:143–150.

Sutherland WHF, Walker RJ, Ball MJ, et al. Oxidation of low density lipoproteins from patients with renal failure or renal transplants. *Kidney Int* 1995;48:227–236.

Wanner C, Bartens W, Walz G, et al. Protein loss and genetic polymorphism of apolipoprotein(a) modulate serum lipoprotein(a) in CAPD patients. *Nephrol Dial Transplant* 1995;10:75–81.

Webb AT, Brown EA. Prevalence of symptomatic arterial disease and risk factors for its development in patients on continuous ambulatory peritoneal dialysis. *Perit Dial Int* 1993;13(Suppl 2):S406–S408.

Requirements for Protein, Calories, and Fat in the Predialysis Patient

Bradley J. Maroni

GOALS OF NUTRITIONAL THERAPY

When the diet exceeds the daily protein requirement, the excess is degraded to urea and other nitrogenous wastes eliminated primarily by the kidney. Moreover, foods that are rich in protein also contain hydrogen ions, phosphates, and other inorganic ions that must be excreted by the kidney. Therefore, when chronic renal failure (CRF) patients consume excessive dietary protein, nitrogenous wastes and inorganic ions accumulate, resulting in the clinical and metabolic disturbances characteristic of uremia. This is the basis for the observation that restricting dietary protein (and phosphorus) can ameliorate many symptoms of uremia as well as some of its metabolic complications (e.g., metabolic acidosis, insulin resistance, secondary hyperparathyroidism). Unless nutritional therapy is tailored to the patient's requirements and monitored to ensure dietary adequacy, protein or energy stores may be depleted.

The goals of nutritional therapy are 1) to prescribe a diet sufficient to prevent malnutrition; 2) to diminish the accumulation of nitrogenous wastes and metabolic disturbances characteristic of uremia; and 3) to slow the progression of renal failure.

ASSESSING PROTEIN REQUIREMENTS

Nitrogen Balance and Protein Requirements

Despite its limitations, nitrogen balance remains the gold standard for assessing dietary protein requirements. When defining the protein requirement, a realistic intake of energy must be prescribed because for any intake of nitrogen, supplemental calories improve nitrogen balance. Conversely, subjects consuming a marginal intake of protein are at risk of catabolizing body protein stores if the energy intake is inadequate.

In healthy adults performing moderate physical activity and consuming sufficient (but not excessive) calories, the average protein requirement is ~0.6 g protein/kg/day. The "safe level of intake" (i.e., defined as the average requirement plus two standard deviations) is ~0.75 g protein/kg/day; this amount meets the protein requirements of ≥97.5% of normal adults.

The recommended protein intake for CRF patients has been equated with the average intake necessary to achieve neutral nitrogen balance (e.g., ~0.6 g protein/kg/day). Despite concern that the "average" requirement may not be adequate for all patients, long-term follow-up of CRF patients consuming low-protein diets indicates that nutritional status can be maintained (see later).

MECHANISMS RESPONSIBLE FOR
NEUTRAL NITROGEN BALANCE

Normal Subjects

In Western societies, individual protein intake is usually well above the daily requirement (i.e., 1 to 2 g protein/kg/day). Because dietary protein (and amino acids) in excess of the daily requirement is not stored, the principal response to a surplus of dietary protein is a marked increase in amino acid oxidation. Nitrogen derived from amino acid catabolism is converted to waste nitrogen (principally urea) and eliminated, primarily by the kidney. In contrast, the principal mechanism for successful adaptation to a low, but adequate, intake of protein is a dramatic reduction in amino acid oxidation, resulting in more efficient utilization of dietary essential amino acids (EAA; see Chapter 1). Waste nitrogen excretion declines so that nitrogen balance is neutral (i.e., nitrogen intake equals output) with the lower protein intake. If the protein intake is below the minimum daily requirement, amino acid catabolism does not decrease further and nitrogen balance becomes negative, with loss of lean body mass.

Protein turnover (i.e., protein synthesis and degradation) is a dynamic process resulting in the remodeling of ~280 g of body protein per day. In response to fasting, body protein stores (principally skeletal muscle) are degraded and the amino acids used in the liver for gluconeogenesis. During feeding, body protein stores are replenished and anabolism (i.e., protein synthesis > protein degradation) takes place because of an inhibition of whole-body protein degradation; there may also be an increase in protein synthesis. If the diet is nutritionally adequate, the net response over 24 hours is a neutral (or positive) nitrogen balance with preservation of body protein stores. Thus, in healthy adults, successful adaptation to dietary protein restriction involves 1) suppression of EAA catabolism, and 2) postprandial (after feeding) inhibition of whole-body protein degradation and perhaps a stimulation of protein synthesis.

Chronic Renal Failure Patients

It is important to show that low-protein diets can be used safely in patients with progressive CRF, because avoiding malnutrition is a primary goal of nutritional therapy. Fortunately, even patients with advanced CRF (glomerular filtration rate [GFR] ~10 to 15 ml/minute) can maintain lean body mass during long-term therapy with a low-protein diet. CRF patients are able to activate the same adaptive responses to dietary protein restriction as normal subjects, namely, a postprandial suppression of whole-body protein degradation and a dramatic inhibition of amino acid oxidation (Fig. 7-1). When measured after at least 1 year of therapy with a low-protein diet (range, 12 to 24 months), these same adaptive responses persisted, indicating that the compensatory responses to dietary protein restriction are sustained during long-term therapy. Further evidence that low-protein diets are safe in CRF patients is provided by the finding that serum proteins, anthropometric values, and nitrogen balance remained normal during long-term therapy (Fig. 7-2).

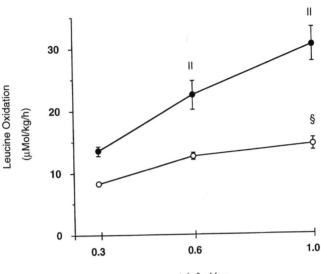

Fig. 7-1. The rates of amino acid (leucine) oxidation measured in chronic renal failure (CRF) patients consuming either a very–low-protein diet (VLPD) supplemented regimen (identified as 0.3) or, alternatively, 0.6 or 1.0 g protein/kg/day. Leucine oxidation rates were measured during fasting (open circles) and feeding (closed circles). Results are expressed as mean ±SE. By analysis of variance, feeding stimulates leucine oxidation during all three dietary regimens ($P < 0.001$). §$P < 0.005$, compared with a fasting leucine oxidation value for 0.28 g protein/kg/day. ‖$P < 0.001$, compared with the feeding leucine oxidation value for 0.28 g protein/kg/day. (From Masud T, Young V, Chapman T, et al. Adaptive responses to very low protein diets: first comparison of ketoacids to essential amino acids. *Kidney Int* 1994;45:1182–1192, with permission.)

The Modification of Diet in Renal Disease Study was the largest prospective trial to evaluate the impact of dietary protein restriction on nutritional status and the progression of renal failure (see Chapter 11). In this study, there were some minor, albeit statistically significant changes in some nutritional parameters in the low-protein diet groups (i.e., an increase in serum albumin and a decrease in serum transferrin and anthropometric values). Notably, these abnormal values stabilized after the first few months of therapy, and average values for the low-protein diet groups remained within the normal range. Most important, a low protein intake was not associated with a higher rate of nutritional stop points, hospitalizations, or death.

Is Dietary Protein Restriction Safe in the Nephrotic Syndrome?

Until recently, it was recommended that patients with the nephrotic syndrome (i.e., proteinuria >3 g/day) consume a high-

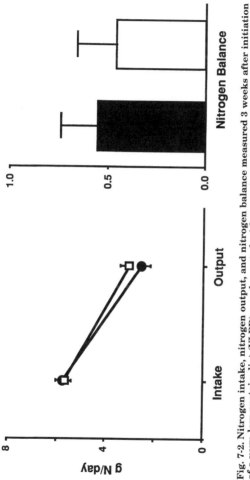
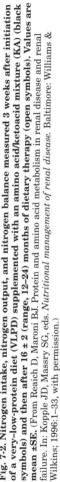

Fig. 7-2. Nitrogen intake, nitrogen output, and nitrogen balance measured 3 weeks after initiation of a very-low-protein diet (VLPD) supplemented with an amino acid/ketoacid mixture (KA) (black symbols) and then after 16 ± 2 (range, 12–24) months of dietary therapy (open symbols). Values are mean ±SE. (From Reaich D, Maroni BJ. Protein and amino acid metabolism in renal disease and renal failure. In: Kopple JD, Massry SG, eds. *Nutritional management of renal disease*. Baltimore: Williams & Wilkins; 1996:1–33, with permission.)

protein diet to promote anabolism and to compensate for urinary albumin losses. This recommendation was brought into question when Kaysen and colleagues reported that there is a distinct advantage in restricting dietary protein. When nephrotic patients were fed a diet providing 0.8 g protein/kg/day, urinary albumin excretion decreased and serum albumin increased, compared with results obtained when these same subjects consumed a diet providing 1.6 g protein/kg/day.

We measured nitrogen balance and whole-body protein turnover in healthy control subjects and nephrotic patients consuming 0.8 or 1.6 g protein (the diet was increased by 1 g protein for each gram proteinuria) and 35 kcal/kg body weight per day. In both groups, nitrogen balance was neutral or positive and anabolism was due to a feeding-induced inhibition of whole-body protein degradation and stimulation of protein synthesis. The principal compensatory response to the low-protein diet was a suppression of amino acid oxidation, and this response was identical in both normal subjects and nephrotic patients. Amino acid oxidation also correlated inversely with urinary protein losses, suggesting that proteinuria served as an additional stimulus to conserve amino acids (Fig. 7-3).

A report by Walser and colleagues suggests that an even more restrictive dietary regimen can be used safely in nephrotic patients. When they treated patients with a very–low-protein

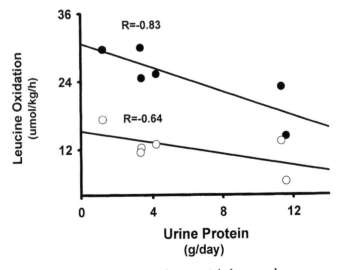

Fig. 7-3. **Relationship between urinary protein losses and leucine oxidation rates measured during fasting (open circles) and feeding (closed circles) while nephrotic subjects consumed a diet providing 0.8 g protein/kg/day (plus 1 g protein/g proteinuria). By linear regression, there was a significant correlation during feeding ($P = 0.04$).** (From Maroni BJ, Staffeld C, Young VR, et al. Mechanisms permitting nephrotic patients to achieve nitrogen equilibrium with a protein-restricted diet. *J Clin Invest* 1997;99:2479–2487, with permission.)

diet (VLPD) providing ~0.3 g protein/kg/day plus a mixture of EAA, serum albumin increased and serum cholesterol and proteinuria decreased. Moreover, in four of six patients whose initial GFR exceeded 30 ml/minute, this dietary regimen resulted in a prolonged remission of nephrosis.

In conclusion, evidence indicates that both nephrotic and nonnephrotic CRF patients can activate normal compensatory responses to a low-protein diet resulting in neutral nitrogen balance and maintenance of lean body mass during long-term dietary therapy.

Metabolic Acidosis and Protein Turnover in Uremia

Metabolic acidosis is a common complication of CRF. Acidosis causes insulin resistance and impaired growth in children and stimulates protein and amino acid catabolism. Metabolic acidosis stimulates protein breakdown by activating the adenosine triphosphate-dependent ubiquitin–proteasome proteolytic pathway in skeletal muscle. Acidosis also activates the rate-limiting enzyme for branched-chain amino acid catabolism in skeletal muscle, branched-chain ketoacid dehydrogenase. Because metabolic acidosis stimulates protein degradation and amino acid oxidation, its catabolic effect could counteract the adaptive responses to a low-protein diet. Indeed, when acidotic CRF patients were fed a low-protein diet, urinary 3-methylhistidine (an index of skeletal muscle protein degradation) and urea nitrogen excretion increased compared with values obtained after correcting acidosis with sodium bicarbonate. Thus, metabolic acidosis is a potentially reversible complication of CRF that stimulates protein catabolism and increases nitrogen requirements. Supplemental alkali (e.g., sodium bicarbonate, potassium or sodium citrate) should be prescribed to correct the serum HCO_3 to ≥ 24 mmol/l. Usually, two or three 650-mg sodium bicarbonate tablets (~8 mEq of sodium and bicarbonate per tablet) given two to three times daily is sufficient for this purpose and is well tolerated.

SPONTANEOUS PROTEIN INTAKE DURING PROGRESSIVE CHRONIC RENAL FAILURE

Concern has been raised that low-protein diets cause malnutrition in CRF patients and it has been suggested that these diets should be used cautiously or not at all. These concerns arise from two observations: 1) there is an association between hypoalbuminemia and increased mortality in hemodialysis patients, and 2) there is evidence of a spontaneous reduction in protein intake and worsening of some indices of nutritional status when CRF patients consume unrestricted diets. In fact, there is evidence that both concerns are misplaced. First, evidence indicates that when properly implemented, low-protein dietary therapy maintains normal values of serum proteins and anthropometrics, and neutral nitrogen balance during long-term therapy (see earlier). Second, hypoalbuminemia in hemodialysis patients appears to be more closely related to an inflammatory response than to an inadequate diet. Third, use of a low-protein diet in the predialysis period does not worsen, and may actually improve survival of CRF patients during the first 2 years after initiation of hemodialysis.

Clearly, proper dietary education of CRF patients is required or they may inadvertently consume meals rich in protein, resulting in the accumulation of nitrogenous wastes and uremic symptoms. In this setting, satiety may actually represent anorexia, so that an inadequate diet increases the risk of malnutrition. In contrast, a planned diet with sufficient protein and energy will maintain nitrogen balance and limit the accumulation of nitrogenous wastes, so that uremic symptoms do not develop and the nutritional status remains normal.

In conclusion, a spontaneous decrease in dietary protein intake in patients with progressive CRF consuming unrestricted diets should not be considered as evidence against the use of low-protein diets. Rather, it is a persuasive argument in favor of restricting dietary protein intake to minimize complications of renal failure while preserving nutritional status.

ASSESSING DIETARY ADEQUACY AND COMPLIANCE

Dietary Adequacy

Successful nutritional therapy requires periodic assessment of dietary adequacy and compliance. Unfortunately, traditional measures of dietary adequacy such as changes in serum albumin or transferrin and anthropometric values are insensitive to an early decrease in nutritional status. Moreover, a dichotomy between changes in anthropometric values and serum proteins can occur—one of these parameters can decline while the other suggests no change in nutritional status. Consequently, no single index is a reliable index of nutritional status. Recognizing these limitations, our approach is to monitor serum albumin, serum transferrin, and anthropometric values serially and to interpret these indices in light of the patient's dietary compliance.

Monitoring Compliance With the Diet Prescription

Protein Intake

In the outpatient setting, compliance with the protein prescription can be estimated using a simple method we devised. To understand this technique (and its limitations), one must recognize that waste nitrogen arising from degraded protein is excreted as urea and nonurea nitrogen (NUN). The urea nitrogen appearance rate (i.e., urea excretion plus accumulation) parallels protein intake, but NUN excretion (e.g., nitrogen in feces and urinary creatinine, uric acid, ammonia) does not vary substantially with dietary protein and averages 0.031 g N/kg/day (Fig. 7-4). When nitrogen balance is neutral (i.e., nitrogen intake equals output), then nitrogen intake (I_N) equals urea nitrogen appearance plus an estimate of NUN losses as 0.031 g N/kg (Table 7-1, formula 2). In the steady state (i.e. blood urea nitrogen and weight are constant), urea nitrogen appearance equals urinary urea nitrogen (UUN) excretion; hence, I_N equals UUN plus 0.031 g N/kg (see Table 7-1, formula 4).

In the example illustrated in Table 7-1, the calculated and prescribed values of protein intake are similar, so we would conclude that the patient is compliant with the protein prescription. If the estimated intake is less than prescribed, the patient should be encouraged to increase his or her protein intake to reach the goal. In contrast, if the estimated intake exceeds that prescribed by

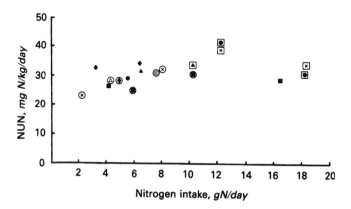

Fig. 7-4. Nonurea nitrogen (NUN) losses measured in normal subjects (closed triangles, circles, and squares) and patients with chronic renal failure being treated with low-protein diets (solid diamond, open circles with cross, open triangle, and solid diamond), by hemodialysis (open circle with solid square and open square with solid triangle), or continuous ambulatory peritoneal dialysis (open square with cross and open square with solid circle). These results indicate that NUN losses (i.e., nonurea urinary nitrogen plus fecal nitrogen) are relatively constant despite large variations in nitrogen intake and renal function. (From Maroni BJ, Steinman TI, Mitch WE. A method for estimating nitrogen intake in patients with chronic renal failure. *Kidney Int* 1985;27:58–65, with permission.)

Table 7-1. Estimating compliance with the dietary protein prescription from the 24-hour urinary urea nitrogen excretion

---

Formulas
1. $B_N = I_N - U - NUN$, where
   NUN = 0.031 g N/kg body weight
2. if $B_N = 0$, then $I_N = U + 0.031$ g N/kg body weight
3. when BUN is unchanging, then $U = UUN$, and
4. $I_N = UUN + 0.031$ g N/kg body weight

Example
A 40-year old woman is seen 1 month after
  instruction in a diet providing 0.6 protein/kg/day
  (i.e., 60 kg × 0.6 protein/kg = 36 g protein).
  Weight: 60 kg; UUN = 4.1 g/day; NUN = 0.031 g N × 60 kg
    = 1.86 g N/day
  if $B_N = 0$, then $I_N = UUN+NUN$
    = 4.1 + 1.86 = 5.96 g N
    = 5.96 g N × 6.25 g protein/g N
    = **37.3 g protein/day**

N, nitrogen; B_N, nitrogen balance (g N/day); I_N, nitrogen intake (g N/day); BUN, blood urea nitrogen; U, urea nitrogen appearance (g N/day); UUN, 24-hour urinary urea nitrogen (g N/day); NUN, nonurea nitrogen (g N/day).

more than 25%, there are two potential explanations: 1) a super-imposed catabolic illness or condition (e.g., gastrointestinal bleed, metabolic acidosis) is increasing waste nitrogen production derived from degradation of body protein stores; or 2) the patient is noncompliant. If a careful evaluation reveals no abnormality, the patient should be referred to the dietitian for counseling. The formula presented in Table 7-2 illustrates another use for the nitrogen balance relationship. If the urea clearance is known, the steady-state blood urea nitrogen expected for a given protein intake (and level of renal function) can be calculated.

Energy Intake

Although a patient's protein intake can be reliably estimated from the 24-hour UUN excretion (see previous discussion), dietary diaries or recall are the only practical methods for assessing energy intake in the outpatient setting. Their accuracy depends on documenting all foods consumed and the portion size as well as the number of days monitored. Despite these efforts, the clinician must remain cautious when interpreting energy intakes derived from food records because subjects tend to underestimate their actual caloric intake. As a compromise, we have used 3-day food diaries obtained every 3 to 4 months to monitor the energy intake of CRF patients treated with low-protein diets.

As with any dietary intervention, the patient and family members responsible for meal preparation should have a clear understanding of the principles on which dietary therapy is based. They should be trained in meal planning and be familiar with the protein contents of various foods so that compliance and nutritional adequacy can be achieved. Meal planning should also take into account the patient's food preferences, but the assistance of a skilled dietitian must be enlisted. The dietitian can provide sample menus to enhance patient satisfaction and assist in monitoring the patient's nutritional status and dietary compliance. Once patients are comfortable with the diet, we typically see them as outpatients every 3 months to 1) calculate protein intake (and hence compliance) from the 24-hour UUN excretion (see

Table 7-2. Relationship between nitrogen balance, urea nitrogen appearance rate and steady-state blood urea nitrogen[*]

Dietary protein (g/day)	I_N-NUN (g N/day)	Steady-state BUN(mg/dl)
80	10.6	123
60	7.4	86
40	3.9	49

where, $BUN = \dfrac{I_N - 0.031 \text{ g N/kg body weight}}{C_{UREA}} \times 100$

N, nitrogen; I_N, nitrogen intake (16% of protein intake); BUN, blood urea nitrogen; NUN, non-urea nitrogen, which averages 0.031 g N/kg/day; C_{UREA}, urea clearance (l/day).
[*]Calculated for a 70-kg person with a urea clearance of 6 ml/minute (8.6 l/day).

Table 7-1); 2) estimate caloric intake from food recall/diaries; 3) monitor serum albumin, transferrin, and anthropometric values; and 4) use these parameters to provide the patient with feedback regarding dietary adequacy and compliance.

PROTEIN REQUIREMENTS OF PREDIALYSIS PATIENTS

Two dietary regimens have been used to treat patients with progressive CRF: 1) a conventional low-protein diet providing ~0.6 g protein/kg/day; or 2) a VLPD containing ~0.3 g protein/kg/day, supplemented with a mixture of EAA or their nitrogen-free ketoanalogs (i.e., ketoacids [KA]). Because energy expenditures (and hence energy requirements) of CRF patients are comparable to those of normal subjects, 35 kcal/kg/day is usually recommended (see later).

Conventional Low-Protein Diet

Early studies of CRF patients suggested that they could achieve neutral nitrogen balance while consuming ~0.3 g protein/kg/day. This intake represents an intake ~4 SDs below the average requirement for normal subjects, and the results were attributed to reutilization of nitrogen derived from urea degradation to synthesize amino acids and, ultimately, protein. It is now recognized that nitrogen derived from urea does not contribute substantially to protein nutrition in uremia. More recent studies indicate that predialysis CRF patients require ~0.60 g protein/kg/day, an intake similar to the average requirement for normal subjects. To ensure an adequate intake of EAA, approximately two thirds of the protein should be "high biologic value" (e.g. eggs, lean meat).

Essential Amino Acid-Supplemented Diet Regimens

Several studies have evaluated the efficacy and acceptability of a VLPD containing 15 to 25 g/day (~0.3 g protein/kg/day) of unrestricted high-quality protein (essentially vegetarian) plus a supplement of EAA. In general, the VLPD/EAA regimen promptly corrects uremic symptoms while maintaining serum proteins, muscle strength, and nitrogen balance during long-term therapy. In most studies, the supplement provided EAA in the proportions recommended for normal subjects (Table 7-3). Despite the apparent success with these EAA mixtures, a supplement based on the requirements for normal subjects may not be optimal because 1) specific defects in amino acid metabolism have been identified in patients with renal failure; 2) plasma and intracellular concentrations of amino acids in uremic patients differ markedly from normal subjects; and 3) during dietary protein restriction, plasma amino acid levels change in a pattern different from that observed in normal subjects.

For instance, even though tyrosine is not considered an EAA, its synthesis from phenylalanine is impaired in uremia, suggesting that a supplement of tyrosine should be provided. When CRF patients were fed a diet lacking histidine, plasma levels rapidly declined and the patients manifested a syndrome characterized by malaise, an erythematous scaling rash, and negative nitrogen balance. Because supplemental histidine rapidly corrected these abnormalities, histidine should be considered an EAA in uremic patients. Perhaps serine should also be included in the supple-

Table 7-3. Composition of a mixture of amino acids or ketoacid/amino acids given as a supplement to a very-low-protein diet and used to treat patients with chronic renal failure

	Daily intake	
	g/day	g N/day
Composition of amino acid mixture*		
L-Histidine	1.65	0.447
L-Isoleucine	2.10	0.224
L-Leucine	3.30	0.353
L-Lysine	2.40	0.460
L-Methionine	3.30	0.310
L-Phenylalanine	3.30	0.280
L-Threonine	1.50	0.176
L-Tryptophan	0.75	0.103
L-Valine	2.40	0.287
Total	20.70	2.640
Composition of ketoacid mixture "EE"+		
L-Tyrosine	3.62	0.280
L-Threonine	1.78	0.210
L-Ornithine α-ketoisovalerate	1.74	0.196
L-Ornithine α-ketoisocaproate	1.84	0.196
L-Ornithine (R,S) α-keto-B-methylvalerate	1.84	0.196
L-Lysine α-ketoisovalerate	1.84	0.196
L-Lysine α-ketoisocaproate	1.94	0.196
L-Lysine (R,S) α-keto-B-methylvalerate	1.94	0.196
L-Histidine α-ketoisocaproate	1.14	0.112
Calcium D,L α-hydroxy-γ-methylthiobutyrate	0.34	0
Total	18.02	1.778

g N/day, grams of nitrogen per day.
*From Alvestrand A, Furst P, Bergstrom J. Plasma and muscle free amino acids in uremia: influence of nutrition with amino acids. *Clin Nephrol* 1982;18:297–305; and Noree L-O, Bergstrom J. Treatment of chronic uremic patients with protein-poor diet and oral supply of essential amino acids. II. clinical results of long-term treatment. *Clin Nephrol* 1975;3:195–200.
+From Mitch WE, Abras E, Walser M. Long-term effects of a new ketoacid-amino acid supplement in patients with chronic renal failure. *Kidney Int* 1982;22:48–53; and Walser M. Clinical nutrition cases: effect of ketoacid diets in chronic renal failure. *Nutrition Reviews* 1987;45:305–308. Reprinted from Table 8-2 in Maroni BJ. Protein, calories and fat in the predialysis patient. In: Mitch WE, and Klahr S, eds. *Nutrition and the kidney.* 2nd ed. Boston: Little, Brown and Company, 1993;185–212.

ment because it is synthesized primarily in the kidney and plasma levels are low in most patients with renal failure.

Supplements have been tested where the proportions of EAA were modified to include tyrosine and histidine plus a higher proportion of valine. In response to this modified VLPD/EAA regimen, intracellular concentrations of these amino acids normalized and long-term nitrogen balance improved.

Ketoacid-Supplemented Diet Regimens

Several studies have demonstrated that a VLPD supplemented with a mixture of the nitrogen-free ketoanalogs (KA) of EAA reduces uremic symptoms while maintaining serum proteins, anthropometric values, and nitrogen balance during long-term therapy. In the formulation illustrated in Table 7-3, the KA of branched-chain amino acids are provided as salts of basic amino acids (lysine, ornithine, and histidine). In addition, tyrosine and a small amount of threonine and the hydroxy-analog of methionine are provided, but tryptophan and phenylalanine are omitted. When given to patients with severe CRF (average GFR, 4.8 ml/minute) consuming a diet providing 20 to 25 g of mixed-quality protein, urea nitrogen appearance decreased, nitrogen balance remained neutral, and body weight, serum albumin, and transferrin were maintained for 4 to 19 months. A direct comparison of a VLPD providing 0.28 g protein kg/day plus either an isomolar mixture of EAA or KA revealed that either of the diets yielded neutral nitrogen balance even though the KA-based regimen contained ~15% less nitrogen; nitrogen balance with the VLPD/KA diet was due to a greater decrease in urea nitrogen appearance.

The VLPD/KA regimen also improves clinical and biochemical evidence of secondary hyperparathyroidism. Decreased plasma phosphate, alkaline phosphatase, and parathyroid hormone and increased plasma calcium and 1,25-dihydroxycholecalciferol levels as well as amelioration of renal osteodystrophy have been reported. Although the improvement seen with this regimen is likely due in part to the corresponding reduction in dietary phosphorus, inhibition of phosphate absorption may also contribute; calcium salts of KA appear to be as effective in binding dietary phosphorus as $CaCO_3$.

Improvement in metabolic acidosis is an obvious consequence of less hydrogen ion generation from the metabolism of dietary phosphate- and sulfur-containing amino acids. Lessening the catabolic influence of acidosis may also explain part of the beneficial effect of protein-restricted diets on nitrogen metabolism in renal failure. Evidence also suggests that the KA-based regimen improves glucose intolerance in uremia by increasing tissue sensitivity to insulin: fasting hyperglycemia and insulin resistance improved in children treated with this regimen.

In summary, long-term treatment of patients with the VLPD/KA regimen has been shown to maintain nutrition while reducing uremic symptoms and metabolic complications of CRF (e.g., metabolic acidosis, insulin resistance, and secondary hyperparathyroidism). Unfortunately, in contrast to Europe and Japan, KA supplements are not available in the United States. In addition, neither an EAA nor a KA supplement have any nutritional benefit in CRF subjects eating more than the minimal amount of protein (i.e., >35 to 40 g/day); the excess EAA or KA are simply oxidized.

DIETARY PROTEIN PRESCRIPTION

Despite many provocative observations, it has not been proven that dietary protein (or phosphorus) restriction slows the progression of renal failure in humans (see Chapter 10). A reasonable approach is to emphasize control of hypertension initially, aiming for a blood pressure ≤125/75 mm Hg in patients with proteinuria >1 g/day. In proteinuric patients, more aggressive blood pressure control is associated with a slower rate of progression. Angiotensin-converting enzyme inhibitors should be considered first-line therapy because the rate of progression of renal disease is ~50% slower with these agents in both diabetic and nondiabetic patients. In motivated patients who are progressing despite hypertensive control, dietary protein restriction is recommended.

The recommended protein intake for CRF patients is based on 1) the degree of renal insufficiency, 2) the presence of progressive renal failure, 3) the level of proteinuria, and 4) whether glucocorticoids are prescribed. Specific dietary recommendations for patients with diabetic nephropathy are discussed in Chapter 7 and the impact of glucocorticoid therapy on the protein requirements of renal transplant recipients is reviewed in Chapter 14. Consequently, this discussion is limited to the management of predialysis CRF patients with or without the nephrotic syndrome.

Mild Chronic Renal Failure

There are essentially no scientific data to indicate whether dietary protein restriction is beneficial in patients with mild renal insufficiency (GFR >60 ml/minute). These patients typically have serum creatinine levels <2 mg/dl, and unless there is a coexisting systemic illness, they are asymptomatic. The patient should be informed that at this level of renal function, low-protein diets are not typically recommended unless there is evidence of a progressive decline in renal function. Instead, therapy should be directed at controlling hypertension and other coexisting problems, such as edema and hyperlipidemia. If the patient desires to institute dietary protein restriction, the recommendations outlined in the subsequent section and Table 7-4 can be initiated. Although dietary modification requires substantial commitment, it can be stated that when properly implemented and monitored, these dietary regimens are safe.

Moderate Chronic Renal Failure

Typically, dietary therapy in the patient with moderate CRF (GFR 25 to 60 ml/minute) is initiated with a conventional low-protein diet providing ~0.6 g protein/kg/day, of which approximately two thirds is provided as high–biologic-value protein (e.g., meat, fish, eggs; see Table 7-4). An advantage of the conventional low-protein diet is that the protein requirement can be achieved using traditional foods.

In patients who progress while consuming the conventional low-protein diet, an essentially vegetarian diet containing ~0.3 g protein/kg/day (~15 to 25 g/day) supplemented with a mixture of

Table 7-4. Recommended intakes of protein, energy and phosphorus for patients with chronic renal failure or the nephrotic syndrome

	Protein (g/kg/day)	Energy[*] (kcal/kg/day)	Phosphorus[+] (mg/kg/day)
Chronic renal failure GFR (ml/min)			
>60	Protein restriction not usually recommended	≥35	No restriction
25–60	0.6 g/kg/day including ≥0.35 g/kg/day of HBV	≥35	≤10
5–25	1. 0.6 g/kg/day including ≥0.35 g/kg/day of HBV or	≥35	≤10
	2. 0.3 g/kg/day supplemented with EAA or KA	≥35	≤9
Nephrotic syndrome GFR (ml/min)			
<60	1. 0.8 g/kg/day (plus 1 g protein/g proteinuria)	≥35	≤12
	2. 0.3 g/kg/day supplemented with EAA or KA (plus 1 g protein/g proteinuria)[++]	≥35	≤9

HBV, high biologic-value protein; EAA, essential amino acid supplement; KA, amino acid-ketoacid supplement; GFR, glomerular filtration rate.
[*]Energy intake recommended for chronic renal failure patients sustaining moderate activity and consuming limited intakes of protein. Energy intake may be cautiously decreased in obese patients (>120% normal weight) or those who gain undesired adiposity with the recommended intake.
[+]Phosphate binders are often needed to maintain normal serum phosphorus.
[++]See text for discussion.

EAA or, if available, KA, may be considered. Because these supplements provide the daily EAA requirement, more variety in food selections may be possible. However, achieving this level of protein restriction while meeting the patient's energy requirements frequently requires the use of low-protein, high-calorie food products. Fortunately, a plethora of these products are now commercially available. Examples include glucose polymers (Polycose; Ross Laboratories, Columbus, Ohio) added to beverages, high-density oral supplements (Suplena; Ross Laboratories, Columbus, Ohio), and low-protein breads, pastas, and cookies (see Chapter 15).

Phosphorus restriction is an essential component of dietary therapy because limiting phosphorus is the initial step in the management of secondary hyperparathyroidism, and studies in both animals and humans suggest that low-phosphorus diets may retard the rate of progression of renal failure. Because there is a rough correlation between dietary protein and phosphorus content, the requirement for phosphate binders is frequently decreased when dietary protein restriction is used. The rationale for phosphorus restriction is discussed in Chapter 4.

Advanced Chronic Renal Failure

The dietary regimens recommended in the preceding section (and Table 7-4) are also indicated for patients with advanced CRF (GFR 5 to 25 ml/minute). At this level of renal function, these regimens reduce both uremic symptoms and the metabolic complications of CRF and can delay the time until end-stage renal disease. They may also slow the rate of loss of renal function, but this is controversial.

With this degree of renal insufficiency, the use of the VLPD/EAA or KA regimens may have several potential advantages. Because these regimens have a lower nitrogen content than the conventional low-protein diet, less waste nitrogen accumulates and patients with more advanced renal failure can be managed conservatively. Second, dietary phosphorus and the requirement for phosphate binders are lower with the VLPD regimens. If KA are not available, the options are to use the conventional low-protein diet containing ~0.6 g protein/kg/day or a VLPD providing ~0.3 g protein/kg/day plus an EAA supplement (see Table 7-4). Because patients with a GFR <10 ml/minute are at the greatest risk for development of malnutrition, they should be closely monitored to ensure an adequate intake and nutritional status.

Nephrotic Syndrome

Because low-protein diets reduce proteinuria and hypercholesterolemia in nephrosis and because proteinuria is a risk factor for progressive renal insufficiency, dietary protein restriction could be used as adjunctive therapy in nephrotic patients (GFR <60 ml/minute). Indeed, it has been demonstrated that a diet providing 0.8 g protein (plus 1 g protein/g proteinuria) and 35 kcal/kg body weight per day yields neutral nitrogen balance in nephrotic patients. Because nitrogen balance was neutral (or positive) regardless of the level of renal function (i.e., GFR 19 to 120 ml/minute) this regimen should be safe even in patients with advanced renal insufficiency. Several long-term studies also indicate that serum albumin levels remain stable or increase when nephrotic patients are prescribed more restrictive diets providing 0.45 to 0.80 g protein/kg/day. A report by Walser and colleagues showed that a VLPD providing ~0.3 g protein/kg/day supplemented with EAA resulted in a nearly complete remission of the nephrotic syndrome in five patients with GFR >30 ml/minute. Taken together, these studies indicate that dietary protein restriction is safe in patients with the nephrotic syndrome. However, we do not recommend using low-protein diets in nephrotic patients with extremely high levels of proteinuria (>15 g/day) or in patients with catabolic illnesses (e.g., vasculitis, systemic lupus erythematosus) or those receiving catabolic medications (e.g., glucocorticoids), because safety has not been demonstrated in these settings.

End-Stage Renal Failure

When the GFR declines below 5 ml/minute, uremic symptoms may develop despite dietary protein restriction, and anorexia can place the patient at increased risk for malnutrition. It is usually advisable to initiate dialysis or renal transplantation at this stage.

ENERGY METABOLISM IN CHRONIC RENAL FAILURE PATIENTS

Influence of Energy Metabolism on Protein Turnover

Energy intake influences nitrogen metabolism. For example, when the energy intake of CRF patients was varied from 15 to 45 kcal/kg/day while their protein intake remained constant at 0.55 to 0.60 g/kg/day, nitrogen balance became more positive as energy intake increased. Moreover, urea nitrogen appearance correlated inversely with energy intake (Fig. 7-5). Because protein intake remained constant, the decrease in urea nitrogen appearance means that an increase in energy intake improves protein utilization in CRF patients. Conversely, subjects consuming low-protein diets are at risk of catabolizing body protein if their energy intake is inadequate.

Abnormal lipid metabolism can adversely affect protein turnover in CRF. In CRF rats fed ad libitum, body adiposity was subnormal and correlated inversely with muscle protein degradation, suggesting that insufficient lipid stores may adversely affect protein metabolism. With respect to carbohydrate metabolism, lactate production from uremic muscle is highly correlated with protein degradation, suggesting that abnormal regulation of muscle protein turnover may be a consequence of defective glucose utilization. Finally, metabolic acidosis can impair energy metabolism by inducing insulin resistance and impairing triglyceride utilization. These results emphasize the importance of ensuring an adequate caloric intake and correcting metabolic acidosis in CRF patients.

Energy Requirements in Chronic Renal Failure

In CRF patients, energy expenditures (and hence energy requirements) at rest and during exercise are similar to those of healthy subjects. An energy intake of ~35 kcal/kg/day is recommended because this intake can maintain serum proteins, anthropometric values, and nitrogen balance in patients con-

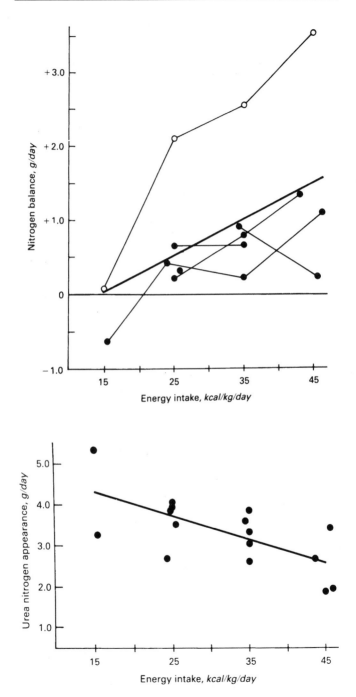

suming protein-restricted diets (see Table 7-4). The energy prescription is commonly calculated using the patient's ideal body weight because actual body weight may overestimate or underestimate energy requirements in obese or malnourished people, respectively. In the elderly, the obese, or patients with undesired weight gain, a lower energy intake may be cautiously prescribed (e.g., ~30 kcal/kg/day).

Energy intake and nutritional status must be monitored regularly. If evidence of energy deficiency (e.g., decreased serum albumin or transferrin, unintentional weight loss, or declining anthropometric values) or positive energy balance (e.g., undesired weight gain or increased skinfold thickness) occurs, the energy intake can be modified accordingly. To improve dietary intake, counseling sessions with the renal dietitian are beneficial. If attempts at increasing energy intake using conventional foods are unsuccessful, a number of high-energy/low-protein products are available (see earlier, and Chapter 15).

ABNORMALITIES IN GLUCOSE AND LIPID METABOLISM

Glucose Metabolism

Uremic subjects exhibit glucose intolerance, fasting hyperglycemia, and hyperinsulinemia. The major abnormality resides in peripheral tissues and is characterized by decreased glucose uptake by skeletal muscle and adipose tissue, both in the basal state and during insulin stimulation. In contrast, hepatic glucose production is normal and suppresses appropriately in response to insulin.

The predominant abnormality appears to lie at some point beyond the interaction of insulin with its receptor (i.e., postreceptor defect). The possibility of a circulating factor causing insulin resistance is suggested by 1) the ability of uremic serum to inhibit insulin-stimulated glucose metabolism, lipogenesis, and amino acid uptake in normal adipocytes and hepatocytes; and 2) improved glucose utilization after dietary protein restriction or hemodialysis. Candidates for this uremic factor include a partially purified peptide and parathyroid hormone.

Prevention or correction of secondary hyperparathyroidism improves glucose tolerance. The defect appears to result from an impairment of insulin secretion, caused by increased calcium entry into pancreatic islet cells. Notably, chronic administration of the calcium channel blocker verapamil normalizes intracellular calcium, insulin secretion, and glucose tolerance.

Exercise has a beneficial effect on glucose intolerance in uremic patients, and in rats with moderate renal insufficiency, a

Fig. 7-5. The correlation between energy intake and (a) nitrogen balance or (b) urea nitrogen appearance in six nondialyzed patients with chronic renal failure (CRF). The heavy diagonal line in both figures represents the least-squares regression equation. As energy intake is increased nitrogen balance becomes more positive (a). Energy intake is inversely correlated with urea nitrogen appearance (b). (From Kopple JD, Monteon FJ, Shaib JK. Effect of energy intake on nitrogen metabolism in nondialyzed patients with chronic renal failure. *Kidney Int* 1986;29:734–742, with permission.)

regular exercise regimen increases insulin sensitivity and responsiveness in muscle. This beneficial effect on glucose metabolism can now be added to the growing list of favorable benefits that exercise imparts on intermediary metabolism.

Lipid Metabolism

Hyperlipidemia is common in uremic patients, with a prevalence of 20% to 70%. The predominant abnormality in non-nephrotic CRF and hemodialysis patients is hypertriglyceridemia, with increased very–low-density lipoproteins (VLDL), decreased high-density lipoprotein (HDL) cholesterol, and normal to low-normal levels of low-density lipoproteins (LDL)—that is, a type IV hyperlipoproteinemia pattern. In addition to uremia, other factors including a genetic predisposition, gender, steroid therapy, and proteinuria can influence the lipoprotein pattern.

Uremic hypertriglyceridemia is due primarily to defective catabolism of triglyceride-rich lipoproteins. Lipoprotein lipase and hepatic triglyceride lipase activity are decreased by uremia, and a circulating inhibitor of lipoprotein lipase has been isolated. The levels of apolipoprotein C-II, the main activator of lipoprotein lipase, have been reported to be decreased in CRF patients. Metabolic acidosis and hyperinsulinemia are associated with uremia, and both depress lipoprotein lipase activity. Finally, secondary hyperparathyroidism may contribute to hypertriglyceridemia in uremia; parathyroidectomized, chronically uremic dogs exhibit normal serum levels of triglycerides, postheparin lipolytic activity, and intravenous fat tolerance. Conversion of triglyceride-rich VLDL to LDL is also defective in patients with CRF, resulting in the accumulation of potentially atherogenic intermediate-density lipoproteins (IDL). Although decreased catabolism of triglyceride-rich lipoproteins is the predominant abnormality, increased triglyceride production also contributes to uremic hypertriglyceridemia. Despite equivalent chylomicron clearance rates, hemodialysis patients exhibit higher fasting serum triglyceride levels than control subjects.

Most patients with the nephrotic syndrome have elevated plasma levels of total, LDL, and VLDL cholesterol, normal or low levels of HDL cholesterol, and normal or elevated triglycerides (i.e., types IIa, IIb, or V hyperlipoproteinemia). Early in the course of the nephrotic syndrome, there is overproduction of VLDL, which is then rapidly catabolized to LDL; LDL clearance may also be impaired, especially in severely nephrotic patients. The most likely explanation for hypertriglyceridemia is decreased clearance of triglyceride-rich VLDL particles.

Previous attempts to identify the signal causing increased lipoprotein synthesis in patients with the nephrotic syndrome suggested that the reduction in plasma oncotic pressure or viscosity acted as a generalized stimulus to hepatic protein synthesis. This viewpoint was challenged by a report that the serum cholesterol concentration may be regulated independently of the rate of albumin synthesis. Rather, serum cholesterol was correlated with the rate of urinary albumin losses. Urinary albumin losses or loss of another liporegulatory substance seem to be responsible for hyperlipidemia in the nephrotic syndrome.

Treatment of Hyperlipidemia

In patients with renal disease, it is unclear whether hyperlipidemia increases the risk of atherosclerosis or whether therapy designed to lower lipid levels is beneficial. Proponents of lipid-lowering therapy cite epidemiologic studies linking an elevated serum cholesterol with accelerated atherosclerosis, and the reduction in coronary artery disease occurring in primary and secondary intervention trials of otherwise healthy subjects.

Despite the lack of conclusive data demonstrating a benefit of lipid-lowering therapy in patients with renal failure, some general guidelines can be provided. Diet modification should remain the initial step in the management of hyperlipidemia. The National Cholesterol Education Program guidelines seem appropriate for hyperlipidemic renal patients. Patients with a total cholesterol >200 mg/dl on two occasions should be instructed in a Step I American Heart Association diet providing <30% of total calories from fat (with <10% of calories from saturated fat) and <300 mg cholesterol daily. People should be encouraged to eliminate other cardiovascular risk factors, such as smoking, obesity, and hypertension. Improved glycemic control in diabetic patients and avoiding excessive alcohol intake would also seem prudent. A lipoprotein profile should be obtained in patients with a total cholesterol >240 mg/dl or between 200 to 239 mg/dl plus two risk factors (i.e., HDL cholesterol <35 mg/dl, documented coronary artery disease or a family history of coronary artery disease before age 55 years, history of cerebrovascular or peripheral vascular disease, diabetes mellitus, severe obesity, male sex, or cigarette smoking). If the LDL cholesterol remains >190 mg/dl (or 160 mg/dl with two risk factors) after 6 months of dietary modification, drug therapy should be considered.

Despite dietary modification, a number of patients (particularly nephrotic and renal transplant patients) continue to have serum cholesterol levels above the desirable range (i.e., LDL cholesterol <130 mg/dl). Because these drugs can be given once daily, are potent, and have a favorable side effect profile, 3-hydroxy-3-methylglutaryl coenzyme A (HMG-CoA) reductase inhibitors should be considered for initial therapy. HMG-CoA reductase inhibitors inhibit cholesterol synthesis, which results in a compensatory increase in hepatic LDL receptor activity; these agents may also decrease hepatic production of LDL cholesterol. The increased LDL receptor activity lowers LDL cholesterol levels by increasing hepatic uptake of LDL and its precursors, IDL and VLDL. The increased removal of IDL and VLDL explains the modest decrease in triglycerides observed with these agents. Although early experience suggested that HMG-CoA reductase inhibitors may be associated with an increased risk of hepatotoxicity and myopathy (and occasionally myoglobinuria) in CRF patients, in general these agents are well tolerated. Besides decreased LDL cholesterol levels, there may be a favorable immunosuppressive effect of HMG-CoA reductase inhibitors in transplant patients. Use of the agents after cardiac transplantation was associated with a decrease in serum cholesterol, acute rejection episodes, and coronary vasculopathy, and an improved 1-year survival rate; a similar benefit on lipids and the frequency of acute rejection episodes has been reported in renal transplant recipients.

In patients refractory to monotherapy, the combination of an HMG-CoA reductase inhibitor with either a bile acid sequestrant or nicotinic acid may be considered. Creatine phosphokinase levels should be monitored when nicotinic acid, gemfibrozil, or cyclosporin A are used concomitantly with HMG-CoA reductase inhibitors because rhabdomyolysis appears to be more common in this setting. Bile acid sequestrants interfere with cyclosporin A absorption and should not be used in transplant patients receiving this immunosuppressive agent. Constipation and abdominal gas are also troublesome side effects and the need for multiple daily dosing may compromise compliance. Probucol has been reported to reduce total and LDL cholesterol in nephrotic patients, although this may be associated with a concomitant reduction in HDL cholesterol. Animal studies suggest that an additional benefit of probucol may relate to its ability to retard the development of atherosclerosis by a mechanism that is independent of its antihyperlipidemic action.

The fibric acids, clofibrate and gemfibrozil, mainly reduce serum triglycerides (LDL cholesterol may actually increase). In view of the increased risk of myopathy reported in nephrotic patients receiving clofibrate, their use in uremic hyperlipidemia seems inadvisable.

CONCLUSION

In summary, the nutritional management of the CRF patient requires a dietary prescription based on each patient's protein and energy requirements. Dietary compliance and nutritional adequacy must be monitored regularly, and the importance of any adequate energy intake cannot be overemphasized. Although successful dietary therapy requires motivation, the opportunity to have some "control" over their illness is welcomed by many patients. Tangible rewards include a reduction in uremic symptoms and metabolic complications and possibly slowing the progression of renal failure.

ACKNOWLEDGMENTS

This work was supported in part by National Institutes of Health grants DK40907, DK49243, and DK45215.

SELECTED READINGS

Coresh J, Walser M, Hill S. Survival on dialysis among chronic renal failure patients treated with a supplemented low-protein diet before dialysis. *J Am Soc Nephrol* 1996;6:1379–1385.

FAO/WHO/UNU. *Energy and protein requirements*. Technical Report Series 724. Geneva: World Health Organization; 1985:1–206.

Goodship THJ, Mitch WE, Hoerr RA, et al. Adaptation to low-protein diets in renal failure: leucine turnover and nitrogen balance. *J Am Soc Nephrol* 1990;1:66–75.

Ikizler TA, Greene JH, Wingard RL, et al. Spontaneous dietary protein intake during progression of chronic renal failure. *J Am Soc Nephrol* 1995;6:1386–1391.

Kaysen GA. Albumin metabolism in the nephrotic syndrome: the effect of dietary protein intake. *Am J Kidney Dis* 1988;12:461–480.

Kaysen GA, Rathore V, Shearer GC, et al. Mechanisms of hypoalbuminemia in hemodialysis patients. *Kidney Int* 1995;48:510–516.

Kopple JD, Levey AS, Greene T, Chumlea WC, Gassman J, Hollinger DL, Maroni BJ, Merrill D, Scherch LK, Shulman G, Wang S, Zimmer GS for the Modification of Diet in Renal Disease Study Group. Effect of dietary protein restriction on nutritional status in the Modification of Diet in Renal Disease study. *Kidney Int* 1997;52:778–791.

Kopple JD, Coburn JW. Metabolic studies of low protein diets in uremia: I. nitrogen and potassium. *Medicine* 1973;52:583–595.

Kopple JD, Monteon FJ, Shaib JK. Effect of energy intake on nitrogen metabolism in nondialyzed patients with chronic renal failure. *Kidney Int* 1986;29:734–742.

Maroni BJ, Staffeld C, Young VR, et al. Mechanisms permitting nephrotic patients to achieve nitrogen equilibrium with a protein-restricted diet. *J Clin Invest* 1997;99:2479–2487.

Maroni BJ, Steinman T, Mitch WE. A method for estimating nitrogen intake of patients with chronic renal failure. *Kidney Int* 1985;27:58–65.

Maschio G, Alberti D, Janin G, et al. Effect of the angiotensin-converting-enzyme inhibitor benazepril on the progression of chronic renal insufficiency. *N Engl J Med* 1996;334:939–945.

Mitch WE, Abras E, Walser M. Long-term effects of a new ketoacid-amino acid supplement in patients with chronic renal failure. *Kidney Int* 1982;22:48–53.

Monteon FJ, Laidlaw SA, Shaib JK, et al. Energy expenditure in patients with chronic renal failure. *Kidney Int* 1986;30:741–747.

Owen WF Jr, Lew NL, Yan Liu SM, et al. The urea reduction ratio and serum albumin concentration as predictors of mortality in patients undergoing hemodialysis. *N Engl J Med* 1993;329:1001–1006.

Peterson JC, Adler S, Burkart JM, et al. Blood pressure control, proteinuria and the progression of renal disease. *Ann Intern Med* 1995;123:754–762.

Reaich D, Channon SM, Scrimgeour CM, et al. Correction of acidosis in humans with CRF decreases protein degradation and amino acid oxidation. *Am J Physiol* 1993;265:E230–E235.

Tom K, Young VR, Chapman T, et al. Long-term adaptive responses to dietary protein restriction in chronic renal failure. *Am J Physiol* 1994;268:E668–E677.

Walser M. Does prolonged protein restriction preceding dialysis lead to protein malnutrition at the onset of dialysis? *Kidney Int* 1993;44:1139–1144.

Walser M, Hill S, Tomalis EA. Treatment of nephrotic adults with a supplemented, very low-protein diet. *Am J Kidney Dis* 1996;28:354–364.

Nutritional Requirements of Diabetics with Nephropathy

Hassan N. Ibrahim, Karl A. Nath, and
Thomas H. Hostetter

Diabetes mellitus and chronic renal insufficiency lead to multiple derangements in intermediary metabolism. Their combination, occurring in the course of diabetic nephropathy, imposes a spectrum of metabolic disturbances that impairs the utilization of nutrients and promotes protein-calorie malnutrition. Dialytic procedures used in the therapy of end-stage diabetic nephropathy, although partially reversing the uremic milieu, incur a loss of nutrients and protein and may contribute to malnutrition in the diabetic patient.

This chapter surveys the metabolic alterations in carbohydrate, protein, and fat metabolism in diabetics with advancing diabetic nephropathy and those undergoing dialytic treatment and the evidence that dietary manipulation may retard the progression of diabetic renal disease. These considerations are used to suggest dietary guidelines for the diabetic patient with renal disease.

METABOLIC DERANGEMENTS IN DIABETIC NEPHROPATHY

To provide an overview of the metabolic disturbances in diabetic nephropathy, the following sections review the alterations in intermediary metabolism arising in diabetes mellitus, the derangements occurring in uremia, and, when available, the specific data regarding derangements in metabolism occurring in the course of diabetic nephropathy.

Glucose Metabolism

The type I insulin-dependent diabetic patient is characterized by a severe deficiency in insulin secretion and a resistance to the cellular uptake of glucose in response to exogenously administered insulin. Patients with type II non–insulin-dependent diabetes mellitus exhibit normal or augmented fasting insulin levels and a resistance in peripheral tissues to the stimulatory effect of insulin on glucose metabolism. In addition, some type II diabetics exhibit a defect in glucose recognition by the β cells of the pancreatic islet. In both insulin-dependent and non–insulin-dependent patients, glucagon levels are increased, relative to insulin levels, or in absolute concentration; the augmented glucagon levels increase hepatic production of glucose. Thus, the characteristic hyperglycemia of the diabetic state involves diminished cellular uptake and utilization of glucose and increased hepatic release of glucose caused by enhanced gluconeogenesis or glycogenolysis.

The mechanisms underlying insulin resistance that occur in diabetes and other states have received much attention and were reviewed in detail. There is renewed interest in the mechanism proposed in 1963 by Randle and colleagues, the so-called glucose–fatty acid cycle, as a factor in the development of insulin resistance. According to this thesis, elevated levels of fatty acids compromise glucose uptake, glucose oxidation, and pyruvate oxidation, the latter through the inhibitory effects of fatty acids on pyruvate dehydrogenase. By such metabolic effects, elevated levels of free fatty acids, as occur in diabetes and obesity, may contribute to the diminished sensitivity to insulin observed in these states.

The uremic state, like diabetes, predisposes patients to fasting hyperglycemia and glucose intolerance. The dominant mechanism accounting for glucose intolerance is peripheral resistance to the effects of insulin, as clearly demonstrated by the data of Smith and DeFronzo (Fig. 8-1). Using the euglycemic insulin clamp technique, these workers constructed in vivo dose–response curves relating total body insulin-mediated glucose metabolism to plasma insulin concentration in chronically uremic and control subjects. With this technique, glucose is infused to maintain the plasma glucose at a constant level as the plasma insulin level is gradually increased with exogenously administered insulin. In the steady state, glucose utilization equals glucose input. The latter is the sum of exogenously administered glucose and endogenously produced glucose, which can be estimated from kinetic studies with tritiated glucose. Uremic subjects exhibit less glucose utilization at all levels of insulin and lower maximal rates of glucose metabolism compared with normal subjects, findings indicative of insulin resistance.

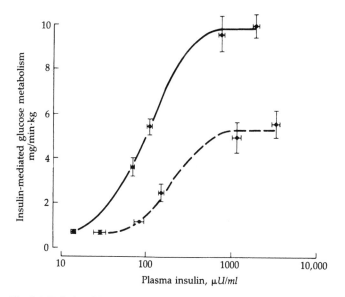

Fig. 8-1. Relationship between insulin-mediated glucose metabolism and plasma insulin concentration in uremic patients (broken line) and in healthy control subjects (solid line). (From Smith D, DeFronzo RA. Insulin resistance in uremia mediated by postbinding defects. *Kidney Int* 1982;22:54. Used with permission from *Kidney International.*)

In nondiabetic uremia, insulin resistance resides at the postreceptor level. For example, adipocytes from uremic subjects display normal insulin binding but diminished glucose uptake and conversion to lipids. The mechanisms accounting for peripheral insulin resistance are unknown and may involve uremic toxins, acidosis, or hormones that are elevated in uremia such as parathyroid hormone (PTH) and glucagon. That the uremic environment per se induces insulin resistance is indicated by in vitro studies demonstrating that tissue utilization of glucose is impaired in the presence of uremic serum. Studies in patients demonstrate that maintenance hemodialysis partially repairs glucose tolerance and increases insulin sensitivity. The reversal of insulin resistance by a low-protein diet suggests that some metabolite generated in the course of altered protein metabolism in uremia may be responsible. The efficacy of protein-restricted diets in ameliorating insulin resistance has been demonstrated in nondiabetic and diabetic preterminal uremic patients. In these patients, the administration of a low-protein diet supplemented with an α-ketoacid mixture leads to increased tissue sensitivity to insulin as measured by the euglycemic clamp technique. In this study, the diets decrease the tissue requirements for insulin in the diabetic patient.

A study by Schmitz specifically examined insulin resistance in uremic diabetic patients. Using a three-step, euglycemic, insulin clamp technique, he demonstrated that sensitivity to insulin, reflected in the glucose infusion rate, was more compromised in nondialyzed, uremic, insulin-dependent subjects than in nondiabetic uremic subjects or in insulin-dependent subjects with normal renal function (Fig. 8-2). Thus, the combined lesions of insulin-dependent diabetes plus uremia impart a degree of insulin resistance that is greater than in either disease state alone. It is interesting that this study also demonstrated that the improvement in insulin resistance in uremic, insulin-dependent diabetic subjects is greater when treated by continuous ambulatory peritoneal dialysis (CAPD) than by hemodialysis. Although CAPD leads to a greater glucose load than hemodialysis, it is unlikely that differences in the glucose delivered account for the differences in insulin sensitivity; a more likely explanation involves the route of insulin delivery in CAPD. Administration of insulin by the intraperitoneal and thus intraportal route, instead of the conventional routes, leads to lower peripheral insulin levels. Peripheral hyperinsulinemia has been increasingly implicated as a cause of insulin resistance. Given these considerations, Schmitz suggested that CAPD, with intraportal delivery of insulin, leads to lower peripheral insulin levels and improved insulin sensitivity.

Other mechanisms besides peripheral insulin resistance contribute to glucose intolerance in the nondiabetic uremic state. DeFronzo and colleagues showed a varying degree of impairment in the insulin secretory response to a glucose load in nondiabetic uremics. Such β-cell dysfunction superimposed on peripheral insulin resistance would exacerbate fasting hyperglycemia and glucose intolerance. Decreased insulin secretion by pancreatic β cells may arise from a defect in glucose metabolism by these cells. Studies by Fadda and colleagues demonstrated that the elevated levels of PTH in uremia lead to increased

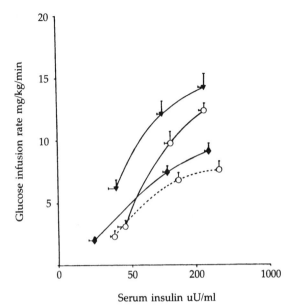

**Fig. 8-2. Relationship between glucose infusion rate
and serum insulin concentration in healthy subjects (solid lines,
closed triangles), in insulin-dependent diabetic subjects with
normal renal function (solid lines, open circles), in nondiabetic
uremic subjects (solid lines, closed diamonds), and in nondialyzed,
uremic, insulin-dependent diabetic patients (broken line, open
circles). Insulin was administered in increasing doses, and
euglycemia was maintained by exogenously administered glucose.
The amount of glucose required to maintain euglycemia over the
last 30 minutes of each insulin infusion represents the glucose
infusion rate and is a measure of tissue sensitivity to insulin.**
(From Schmitz O. Insulin-mediated glucose uptake in non-dialyzed
and dialyzed uremic insulin-dependent diabetic subjects. *Diabetes*
1985;34:1152. Copyright 1985 by American Diabetes Association, Inc.)

intracellular calcium in the β cell, with attendant reductions in
adenosine triphosphate (ATP) levels; glucose metabolism and, in
turn, glucose-triggered insulin secretion are impaired.
Compromised insulin secretion may also reflect decreased levels
of 1,25-dihydroxycholecalciferol that occur in uremia. For example, acute administration of 1,25-dihydroxycholecalciferol to
patients on hemodialysis, in the absence of changes in serum
PTH or calcium levels, increases insulin levels and improves glucose tolerance. This secretory defect, like peripheral resistance,
is also improved with dialysis. These workers also demonstrated
that hepatic glucose uptake and suppression of hepatic glucose
production by insulin are both normal in nondiabetic uremic
subjects, but that hepatic glucose production from gluconeogenesis is increased in nondiabetic uremia. Glucagon most likely is
the stimulus for augmented gluconeogenesis because this hor-

mone is elevated in nondiabetic uremia, and administration of glucagon to uremic subjects evokes a further elevation in plasma glucose. Thus, enhanced gluconeogenesis and impaired insulin secretory response provide additional mechanisms for glucose intolerance in nondiabetic uremia. Because these metabolic derangements occur as primary defects in diabetes, it is likely but not proved that they will be magnified in diabetic uremia; this has been clearly shown for the peripheral resistance to insulin.

Protein Metabolism

Insulin is the major anabolic hormone, promoting cellular uptake of amino acids and protein synthesis while suppressing cellular efflux of amino acids and protein catabolism. Insulin deficiency, not unexpectedly, is associated with increased protein degradation. For example, withdrawal of insulin therapy in diabetic patients and in animals with experimentally induced diabetes is attended by increased urinary nitrogen loss, which can be reversed with restitution of insulin therapy. The withdrawal of insulin therapy in type I insulin-dependent diabetics leads to marked increments in whole-body protein degradation and leucine oxidation. Interestingly, in these patients, albumin synthesis, in all likelihood an insulin-sensitive process, is decreased, whereas fibrinogen synthesis, an acute-phase response, is increased. These observations suggest that the production of albumin is an insulin-dependent process, and indicate the differential effects resulting from a deficiency of insulin on the net synthesis of specific proteins. Different organs may also exhibit varying dependency on the anabolic effects of insulin, as suggested by a study by Nair and colleagues of whole-body protein metabolism in poorly controlled type I diabetics. Surprisingly, rates of both protein synthesis and protein degradation were increased, but protein catabolism exceeded anabolism, resulting in a net loss of total body protein stores. The authors concluded that compensatory increments in protein synthesis occur in viscera such as liver and gut, which are relatively less dependent on the anabolic effects of insulin, but that such increments fail to repair the negative nitrogen balance caused by increased protein degradation.

The tendency toward protein wasting in insulin-deficient diabetic patients may arise, at least in part, from derangements in interorgan transport of amino acids. In normal humans in the postabsorptive state, amino acids, primarily alanine and glutamine, are released from muscle. Alanine is taken up the liver, where it is converted into glucose, whereas glutamine is primarily used in intestine and kidney to generate ammonia.

Alanine released from muscle is formed by the transamination of pyruvate with nitrogen derived from the branched-chain amino acids, leucine, isoleucine, and valine. After a protein meal, this negative nitrogen balance in muscle is reversed; branched-chain amino acids exhibit the greatest postprandial rise in the systemic circulation because the liver has a limited capacity for transamination of branched-chain amino acids compared with most other amino acids. Thus, branched-chain amino acids escape hepatic degradation and appear in the systemic circulation in increased amounts. On the other hand, skeletal muscle has considerable capacity for the uptake and transamination of these branched-chain amino acids. Increased muscle utilization of these amino acids, stimulated by the surge of insulin that follows a protein load in normal subjects, replenishes the nitrogen loss from muscle in the fasting state.

Studies of insulin-dependent diabetics revealed derangements in interorgan amino acid flux. First, in the fasting state, diabetics exhibit a lower arterial concentration of alanine because of increased splanchnic extraction of alanine and subsequent conversion to glucose in the liver. Alanine is siphoned off from muscle and used for hepatic glucose production in increased amounts. Second, fasting levels of all branched-chain amino acids are elevated because of a decrease in their metabolic clearance as a consequence of insulin deficiency. After protein feeding, the expected increase in skeletal muscle uptake of branched-chain amino acids fails to occur in insulin-dependent diabetics. In these subjects, insulin deficiency promotes negative nitrogen balance even in the fed state.

Improved metabolic control with subcutaneous continuous insulin infusion leads to normalization of the branched-chain amino acid levels. Although this effect suggests that the tendency to negative protein balance in skeletal muscle may be corrected with insulin, such conclusions should be tempered by the demonstration that deranged intracellular pools of amino acids persist even after correction of plasma levels of amino acid with insulin therapy, and such intracellular alterations may be a more important determinant of impaired protein synthesis. Such failure of insulin to increase skeletal muscle and whole-body protein synthesis in type I insulin-dependent diabetics occurs even when plasma levels of amino acids are maintained in the normal range. Furthermore, type I insulin-dependent diabetics exhibit defective insulin suppression of leucine-carbon appearance and oxidation as well as proteolysis. Thus, derangements in protein metabolism in insulin-dependent diabetics cannot be ascribed simply to a deficiency of insulin.

Although the specific derangements in protein metabolism in patients with diabetic nephropathy have not been examined, chronic, nondiabetic uremia, like the diabetic state, predisposes to loss of skeletal muscle mass and a tendency toward negative nitrogen balance. That the uremic state per se leads to abnormalities in protein turnover is supported by studies demonstrating a deficient cellular uptake of amino acids and protein synthesis in the presence of uremic serum. Skeletal muscle preparations from chronically uremic rats exhibit an increased efflux of several amino acids, including alanine, glutamine, and tyrosine, compared with control animals, a finding that is consistent with augmented rates of skeletal muscle degradation in chronic uremia.

The mechanisms underlying the abnormal rates of muscle protein turnover in chronic uremia do not appear to involve insulin resistance, unlike the situation in acute experimental uremia, in which insulin resistance has been demonstrated. The capacity for insulin to promote the cellular uptake of amino acids in incubated muscle preparations from chronically uremic animals is intact. Studies in nondiabetic uremic patients demonstrated that although the fasting levels of leucine and valine are reduced, the decline in the concentrations of these branched-chain amino acids after insulin is normal. The uremic state differs from the diabetic state, therefore, in that the cellular uptake of branched-chain amino acids in muscle tissue is intact. It is interesting that peripheral resistance to insulin in experimental chronic uremia can be induced with either starvation or a high-protein diet. These observations may be clinically relevant. A deficient nutrient and caloric intake may promote muscle breakdown by inducing a failure of insulin to suppress proteolysis. On the other hand, high-protein diets could exacerbate the uremic state, not only by providing increased nitrogen but by attenuating the capacity of insulin to suppress muscle breakdown.

Metabolic alterations in uremia that appear to promote protein degradation in muscle include increased levels of PTH and glucagon, assorted uremic toxins, and metabolic acidosis. The importance of metabolic acidosis as a specific stimulus to protein catabolism was demonstrated by the studies of May and colleagues. Skeletal muscle from rats with chronic metabolic acidosis exhibited increased proteolysis but no alteration in protein synthesis. In addition, correction of the acidosis of chronic uremia with alkali therapy prevented the excess proteolysis of uremia. Correction of metabolic acidosis in uremic, nondialyzed patients by bicarbonate supplements has also been shown to improve nitrogen balance. Because several types of metabolic acidosis complicate the diabetic state even in the absence of significant renal dysfunction, acidosis-induced proteolysis may be an important mechanism of muscle wasting throughout the natural history of diabetic nephropathy.

The importance of metabolic acidosis in provoking protein degradation was emphasized by Williams and colleagues. These workers demonstrated that in patients with chronic renal failure (mean glomerular filtration rate [GFR] 12.8 ml/minute) and mild acidosis (mean plasma bicarbonate, 17 mEq/l), dietary protein restriction leads to decreased urinary nitrogen losses but increased skeletal muscle breakdown as reflected by urinary excretion of 3-methylhistidine, if the acidosis is left untreated. However, bicarbonate supplementation, concomitant with dietary protein restriction, that achieves normalization of serum bicarbonate prevents such muscle breakdown (Fig. 8-3).

These findings indicate that persisting metabolic acidosis may overwhelm the metabolic adaptation that preserves nitrogen balance when dietary protein restriction is imposed. Metabolic acidosis may thus prove particularly harmful to protein balance in the diabetic patient on a restricted protein intake.

More recently, Mitch and colleagues (reviewed by Mitch and Goldberg) described the pathway responsible for accelerated proteolysis in catabolic conditions, including acidosis. This has been identified as the ubiquitin–proteasome system. In studies of rats in the fasting state or acidosis, accelerated proteolysis is not inhibited when atrophying muscles are incubated in vitro with agents that block the activity of lysosomal or calcium-activated proteases. However, inhibitors of ATP production eliminate the difference in protein degradation between atrophying and normal muscles. This, at least partially, explains the poor growth of rats with acidosis through this newly described nonlysosomal proteolytic pathway that requires ATP.

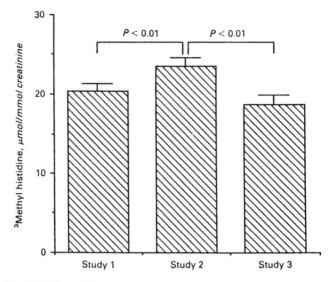

Fig. 8-3. **Effect of dietary protein restriction and dietary protein restriction with concomitant bicarbonate supplementation on skeletal muscle myofibrillar protein degradation as reflected by urinary excretory rates for 3-methylhistidine. Such excretory rates were determined in patients with chronic renal failure and patients with mild metabolic acidosis on an unrestricted protein diet (study 1), after dietary protein restriction only (study 2), and after dietary protein restriction and treatment with sodium bicarbonate, such that the serum bicarbonate was normalized (study 3).** (From Williams B, et al. Metabolic acidosis and skeletal muscle adaptation to low-protein diets in chronic uremia. *Kidney Int* 1991;40:779. Used with permission from *Kidney International*.)

In uremia, alterations in plasma levels of several amino acids in addition to branched-chain amino acids occur. For example, the tyrosine-to-phenylalanine ratio is decreased because of suppressed activity of phenylalanine hydroxylase. In general, nonessential amino acids are elevated, whereas essential acids are decreased. Altered intracellular pools of amino acids, such as decreased valine and tyrosine, have also been recognized in uremia, and in fact appear to correlate more closely with protein synthesis than do alterations in the extracellular amino acid pools. In this regard, the work of Alvestrand and collaborators has proved particularly enlightening. Uremic patients were maintained on one of two dietary regimens for 10 weeks: a low-protein diet supplemented with an essential amino acid preparation containing two to three times the minimum daily requirements for normal humans, or a low-protein diet similarly supplemented with essential amino acids but containing higher amounts of valine and tyrosine. Only the diet with additional valine and tyrosine normalized the intracellular valine concentration, increased the intracellular tyrosine concentration, and improved nitrogen balance. Thus, abnormalities in the intracellular amino acid pools occur in the uremic state and influence nitrogen balance. Interestingly, in patients on maintenance hemodialysis without clinical evidence of protein malnutrition, hemodialysis does not fully correct the abnormal intracellular amino acid profile. Part of the explanation may reside in the persisting acidosis that occurs in hemodialysis patients. Bergstrom and associates found that the predialysis and postdialysis plasma bicarbonate concentrations significantly correlated with muscle content of the branched-chain amino acid valine; thus, uremic acidosis may underlie the abnormalities in branched-chain amino acids. Whether specific abnormalities in amino acid pools occur in diabetic uremia is yet to be addressed.

It is clear, therefore, that multiple derangements in protein metabolism arising in diabetic and uremic states conspire to promote negative nitrogen balance. Additional factors such as proteinuria, extrarenal diabetic complications, and the dialytic procedures used in the treatment of end-stage diabetic nephropathy all threaten the maintenance of neutral nitrogen balance.

Lipid Metabolism

Hyperlipidemia is a common metabolic abnormality in diabetes, with a prevalence ranging from 20% to 70%. The pattern of hyperlipidemia is a mild to moderate hypertriglyceridemia, caused by increased very–low-density lipoproteins (VLDL) and, less commonly, mild hypercholesterolemia. Elevated cholesterol levels may arise from increased concentrations of VLDL, low-density lipoproteins (LDL), or high-density lipoproteins (HDL). Hyperlipidemia in diabetes may follow excessive production rates, diminished degradation rates, or both. In insulin-dependent diabetics, lipoprotein lipase activity is decreased because of insulin deficiency, thereby leading to diminished degradation of triglyceride-rich lipoproteins. Additional abnormalities may exist in the interaction between circulating lipoproteins and lipoprotein lipase. Thus, in insulin-dependent diabetics, hypertriglyceridemia is caused primarily by diminished rates of degradation of serum lipoproteins. In type II diabetic patients, the stimulatory effect of insulin on the hepatic production of VLDL is intact, but the ability of insulin to suppress lipolysis in the periphery is impaired. Consequently, increased hepatic delivery of free fatty acids in the presence of insulin, which can be elevated in type II diabetics, leads to an increased production of VLDL and, therefore, hypertriglyceridemia. In addition, some patients exhibit decreased lipoprotein lipase activity, which may contribute to the hypertriglyceridemia.

Overexpression of human lipoprotein lipase was found to protect diabetic transgenic mice from diabetic hypertriglyceridemia and hypercholesterolemia. Moreover, this same strain of mice was resistant to diet-induced hypertriglyceridemia. These sets of studies suggest that lipoprotein lipase determines not only hydrolysis of triglycerides but lipolytic conversion.

Oxidative modification of LDL confers increased cellular toxicity and atherogenicity. Furthermore, LDL oxidation may occur to a greater extent in diabetes. For example, rats rendered diabetic with streptozotocin had increased oxidation of VLDL and LDL plasma fractions. This oxidation was mitigated by scavenging agents such as vitamin E and probucol without altering hyperglycemia. In addition, the cytotoxicity of the lipid fractions was diminished with scavengers. Whether any such antioxidant therapy will have a role in reducing lipid-associated cardiovascular risk in patients with diabetes is yet to be determined.

High-density lipoprotein cholesterol levels are also abnormal in type I and type II diabetics. Before the initiation of insulin therapy in type I diabetics, HDL cholesterol levels are uniformly decreased; with insulin therapy, HDL levels increase into the normal range. Type I diabetics treated with conventional insulin regimens usually display normal to increased levels of HDL. In type II diabetics, however, several studies have demonstrated decreased HDL cholesterol levels, quite independently of the effects of adiposity and hypertriglyceridemia, factors that are usually inversely correlated with HDL cholesterol. Improved glycemic control in type II diabetics has been reported to elevate HDL cholesterol, at least in some studies. Lipoprotein(a) may represent a risk factor for accelerated atherosclerosis. This particle appears to limit clot lysis and could lead to the basis for an atherosclerotic plaque. In fact, epidemiologic studies have linked the plasma level of lipoprotein(a) directly to cardiovascular risk. An independent role in diabetes has not been established, but studies have suggested that strict glycemic control in type I diabetic subjects lowers the plasma lipoprotein(a) level. Thus, in addition to the effects on other lipoproteins, glycemic control may be beneficial by reducing lipoprotein(a).

As renal disease develops in the diabetic patient, further alterations in lipid metabolism occur. Proteinuria and advanced renal insufficiency are associated with decreased HDL cholesterol levels. In long-standing type I insulin-dependent diabetes, total cholesterol and LDL cholesterol levels are inversely correlated with creatinine clearance. Diabetic patients with albuminuria, even when detectable by dipstick, exhibited lower plasma levels of HDL cholesterol, a lower HDL/LDL cholesterol ratio, and higher plasma levels of triglycerides and total LDL cholesterol compared with control diabetic patients with no detectable albuminuria. The fall in HDL associated with renal failure appears to result from disproportionate reductions in its clearance and production, with diminution of the latter prevailing. Such a pattern of events occurs in nondiabetic uremic patients. Thus, the development of proteinuric nephropathy in diabetic patients leads to increased triglyceride levels and decreased HDL cholesterol.

These alterations in the lipid profile in diabetic nephropathy may arise from several mechanisms. Diminished levels of HDL in all likelihood result from increased urinary loss, given the relatively small molecular size of HDL cholesterol (~60,000 daltons); HDL cholesterol has been demonstrated in the urine of animals with proteinuric renal disease. Diminished levels of HDL promote hyperlipidemia by at least two mechanisms. First, less cholesterol is transported from peripheral tissues to be metabolized in the liver and, second, diminished levels of HDL impair the effectiveness of lipoprotein lipase in degrading VLDL. Not infrequently, nephropathy in both type I and type II diabetics is attended by the nephrotic syndrome, which provides additional mechanisms for elevated serum triglycerides and cholesterol. Diminished plasma oncotic pressure as a consequence of hypoalbuminemia stimulates hepatic albumin synthesis and hepatic production of VLDL. Free fatty acid levels are elevated because of diminished binding to albumin and act to suppress the activity of lipoprotein lipase, thereby diminishing the peripheral catabolism of VLDL. However, in studies of rats with nephrotic syndrome due to experimental glomerulonephritis, the hyperlipidemia was largely attributable to a reduced plasma clearance of lipid due in turn to urinary losses of a lipid-lowering substance. The substance was not identified; it is not lipoprotein lipase. In addition, the activity of the lecithin cholesterol acyltransferase enzyme is diminished in nephrotic syndrome. This enzyme catalyzes the esterification of cholesterol, thereby promoting its transport on HDL to the liver; also, lecithin cholesterol acyltransferase is required for the synthesis of HDL. In summary, the hyperlipidemia of diabetic nephropathy and the nephrotic syndrome results from multiple metabolic abnormalities that promote increased synthesis and decreased removal of serum triglycerides and cholesterol.

Acid–Base Metabolism

The diabetic state is frequently complicated by several forms of metabolic acidosis; as discussed previously, acidosis promotes proteolysis. Diabetic ketoacidosis is characterized by increased lipolysis and free fatty acids, yielding increased amounts of acetoacetic acid and β-hydroxybutyric acid. Systemic acidosis stimulates renal ammoniagenesis and the urinary excretion of ammonium. In severe diabetic ketoacidosis, acid excretion in the form of ammonium may be as high as 500 mEq/day; this causes nitrogen depletion and, together with the proteolytic effect of acidosis per se, can cause negative nitrogen balance.

Diabetes mellitus is the disease most frequently associated with type IV renal tubular acidosis (RTA). Diabetic type IV RTA usually occurs in the setting of mild to moderate renal insufficiency, with acidosis and hyperkalemia disproportionately severe for the reduction in GFR. Hypoaldosteronism, at least in part a consequence of hyporeninism, accounts for the failure of potassium secretion by the distal nephron, and hyperkalemia, by suppressing ammoniagenesis, compromises the renal acid excretory capacity, thereby causing systemic acidosis. Other factors contributing to hyperkalemia include hyperglycemia, insulinopenia, and hypoaldosteronism, all of which decrease translocation of potassium from the extracellular to the intracellular space. The mechanisms for hyporeninemia are complex, and include suppression of renin secretion caused by increased extracellular fluid volume, defective sympathetic drive to renin secretion, deficient production of prostaglandins, and destruction of the renin secretory cells in the afferent arteriole from diabetic vascular disease. The development of type IV RTA in diabetes predisposes the patient to protein malnutrition, not only because of the effects of systemic acidosis but because of hyperkalemia, which has been reported to increase nitrogen catabolism.

With advancing diabetic nephropathy, failure of acid excretion becomes apparent with a GFR <40 ml/minute. This constitutes yet another cause for metabolic acidosis in diabetes. Finally, long-standing diabetes is not infrequently complicated by bowel dysfunction, leading to an intestinal loss of bicarbonate, thereby imposing a nonanion-gap metabolic acidosis.

Thus, several types of metabolic acidosis complicate the course of diabetic nephropathy. Acidosis not only may promote proteolysis but may represent an important pathogenetic mechanism in the development of diabetic renal disease. Renal ammoniagenesis is stimulated by acidosis, and excessive renal ammoniagenesis accompanied by elevated renal cortical ammonia levels can trigger the alternative complement pathway, thereby releasing multiple inflammatory mediators. In two models of experimental renal disease, ammonia-triggered, complement-mediated tissue injury has been identified as a pathway for ongoing renal damage. The frequent occurrence of metabolic acidosis in diabetes mellitus and the recognition that acidosis provokes renal injury by stimulating ammonia production raise the possibility that metabolic acidosis may propagate renal injury in diabetic nephropathy.

RETARDING THE PROGRESSION OF DIABETIC NEPHROPATHY

Effect of Glycemic Control

The most direct test of the role of glycemic control on the development of nephropathy was the prospective study of the effects of different levels of glucose control on the development of kidney disease. This was accomplished by a large multicenter study, the Diabetes Complication and Control Trial. In this study of 1400 patients with either newly diagnosed diabetes or incipient diabetic nephropathy, patients were randomly assigned to either of two treatment groups: intensive insulin therapy or less rigorous control. The intensively treated group had a plasma hemoglobin A_{1C} level of 7 mg/dl, and those in the less intensive regimen had a level of 9 mg/dl. Intensive glucose control resulted in a reduction in the progression to diabetic nephropathy (defined as the appearance of microalbuminuria) of about 50% compared with the standard therapy. The incidence of nerve and eye damage was also lessened with rigorous treatment. In other subjects, there was a similar reduction in the rate of progression from microalbuminuria to macroalbuminuria. Thus, this major trial demonstrates the beneficial effects of intensive glycemic control. Short-term studies have also demonstrated beneficial effects of glycemic control on several parameters associated with diabetic nephropathy. For example, intensive insulin therapy can normalize the elevated GFR and renal hypertrophy found at an early stage of diabetes. In incipient diabetic nephropathy, intensive insulin therapy can decrease microalbuminuria. Finally, definitive treatment of the diabetic state with pancreas transplantation can decrease the development of lesions, in particular, mesangial expansion in the transplanted kidney. Long-term follow-up of these patients is needed to confirm the ultimate outcome of these regimens on the development of end-stage renal disease. In experimental models, intensive insulin therapy has been demonstrated to prevent the development of nephropathy and to ameliorate established nephropathy.

Sustained hyperglycemia may injure tissues through multiple pathways, in particular, the fostering of a prooxidant milieu. Clinical studies have demonstrated increased amounts of lipid peroxidation products (a marker of oxidative stress) in plasma, and a proclivity to diabetic complications such as retinopathy in patients with indices of heightened oxidative stress. Indeed, many of the biochemical effects resulting from sustained hyperglycemia perturb the redox state of tissues, promoting a prooxidative environment. As demonstrated by the studies of Wolff and collaborators, glucose, in the presence of transition metals, undergoes autooxidative reactions, thereby giving rise to reactive oxygen species. Generation of reactive species by glucose autooxidation may in turn denature macromolecules such as structural and enzymic proteins and DNA. Glucose in its straight-chain configuration behaves as an aldehyde and glycates proteins and DNA; protein glycation fosters an oxidative milieu not only by impairing antioxidant enzymes such as superoxide dismutase, but by generating reactive oxygen after the glycation process. Another oxidant-related pathway that operates in sustained hyperglycemia is excessive generation of sorbitol. Although excess accumulation of sorbitol may be injurious to tissues through an osmotic effect, increased generation of sorbitol can reduce the availability of reduced nicotinamide adenine dinucleotide phosphate (NADPH) in tissues and compromise the capacity of the glutathione peroxidase system to catabolize hydrogen peroxide generated in the course of oxidative metabolism. These observations offer the possibility that dietary manipulations that are antioxidant in nature may decrease diabetic complications such as nephropathy. Indeed, the administration of vitamin E supplements to insulin-dependent diabetics reduces protein glycation independently of changes in plasma glucose. Fostering a prooxidant state in the kidney by a diet deficient in antioxidants induces renal damage, whereas pyruvate, an α-ketoacid that avidly scavenges hydrogen peroxide, protects against the increase in capillary permeability induced by hyperglycemia.

Effect of Dietary Protein Restriction

There is firm evidence that dietary protein restriction retards renal injury in experimental models of renal disease, including diabetic nephropathy. Zatz and colleagues varied levels of protein intake in rats with streptozotocin-induced diabetes. Animals fed on the lower-protein diet exhibited decreases in kidney weights, single-nephron glomerular filtration and plasma flow rates, and glomerular transcapillary hydraulic pressure gradients. In addition, the authors found markedly lower rates of albumin excretion and significantly less evidence of glomerular sclerosis. They concluded that decreased dietary protein mitigates renal injury in experimental diabetic nephropathy by hemodynamically mediated mechanisms, as has been demonstrated with dietary protein restriction in several other experimental disease models. Specifically, the high glomerular capillary pressures and flows characteristic of diabetes were augmented by excess dietary protein, and the resultant glomerular hypertension, hyperfiltration, and hyperperfusion were injurious to the microcirculation.

The long-term effects of dietary protein restriction have been tested in patients with a variety of renal diseases. A meta-analysis of these trials concluded that low-protein diets are effective in attenuating the progression of renal disease. Unfortunately, diabetic renal disease was relatively underrepresented in most of these studies. However, investigation of dietary protein restriction exclusively in diabetic patients also showed beneficial results. Specifically, Zeller and colleagues conducted a prospective, randomized trial of type I diabetics with overt proteinuria. The subjects assigned to the lower-protein diet had approximately one fourth the rate of decline in GFR of those on the controlled diet when studied over a period of at least 12 months and for an average of 35 months. The protein restriction was prescribed as 0.6 g protein/kg body weight/day, but patients averaged approximately 0.72 g/kg/day, as judged by nitrogen excretion rates. The control subjects ate at an average of 1.08 g/kg/day (Fig. 8-4A). In another study by Walker and associates, the rates of progressive decay in GFR were compared in a group of type I diabetics during a period of normal protein intake and then during a period of restriction to 0.6 g/kg/day. As with the study of Zeller and colleagues, the rate of decline was reduced to about one fourth of the baseline rate when protein restriction was imposed. In both investigations, changes in blood pressure or hemoglobin A_{1C} were not noted. Thus, protein restriction by some effect other than control of arterial hypertension or glycemia seems to reduce the rate of progression of diabetic renal disease.

Dietary protein restriction below 0.6 g/kg body weight, in conjunction with supplementation with essential amino acids or ketoacid analogs of essential amino acids, has been used in an attempt to retard the progression of chronic renal disease. Because 0.6 g protein/kg body weight represents the approximate minimum daily protein requirement for a normal person as well as for a person with renal insufficiency, dietary protein restriction below this level necessitates supplementation with essential amino acids and their ketoacid analogs. Essential amino acids are the most efficiently utilized sources of nitrogen; when supplemented in the diet, they widen the selection of foods by reducing the need for high–biologic-value protein. Ketoacid analogs of essential amino acids are the carbon skeleton of the amino acid without the nitrogen. There are uncontrolled studies demonstrating that these regimens reduce the progression of renal disease. Although their role in diabetic nephropathy requires investigation, there is little reason to believe that the renal effect of these regimens will be different from that in other chronic nephropathies; however, this has not been proved.

In addition to potential benefits in established nephropathy, data suggest that dietary protein restriction, in microalbuminuric insulin-dependent diabetics with high GFR, reduces these rates to the normal range and decreases the rates of albumin excretion. These findings raise the possibility that dietary protein restriction for diabetic patients with predictive indices of impending overt nephropathy might reduce the risk of such a complication. This possibility awaits testing.

The results of the Modification Diet in Renal Disease (MDRD) trial have become available. This prospective, randomized, controlled study with a mean follow-up of 2.2 years evaluated the

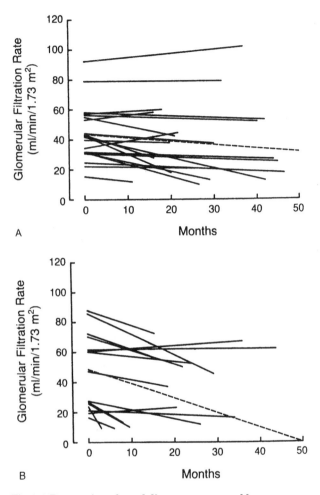

Fig. 8-4. Progression of renal disease as measured by
the rate of decline of glomerular filtration rate in patients with
diabetic nephropathy maintained on a low-protein, low-phosphorus
diet (A) and in patients with diabetic nephropathy with a normal
intake of protein and phosphorus (B). (Reprinted, by permission of
The New England Journal of Medicine. From Zeller K, et al. Effect of
restricting dietary protein on the progression of renal failure in patients
with insulin-dependent diabetes mellitus. *N Engl J Med* 1991;342:78.)

effects of low-protein diet and phosphorus intake together with blood pressure control on the progression of chronic renal disease of different etiologies. Only a small number of patients had type II diabetes. Type I diabetes patients were excluded.

Patients were stratified into two studies based on their GFR: in study 1, 585 patients with a GFR of 25 to 50 ml/minute were randomized to receive either a protein diet of 1.3 g/kg/day or a low-protein diet of 0.58 g/kg/day. The 255 patients who entered study 2 had a GFR of 13 to 24 ml/minute and were randomized to either a low-protein diet as in study 1 or a very–low-protein diet of 0.28 g/kg/day with a ketoacid–amino acid supplement. Patients in both studies were also randomized to receive blood pressure interventions designed to achieve either a mean arterial pressure of 107 mm Hg or low mean arterial pressure of 92 mm Hg. Blood pressure control was achieved using an angiotensin-converting enzyme (ACE) inhibitor with or without a diuretic, followed by the addition of a calcium channel blocker or other medications as needed.

In the MDRD trial, diabetic subjects were not analyzed as a separate group. Based on the rate of GFR as the primary outcome, however, no clearcut difference in the overall mean rate of decline was observed between the diet or blood pressure groups of either study.

However, a meta-analysis by Pedrini and colleagues of randomized, controlled studies of diabetic and nondiabetic renal disease (total of 10 studies) showed that dietary protein restriction slows the progression of kidney disease in both types of renal disease. The small number of diabetic patients included in the analysis and the varied study designs led these investigators to hesitate to recommend a low-protein diet for diabetics. It was thought, however, that those with progressive proteinuria despite good glycemic control and the use of ACE inhibitors should be tried on a low-protein diet, with calories lost replaced by complex carbohydrates.

Effect of Dietary Lipid

There is considerable interest in the role of dietary lipids in progressive renal injury. The mechanisms through which elevated levels of lipoproteins or cholesterol provoke glomerulosclerosis are considered akin to the pathways incriminated in atherogenesis, and include injury to the endothelium; the release of vasoconstrictive, mitogenic, and thrombogenic substances; the discharge of chemoattractant substances; and the recruitment and activation of macrophages, which in turn inflict damage on the glomerulus or vessel wall. Of particular relevance to diabetes is the demonstration that strategies that reduce plasma lipid or cholesterol reduce renal damage in the obese Zucker rat, a hyperlipidemic model that bears many similarities to type II diabetes. Few studies are available in which sustained alterations in dietary lipid have been examined for changes in the pathogenesis of diabetic nephropathy. The retrospective analysis by Mulec and colleagues indicated that serum cholesterol is a significant determinant of the rate of decline of renal function in patients with diabetic nephropathy. A randomized, prospective study of a linoleic-enriched diet was undertaken in diabetics with a urinary albumin excretion rate in the range 10 to 200 mg/minute (the upper limit of normal to dipstick-positive albumin excretion). Subjects were instructed to increase their intake of linoleic acid and decrease the intake of saturated fats. In patients with a high linoleic acid intake, the GFR remained constant over a 2-year period, whereas patients eating their usual diet exhibited a decline in GFR. However, urinary albumin excretion rose quite significantly in patients eating the high-linoleic diet but was unchanged in patients on their usual diet. The long-term outcome of such dietary manipulation on diabetic nephropathy is difficult to predict at this time.

THE DIABETIC DIET FOR PROGRESSIVE DIABETIC NEPHROPATHY

Calories, Carbohydrate, Fat

"The primary desired outcome of nutrition self management training is to assist persons with diabetes in making changes in nutrition and exercise habits that will improve nutrition skills, status and diabetes self management" (Franz and colleagues, 1994). Goals of nutritional management include:

1. Maintenance of near-normal blood glucose level by balancing food intake with insulin or hypoglycemic agents
2. Achievement of optimal lipid levels
3. Provision of adequate calories for maintaining or attaining reasonable weight for adults
4. Prevention, delay, or treatment of nutrition-related risk factors and complications

There is no evidence that the nutritional requirements of diabetics with early renal insufficiency differ in any significant way from those of diabetics without nephropathy (Table 8-1). The first consideration, determining the caloric requirement for a given patient, should be geared toward the attainment of ideal body weight. In this regard, there are significant differences between type I and type II diabetics. Most type I diabetics are underweight when first diagnosed; a significant number remain so when diabetic nephropathy appears. Type II diabetics are almost invariably obese, and obesity itself is considered a significant factor in the genesis of many of the metabolic abnormalities in these patients. Caloric restriction and weight loss markedly improve or even correct glucose intolerance, reduce hypertriglyceridemia, and elevate HDL cholesterol levels. Thus, decreased caloric intake is usually required for type II diabetics, but for type I diabetics, caloric intake should be adjusted so that an ideal body weight is attained. For insulin-dependent diabetics, food intake, physical activity, and the schedule of insulin administration should be regular to achieve good metabolic control and avoid unpredictable swings in blood glucose.

Although the preceding recommendations are in general well accepted, the relative proportions of calories that should be contributed by carbohydrate and fat in the diabetic patient are controversial. The incontrovertible evidence gathered since the early 1960s that the major cause of morbidity and mortality in diabetes mellitus arises from macrovascular and microvascular disease, and the emerging evidence that the propensity toward such vascular disease may be linked to dietary fat intake, led the

Table 8-1. Recommended dietary changes during the course of diabetic nephropathy

Stage of Disease	Carbohydrate	Fat	Protein
Preclinical nephropathy	50%–60%; high fiber (up to 40 g/d)	~30; <10% saturated fat; 6%–8% polyunsaturated; cholesterol <350 mg/d	~20% (1.0–1.5 g/kg)
Progressive nephropathy	60%; high fiber (up to 40 g/d)	~30%; <10% saturated fat; 6%–8% polyunsaturated; cholesterol <350 mg/d	~10% (0.6 g/kg); high biologic value; additional protein to replace urinary loss of protein. During intercurrent catabolic stress protein intake liberalized to 1.2–1.5 g/kg; hyperalimentation may be required
End-stage renal disease			
Hemodialysis	50%–60%; low glycemic index; high fiber	~30%; <10% saturated fat; 6%–8% polyunsaturated; cholesterol <350 mg/d	~20% (1.2–1.5 g/kg)
Peritoneal dialysis	35%–40% (oral); ~15% (peritoneal)	~30%	~20% (1.2–1.5 g/kg)

American Diabetes Association in 1979 to recommend that carbohydrate intake should be increased to account for up to 60% of total energy intake, whereas intake of fat and, in particular, saturated fatty acids should be decreased. Carbohydrate sources that are considered less likely to raise blood glucose (foods possessing a lower glycemic index) should be encouraged at the expense of foods that are more likely to do so. In addition, glucose and glucose-containing simple sugars such as sucrose, which traditionally have been restricted, have more recently been recommended in modest quantities.

The recommendation to alter carbohydrate intake was based on studies, such as those of Simpson and associates, that demonstrated that in both insulin-dependent and non–insulin-dependent diabetics, a relatively high-carbohydrate diet (up to 60% of caloric intake as carbohydrate, compared with 40%) led to lower plasma glucose levels as well as lower plasma cholesterol levels in both type I and type II diabetics. Liberalization of carbohydrate and restriction of fat intake not only lowered plasma levels of cholesterol but led to better glycemic control. In addition, simple and complex carbohydrate foods elicited such variability in blood glucose responses that differentiating between simple and complex carbohydrates did not necessarily correlate with specific postingestion glycemic profiles. These findings led Jenkins and colleagues to suggest that the glycemic index rather than the distinction between simple and complex carbohydrates be used to classify carbohydrate-containing foods, and that diabetic diets should be formulated from carbohydrate sources with low glycemic indices. Finally, the addition of simple sugars such as sucrose, as demonstrated by Bantle and coworkers, did not necessarily aggravate glycemic control in diabetic subjects, as was previously widely believed.

Reaven questioned the validity of these recommendations, arguing that the evidence of improved glycemic control from high-carbohydrate diets is far from convincing. Such studies are relatively short term, he said, and changes observed may be a reflection of the dietary fiber rather than the high-carbohydrate content per se. Reaven also questioned the usefulness of the glycemic index. Although recognizing that the postprandial glucose profile after a carbohydrate load depends on the specific carbohydrate-enriched food ingested, he pointed out that there is no evidence indicating that the incorporation of carbohydrates with different glycemic indices into daily menus for the diabetic patient would lead to improved glycemic control. Finally, he presented data that the chronic ingestion of sucrose by type II diabetics worsens glycemic control and increases total plasma triglyceride and VLDL concentrations.

Other investigators have expressed similar views to those of Reaven, and also emphasize that a high-carbohydrate, low-fat diet reduces LDL cholesterol and elevates plasma triglycerides and lowers HDL cholesterol. They contend that the evidence marshaled in support of the belief that a high-carbohydrate, low-fat diet per se exerts beneficial effects on carbohydrate and lipid metabolism is confounded by improper controls and a failure to assess adequately the effect of differences in dietary fat, and cholesterol or fiber content. Relevant to this viewpoint is the study by Garg and colleagues, which compared the effects of a diet high in carbohydrate to one high in monounsaturated fats in patients with non–insulin-dependent diabetes. For 4 weeks, the patients ate a diet containing 25% of energy as fat and 60% as carbohydrate (predominantly complex carbohydrate) or a diet containing 50% fat (33% of total energy supplied in the form of monounsaturated fatty acids) and 35% carbohydrate; the diets were controlled for simple carbohydrates and fiber. The diet high in monounsaturated fatty acids reduced the insulin requirement and led to lower plasma glucose levels, lower levels of plasma triglycerides and VLDL cholesterol, and higher levels of HDL cholesterol. Others also indicated that saturated fat can be safely replaced by a mixture of monounsaturated and polyunsaturated fatty acids. These results suggest that it is not necessary to resort to high intakes of complex carbohydrates when attempting to avoid the deleterious effects of a high fat intake; simply replacing saturated fat by monounsaturated or a mixture of monounsaturated and polyunsaturated fat can achieve the same goal and may, in fact, be preferable by producing a more desirable effect on carbohydrate and lipid metabolism.

Dietary fiber influences carbohydrate metabolism through several mechanisms: 1) it delays gastric emptying time and decreases intestinal absorption of carbohydrate; 2) it leads to diminished plasma levels of glucagon and stimulates secretion of somatostatin, a hormone that inhibits the glucose uptake from the gastrointestinal tract; 3) it appears to increase insulin sensitivity; and 4) it has been shown to reduce hyperlipidemia. The importance of a high-fiber diet in diabetics with chronic renal failure was emphasized by Parillo and coworkers. A high-carbohydrate, high-fiber diet improved glycemic control and reduced serum cholesterol concentration compared with a high-fat diet with a relatively low fiber content. Because these effects were not observed in a similar diabetic population fed an increased carbohydrate intake without increments in dietary fiber, Parillo and coworkers. ascribed such beneficial effects to fiber content alone.

Few would dispute that the caloric intake designed to achieve ideal body weight is a basic requirement, however, and for diabetics who require insulin, a standardized daily food intake regimen that takes into account the level of physical activity, diet composition, and insulin schedule should be formulated. Whether the diet should include 50% or 60% caloric intake in the form of carbohydrate, with proportionately lowered amounts of fat, cannot be clearly answered from the available literature. It seems prudent, however, to recommend carbohydrate food sources with a relatively high fiber content and less saturated fatty acids and lower amounts of cholesterol in dietary fat. The current guidelines of the American Diabetic Association recommend up to 60% energy intake as carbohydrate and less than 30% caloric intake as fat; saturated fat should be less than 10%; polyunsaturated fat, 6% to 8%; and the remainder should be unsaturated fat. Cholesterol intake should not exceed 300 mg/day, whereas high fiber intake, up to 40 g/day, should be encouraged.

Although the dietary management of hypertriglyceridemia has not been specifically addressed in diabetic nephropathy, several studies have demonstrated that reductions in serum triglycerides in nondiabetic patients with renal insufficiency can be achieved by dietary manipulation. In the study by Sanfelippo and associates, 12 subjects with moderate to advanced chronic renal failure complicated by hypertriglyceridemia were subjected to restriction in dietary carbohydrate from 50% to 35% of total calories, with an increase of dietary fat from 40% to 50%. The carbohydrate-restricted diet also contained a higher proportion of polyunsaturated/saturated fatty acids. When studied over a relatively short period of 11 days, the carbohydrate-restricted diet led to a reduction in fasting plasma triglyceride levels and in triglyceride production rates. In a similar patient population, restriction of carbohydrate intake while maintaining the same ratio of polyunsaturated/saturated fatty acids also reduced serum triglyceride levels. An increase in intake of polyunsaturated relative to saturated fatty acids without altering total carbohydrate, fat, protein, and caloric intake in nonnephrotic, nondialyzed patients with underlying glomerulopathy not only lowers serum triglycerides but elevates the HDL cholesterol ratio. Finally, many studies in diabetic and nondiabetic subjects have reported significant decrements in fasting total and LDL cholesterol levels, with maintenance of fasting HDL cholesterol concentrations after brief or chronic consumption of certain soluble fibers, usually in amounts exceeding 20 g/day. Oat bran, various gums, and psyllium appear to be more effective than wheat bran in lowering cholesterol (reviewed in Franz and colleagues).

Thus, hypertriglyceridemia caused by chronic uremia may be lowered by restricting dietary carbohydrate and increasing the relative amount of polyunsaturated versus saturated fatty acids, as well as increasing dietary fiber. Although these dietary manipulations have been studied in the short term only and have not been applied in diabetic nephropathy, they should be considered for diabetics in whom hypertriglyceridemia develops in the course of renal disease. If there is unacceptable response to an adequate trial of diet, exercise, and improved glucose control, lipid-lowering agents should be started.

As renal insufficiency progresses, resistance of glucose metabolism to insulin develops in peripheral tissues. This resistance is usually compensated for by decreased metabolic clearance of insulin by the failing kidney, and insulin requirements may not change significantly. With more advanced nephropathy, hypoglycemia has been observed in insulin-dependent diabetics; metabolism of insulin by the failing kidney may be so impaired that it more than compensates for the peripheral resistance to insulin. A propensity toward hypoglycemia may be compounded by deficient nutrient intake. Such patients require a reduction in insulin dosages and liberalization of carbohydrate intake.

Protein

Protein comprises the remaining 15% to 20% of caloric intake. As discussed, there is firm experimental evidence that the imposition of dietary protein restriction early in the course of experimental diabetic nephropathy retards the progression of renal injury, and there is evidence from clinical studies that the same may be true of human renal disease. Because diabetic nephropathy is invariably progressive, dietary protein restriction and effective control of systemic arterial pressure (especially with ACE inhibitors) are the only two therapeutic modalities available to the clinician to retard the decline of renal function in diabetic renal disease. Given these considerations, it is difficult not to recommend a trial of dietary protein restriction early in the course of diabetic nephropathy (see Table 8-1). Two therapeutic regimens are available. The first involves dietary protein restriction to the minimum amount that is consistent with maintenance of nitrogen balance in chronic renal failure, that is, 0.55 to 0.60 g protein/kg body weight, with more than 75% of protein of high biologic value. In general, patients with diabetic nephropathy tolerate such protein restriction without evidence of protein depletion. Proteins are considered of high biologic value if they contain large amounts of essential amino acids (e.g., eggs, fish, and poultry); proteins of low biologic value include vegetables and cereals. The second regimen restricts dietary protein to 20 to 25 g of mixed–biologic-value protein supplemented by essential amino acids (10 to 15 g/day). With both regimens, the dietary protein should be increased to replace any urinary protein losses. Proteinuria may increase with progressive decline in renal function.

Of special interest is the observation that there is a distinct renal response in normotensive, nonproteinuric type I diabetics to a vegetable protein diet compared with an animal protein diet. GFR, renal plasma flow, and fractional clearance of albumin were lower with vegetable protein. These two distinctly different responses may stem from the differences in plasma amino acid levels or the much higher level of insulin-like growth factor-I.

If dietary protein restriction is undertaken, careful periodic monitoring of the patient's overall nutritional status is essential. This is particularly important given the propensity of diabetic patients toward development of negative nitrogen balance, not only because of metabolic derangement and urinary protein loss but because of failure to comply with the prescribed diet or essential amino acid supplementation. Anorexia and other symptoms caused by diabetic gastroenteropathy can contribute to decreased dietary intake, and gastrointestinal abnormalities associated with the uremic state may lead to diminished absorption of amino acids and small peptides. Finally, with advancing uremia there is an increased incidence of gastrointestinal bleeding, which depletes body stores of hemoglobin. The patient's weight should be closely followed, with careful attention to the presence of edema, which may obscure changes in lean body mass. In addition, measurements of plasma proteins, such as albumin, transferrin, and complement, and the lymphocyte count are useful to detect protein malnutrition.

Another important consideration if dietary protein is restricted is that the intake of carbohydrate and fat should be increased to make up for the deficit in caloric intake. It is essential that a caloric intake that achieves ideal body weight be maintained. An inadequate intake of calories can stimulate catabolism of body protein stores, thereby contributing to protein-calorie malnutrition. An increase in carbohydrate and fat in the protein-restricted diet may necessitate adjustments in the insulin schedule to achieve good glycemic control.

With advanced nephropathy, the rationale for protein restriction includes the alleviation of uremic symptoms. Diabetics often exhibit uremic symptoms out of proportion to the degree of GFR reduction. Nausea and vomiting may be so severe at this stage that oral intake of calories and nutrients may be significantly impaired. Rather than persist with protein restriction and incur the risk of development of protein-calorie malnutrition, it is often advisable to initiate dialysis and thereby reduce uremic symptoms so that oral nutrient intake can be improved.

HYPERTENSION AND DIABETES

The relationship between diabetes and hypertension has been well described. The high prevalence of hypertension in non–insulin-dependent diabetes, even at the time of diagnosis, may reflect an association between insulin resistance and essential hypertension. Because this insulin resistance not only contributes to hypertension but worsens hyperlipidemia, encouragement of weight loss and exercise is probably the most important step to take for blood pressure management. The association of hypertension with diabetes exists even in the absence of obesity in both type I and type II diabetes. In people with diabetes, the risk for macrovascular complications associated with hypertension and the increased risk with increasing blood pressure occurs to the same degree as in nondiabetic people. However, in people with diabetes, the presence of any degree of hypertension doubles the risk for atherosclerotic events. These relationships are most evident in people with type II diabetes. In people with diabetic nephropathy, the presence of hypertension is associated with a more rapid progression of nephropathy.

Several diet-related interventions may be considered in the treatment of patients with diabetes and hypertension. The benefits of these interventions are due to the effects of nutrition therapy on hypertension in both nondiabetic and diabetic subjects. Interventions with evidence of benefit include weight reduction, sodium restriction, and restricted alcohol intake. These recommendations are made in conjunction with a recommendation for regular exercise. A number of other nutrients (i.e., potassium and calcium) have also been evaluated and may have benefit in some patients with diabetes and hypertension (reviewed in American Diabetes Association, 1993).

HEMODIALYSIS

The major dietary change required in diabetics with the commencement of hemodialysis is an increase in dietary protein. This is necessary because the dialytic procedure itself predisposes toward net negative nitrogen balance; chronic hemodialysis patients exhibit negative nitrogen balance on days of dialysis even on a high protein intake (1.4 g/kg/day). However, a high protein intake (1.4 g/kg/day) but not a low-protein diet (0.5 g/kg) leads to a cumulative positive nitrogen balance. A minimum protein intake of 1.2 g/kg/day containing more than 60% high–biologic-value protein has been recommended. The catabolic stress imposed by hemodialysis was underscored by Löfberg and colleagues. They demonstrated that after a single hemodialysis session, plasma levels of most amino acids decrease, as do the muscle content of alanine, the ribosome concentration per DNA in muscle, and the relative amounts of polyribosomes in muscle. The mechanisms by which dialysis promotes protein catabolism include the effects of cytokines stimulated by dialysis; amino acid and peptide loss, estimated at 1 to 2 g/hour of hemodialysis; and blood loss associated with the dialytic procedure. Blood losses induced by regular dialysis may vary between 1 and 3 l/year, depending on the type of dialyzer used, the frequency and volume of blood sampling, and blood loss at the puncture sites. Gastrointestinal blood loss may significantly contribute to total blood loss in hemodialysis patients, averaging 2 to 3 l/year. Thus a patient undergoing hemodialysis for 1 year can lose a volume of blood that is equivalent to the circulating blood volume of a normal 70-kg man, that is, 5 to 6 l. The availability of erythropoietin and its efficacy in diabetics with renal insufficiency should successfully combat anemia in diabetics with renal insufficiency.

Protein catabolism associated with hemodialysis may also be increased if calorie intake is inadequate; a minimum intake of 35 kcal/kg is necessary for patients undergoing hemodialysis to remain in neutral nitrogen balance. For the reasons reviewed previously, caloric intakes in diabetic patients may be suboptimal and the clinician should be vigilant for signs of protein-calorie malnutrition once hemodialysis is commenced. Protein-calorie requirements would be increased in the presence of such catabolic stresses as intercurrent infections, diabetic acidosis, and added gastrointestinal blood loss.

Similar to nondiabetic patients undergoing hemodialysis, the carbohydrate intake of the diabetic hemodialysis patient should be 50% to 60%; for the reasons discussed previously, carbohydrates with a relatively low glycemic index and a relatively high fiber content are desirable. It is important to achieve good glycemic control in diabetic patients, not only to maintain adequate nutrition, but to avoid the excessive interdialytic weight gain associated with moderate to severe hyperglycemia. Hypertonicity associated with hyperglycemia stimulates thirst, thereby leading to increased fluid intake, which gives rise to volume-dependent hypertension and may precipitate pulmonary edema. Control of hyperglycemia also avoids the risk of hyperkalemia secondary to shifts of potassium from the intracellular to the extracellular space. Insulin requirements may be reduced after the initiation of dialysis because partial correction of the uremic milieu leads to improved sensitivity to insulin. On the other hand, because increased insulin requirements after the initiation of dialysis are also reported, insulin therapy must be individualized.

In addition to the control of hyperglycemia, avoidance of hypoglycemia is an important nutritional consideration. Autonomic dysfunction has been reported to worsen in diabetics on dialysis, which may contribute to a blunted response to hypoglycemia. A lack of full awareness by the diabetic of severe hypoglycemia may lead to seizures and cerebral insults. The dialytic procedure itself may contribute to this attenuated response to hypoglycemia. On the days of dialysis, therefore, insulin-dependent diabetics who exhibit a tendency toward hypoglycemia should decrease their dose of insulin or take a carbohydrate snack before dialysis.

Alterations in the relative proportions of carbohydrates and fats should be considered in the management of hypertriglyceridemia in diabetic patients undergoing dialysis. Studies by

Sanfelippo and colleagues demonstrated in nondiabetic hemodialysis patients that a reduction in carbohydrate from 50% to 35% of total calories and an increase in dietary fat from 40% to 50% without changing protein or total calories over a 10-day period led to a reduction in plasma triglyceride regardless of the relative proportions of polyunsaturated/saturated fatty acids in these diets. Gokal and associates demonstrated that a diet with increased carbohydrate, decreased total fat and cholesterol, and an increased ratio of polyunsaturated/saturated fatty acids reduced plasma triglyceride levels in hemodialysis patients after 1 month of follow-up and again after 30 months. Finally, there has been interest in the effect of eicosapentaenoic acid supplements on lipids and platelet function in hemodialysis patients. Dietary supplementation for 8 weeks with purified fish oil, an enriched source of eicosapentaenoic acid, led to a reduction in triglycerides, rise in HDL cholesterol, and reduction in platelet aggregability and mean arterial pressure in hemodialysis patients. From these studies, it seems reasonable to attempt to achieve strict glycemic control, restrict saturated fatty acids, and increase the intake of polyunsaturated fatty acids in diabetic dialysis patients with hypertriglyceridemia.

CONTINUOUS AMBULATORY PERITONEAL DIALYSIS

The initiation of CAPD in uremic diabetic patients also requires an increased intake of dietary protein. CAPD is attended by significant losses of protein and amino acids, estimated at 8 to 10 g/day and 1 to 3 g/day, respectively. Peritoneal loss of protein, as measured by peritoneal clearances of albumin, transferrin, immunoglobulin G, C3, and α_2-macroglobulin, is greater in diabetic than in nondiabetic uremic patients and may place diabetics at risk for development of negative nitrogen balance. The increased loss of immunoglobulin and complement may also increase the susceptibility of the diabetic patients to infections and compound the tendency toward protein wasting. As in the nondiabetic population, peritonitis in diabetics exacerbates peritoneal loss of protein. In their detailed analysis of the kinetics of protein loss during CAPD, Kagan and associates demonstrated that the clearance of relatively large proteins such as albumin and immunoglobulin G is continuous throughout a 6- to 8-hour dwell period of dialysis, unlike molecules of small or intermediate size, which exhibit markedly decreased clearance after the first hour of dialysis. Indeed, these authors suggested that a continuous cycling peritoneal dialysis regimen (six 1-hour cycles) should be substituted for a CAPD regimen (three 8- or 4-hour cycles) in patients in whom protein loss is particularly likely to occur. These considerations are particularly germane to the diabetic population, which is prone to protein malnutrition.

On the basis of nitrogen balance studies, the recommended protein intake for the CAPD population is 1.2 to 1.4 g/kg body weight. In a study by Blumenkrantz and colleagues, CAPD patients maintained on adequate caloric intake exhibited neutral nitrogen balance on a protein intake of 0.98 g/kg body weight but a positive nitrogen balance on 1.4 g/kg body weight. The relationship between nitrogen balance and protein intake in this study is shown in Fig. 8-5. Nitrogen balance improved as protein intake increased until the protein intake reached 1.1

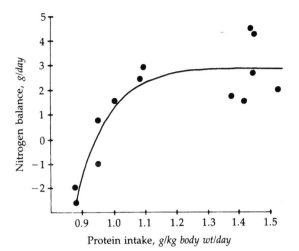

Fig. 8-5. Relationship between nitrogen balance and dietary protein intake in patients with end-stage renal disease undergoing continuous ambulatory peritoneal dialysis. With increasing protein intake, nitrogen balance improves and is neutral at approximately 1.0 g/kg body weight/day. (From Blumenkrantz MJ, et al. Metabolic balance studies and dietary protein requirements in patients undergoing continuous ambulatory peritoneal dialysis. *Kidney Int* 1982;22:849. Used with permission from *Kidney International*.)

g/kg/day. Above this level, there was no further increase in nitrogen balance with increasing protein intake. To allow for the variability in protein requirements in individual patients, a minimum value of 1.2 g/kg body weight is usually recommended. Maintenance of nitrogen balance on such dietary regimens necessitates an adequate daily energy intake, estimated to be 35 to 42 kcal/kg, depending on the activity of the patient.

A portion of the daily carbohydrate intake in CAPD patients is provided by dextrose absorbed from the peritoneal cavity. This varies, of course, depending on the concentration of the dialysate solution (1.5% vs. 4.25% dextrose) and the frequency of exchanges, and has been estimated to be between 100 and 200 g of dextrose per day. The addition of insulin to the peritoneal dialysis fluid allows efficient utilization of absorbed glucose and, indeed, has been considered an important mechanism by which peripheral resistance to insulin is improved in uremic diabetics undergoing CAPD. Absorbed glucose represents approximately 15% of the total caloric intake. Consequently, the oral intake of carbohydrate should provide an additional 35% of the total caloric intake. For the reasons outlined, dietary carbohydrate sources should have a relatively low glycemic index and a relatively high fiber content. Fat comprises the remaining 35% of caloric intake and should contain a higher proportion of polyunsaturated than saturated fatty acids.

The absorbed glucose load during peritoneal dialysis may exacerbate hypertriglyceridemia in the diabetic patient. Indeed, problems associated with glucose as an osmotic agent have led to the investigation of other osmotically active agents such as amino acids for use in CAPD. Parenthetically, one study over a 6-month period examined the effects of a dialysis solution using amino acids as the osmotic agent and concluded that such solutions were effective in achieving adequate dialysis, were relatively nontoxic, did not adversely affect the peritoneal membrane, induced a positive nitrogen balance, and were associated with a reduction in plasma cholesterol and triglycerides. The development of hypertriglyceridemia in diabetic patients is usually maximal during the first 6 months after the initiation of CAPD, and the condition tends to subside with good glycemic control. Peritoneal absorption of glucose can be minimized by decreasing the number of exchanges with 4.25% dextrose. By judiciously restricting the dietary intake of salt and water, the need for ultrafiltration with 4.25% dextrose can be reduced. Unfortunately, restricting carbohydrate intake below 35% of total calories is not feasible for treating hypertriglyceridemia because such restriction severely compromises the palatability of the diet.

The multiple medical problems of patients with long-standing diabetes, as reviewed previously, make the task of maintaining adequate nutrition a difficult one. Caloric intakes in diabetic patients undergoing CAPD, as in patients undergoing hemodialysis, are frequently below the recommended amount. Anorexia, nausea, and vomiting in diabetic patients are sometimes exacerbated with CAPD. Frequent small-volume feedings preceded by metoclopramide often help. Inadequate oral intake in such patients may become severe enough to necessitate hyperalimentation. Catabolic stress arising from a wide variety of intercurrent illnesses may also necessitate parenteral nutritional support.

ACKNOWLEDGMENT

The authors thank Becky McClung for her expert secretarial assistance.

SELECTED READINGS

Alvestrand A, Furst P, Bergstrom J. Plasma and muscle free amino acids in uremia: influence of nutrition with amino acids. *Clin Nephrol* 1982;18:297.

American Diabetes Association. Glycemic effects of carbohydrates. *Diabetes Care* 1984;7:607.

American Diabetes Association. Special report: principles of nutrition and dietary recommendations for individuals with diabetes mellitus. *Diabetes* 1979;28:1027.

American Diabetes Association. Nutritional recommendations and principles for individuals with diabetes mellitus. *Diabetes Care* 1992;15(Suppl 2):21.

American Diabetes Association. Treatment of hypertension in diabetes (consensus statement). *Diabetes Care* 1993;16:1394–1401.

Aparido M, et al. Effect of a ketoacid on glucose tolerance and tissue insulin sensitivity. *Kidney Int* 1989;36:S231.

Appel GB, et al. The hyperlipidemia of the nephrotic syndrome. *N Engl J Med* 1985;312:1544.

Attman PO, et al. Protein-reduced diet in chronic renal failure. *Clin Nephrol* 1983;19:217.

Avram MM, et al. The natural history of diabetic nephropathy: unpredictable insulin requirements a further clue. *Clin Nephrol* 1984;21:36.

Bantle JP, et al. Postprandial glucose and insulin responses to meats containing different carbohydrates in normal and diabetic subjects. *N Engl J Med* 1983;309:7.

Baynes JW. Role of oxidative stress in development of complications in diabetes. *Diabetes* 1991;40:405.

Bennet WM, et al. Inability to stimulate skeletal muscle or whole body protein synthesis in type I (insulin-dependent) diabetic patients by insulin-plus-glucose during amino acid infusion: studies of incorporation and turnover of tracer L-[1-^{13}C] leucine. *Diabetologia* 1990;33:43.

Bergstrom J, Alvestrand A, Fürst P. Plasma and muscle free amino acids in maintenance hemodialysis patients without protein malnutrition. *Kidney Int* 1990;38:108.

Blumenkrantz MJ, et al. Metabolic balance studies and dietary protein requirements in patients undergoing continuous ambulatory peritoneal dialysis. *Kidney Int* 1982;21:849.

Blumenkrantz MJ, Salusky IB, Schmidt RW. Managing the nutritional concerns of the patient undergoing peritoneal dialysis. In: Nolph KD, ed. *Peritoneal dialysis.* Boston: M. Nijhoff; 1985:345.

Boctor DL, Jenkins DJA. Trends in dietary management of diabetes mellitus: an update. In: Alberti KGMM, Krall LP, eds. *The diabetes annual / 6.* Amsterdam: Elsevier Science; 1991:105.

Borah MF. Nitrogen balance during intermittent dialysis therapy of uremia. *Kidney Int* 1978;14:491.

Borghi L, et al. Plasma and skeletal muscle free amino acids in type I, insulin-treated diabetic subjects. *Diabetes* 1985;34:812.

Bruno M, et al. CAPD with an amino acid dialysis solution: a long-term cross-over study. *Kidney Int* 1989;35:1189.

Cahill GH. Physiology of insulin in man. *Diabetes* 1971;20:785.

Ceriello A, et al. Vitamin E reduction of protein glycosylation in diabetes: new prospect for prevention of diabetic complications? *Diabetes Care* 1991;14:68.

Cernacek P, Spustova V, Dzurik R. Inhibitor(s) of protein synthesis in uremic serum and urine: partial purification and relationship to amino acid transport. *Biochem Med* 1982;27:305.

Chase HP, et al. Glucose control and the renal and retinal complications of insulin-dependent diabetes. *JAMA* 1989;261:1155.

Cohen SL, et al. The mechanism of hyperlipidemia in nephrotic syndrome: role of low albumin and the LCAT reaction. *Clin Chim Acta* 1980;104:393.

Coulaton AM, et al. Deleterious metabolic effects of high carbohydrate, sucrose-containing diets in patients with non-insulin dependent diabetes mellitus. *Am J Med* 1987;82:213.

Davies RW, et al. Proteinuria, not altered albumin metabolism, affects hyperlipidemia in the nephrotic rat. *J Clin Invest* 1990; 86:600.

De Feo P, Gaisano MG, Haymond MW. Differential effects of insulin deficiency on albumin and fibrinogen synthesis in humans. *J Clin Invest* 1991;88:833.

DeFronzo RA. Hyperkalemia and hyporeninemic hypo-aldosteronism. *Kidney Int* 1980;17:118.

DeFronzo RA, Beckles AD. Glucose intolerance following chronic metabolic acidosis in man. *Am J Physiol* 1979;236:E328.

DeFronzo RA, Felig P. Amino acid metabolism in uremia: insights gained from normal and diabetic man. *Am J Clin Nutr* 1980; 33:1378.

DeFronzo RA, Smith D, Alverstrand A. Insulin action in uremia. *Kidney Int Suppl* 1983;16:8102.

DeFronzo RA, et al. Glucose intolerance in uremia: quantification of pancreatic beta cell sensitivity to glucose and tissue sensitivity to insulin. *J Clin Invest* 1978;62:425.

DeFronzo RA, et al. Insulin resistance in uremia. *J Clin Invest* 1981; 67:563.

deMendoza SG, et al. High density lipoproteinuria in nephrotic syndrome. *Metabolism* 1976;25:1143.

The Diabetes Control and Complication Trial Research Group. The effect of intensive treatment of diabetes on the development and progression of long term complications in insulin-treated diabetes mellitus. *N Engl J Med* 1993;329:977.

Dornan TL, et al. Long-term dietary treatment of hyperlipidaemia in patients treated with chronic haemodialysis. *Br Med J* 1980; 281:1044.

Dornan TL, et al. Low density lipoprotein cholesterol: an association with the severity of diabetic retinopathy. *Diabetologia* 1982;22: 1675.

Dullaart RPF, et al. Long-term effects of linoleic-acid-enriched diet on albuminuria and lipid levels in type 1 (insulin-dependent) diabetic patients with elevated urinary albumin excretion. *Diabetologia* 1992;35:165.

Fadda GZ, et al. On the mechanism of impaired insulin secretion in chronic renal failure. *J Clin Invest* 1991;87:255.

Falchuk KR, et al. The digestive system and diabetes. In: *Joslin's diabetes mellitus*. Philadelphia: Lea & Febiger; 1985:817.

Feingold KR, Siperstein MD. Diabetic vascular disease. *Adv Intern Med* 1986;31:309.

Feldt-Rasmussen B, et al. Kidney function during 12 months of strict metabolic control in insulin-dependent diabetics with incipient nephropathy. *N Engl J Med* 1986;314:665.

Feldt-Rasmussen, B, et al. Effect of improved metabolic control on loss of kidney function in type 1 (insulin-dependent) diabetic patients: An update of the Steno studies. *Diabetologia* 1991; 34:164.

Felig P. Amino acid metabolism in man. *Annu Rev Biochem* 1975; 44:993.

Fioretto P, et al. Effects of pancreas transplantation on glomerular structure in insulin-dependent diabetic patients with their own kidneys. *Lancet* 1993;342:1193.

Fouque D, et al. Controlled low protein diets in chronic renal insufficiency: meta-analysis. *Br Med J* 1992;304:216.

Franz M, Bantle J, Horton E, et al. Nutrition principles for the management of diabetes and related complications. *Diabetes Care* 1994;17:490–518.

Friedman EA, Delano BG. Recombinant human erythropoietin in the diabetic patient. *Semin Nephrol* 1990;10:(Suppl 1):35.

Fuh MMT, et al. Effect of chronic renal failure on high-density lipoprotein kinetics. *Kidney Int* 1990;37:1295.

Fujioka S, Matsuzawa Y, Tokunaga K, et al. Contributions of intraabdominal fat accumulation to the impairment of glucose and lipid metabolism in human obesity. *Metabolism* 1987;36:54–59.

Garber AJ. Skeletal muscle protein and amino acid metabolism in experimental chronic uremia in the rat. *J Clin Invest* 1978; 62:623.

Garg A, et al. Comparison of a high-carbohydrate diet with a high-monounsaturated fat diet in patients with non-insulin-dependent diabetes mellitus. *N Engl J Med* 1988;319:829.

Gillum RF. The association of body fat distribution with hypertension, hypertensive heart disease, coronary heart disease, diabetes and cardiovascular risk factors in men and women aged 18–79 years. *J Chronic Dis* 1987;40:421.

Ginsberg HN. Lipoprotein physiology in nondiabetic and diabetic states. Relationship to atherogenesis. *Diabetes Care* 1991;14: 839.

Giordano C, et al. Prevention of diabetic nephropathy by low-protein alimentation. In: Friedman EA, L'esperance EA, eds. *Diabetic renal–retinal syndrome.* Vol 3. New York: Grune & Stratton; 1986:201.

Gokal R, et al. Dietary treatment of hyperlipidemia in chronic hemodialysis patients. *Am J Clin Nutr* 1978;31:1915.

Goldberg RB. Lipid disorders in diabetes. *Diabetes Care* 1981;4:561.

Goodship THM, et al. Adaptation to low-protein diets in renal failure: leucine turnover and nitrogen balance. *J Am Soc Nephrol* 1990;1:66.

Haffner SM, Stern MP, Hazuda HP, et al. Role of obesity and fat distribution in non-insulin-dependent diabetes mellitus in Mexican Americans and non-Hispanic whites. *Diabetes Care* 1986;9:153.

Haffner SM, Tuttle KR, Rainwater DL. Decrease of lipoprotein(a) with improved glycemic control in IDDM subjects. *Diabetes Care* 1991;14:302.

Harter HR, et al. Effects of reduced renal mass and dietary protein intake on amino acid release and glucose uptake by rat muscle in vitro. *J Clin Invest* 1979;64:513.

Heidbreder E, Schafferhans K, Heidland A. Autonomic neuropathy in chronic renal insufficiency: comparative analysis of diabetic and nondiabetic patients. *Nephron* 1985;41:50.

Hollenbeck CB, Coulston AM. Effects of dietary carbohydrate and fat intake on glucose and lipoprotein metabolism in individuals with diabetes mellitus. *Diabetes Care* 1991;14:774.

Holliday MA, et al. Effect of uremia on nutritionally induced variations in protein metabolism. *Kidney Int* 1977;11:236.

Holman RR, et al. Prevention of deterioration of renal and sensory-nerve function by more intensive management of insulin-dependent diabetic patients: a two-year randomized prospective study. *Lancet* 1983;1:204.

Hostetter TH. Diabetic nephropathy. *N Engl J Med* 1985;312:642.

Hostetter TH. Diabetic nephropathy. In: Brenner BM, Rector FC Jr, eds. *The kidney.* 4th ed. Philadelphia: WB Saunders; 1991:1695.

Hostetter TH, Rennke HG, Brenner BM. The case for intrarenal hypertension in the initiation and progression of diabetic and other glomerulopathies *Am J Med* 1982;72:375.

Jenkins DJA, et al. Glycemic index of foods: a physiologic basis for carbohydrate exchange. *Am J Clin Nutr* 1981;34:362.

Jennings PE, et al. The relationship of oxidative stress to thrombotic tendency in type I diabetic patients with retinopathy. *Diabet Med* 1991;8:860.

Jiang Z-Y, Woollard ACS, Wolff SP. Hydrogen peroxide production during experimental protein glycation. *FEBS Lett* 1990;268:69.

Kagan A, et al. Kinetics of peritoneal protein loss during CAPD: I. different characteristics for low and high molecular weight proteins. *Kidney Int* 1990;37:971.

Kalkhoff RK, Hartz AH, Rupley D, et al. Relationship of body fat distribution to blood pressure, carbohydrate tolerance and plasma lipids in healthy obese women. *J Lab Clin Med* 1983; 102:621.

Kasiske BL, et al. Treatment of hyperlipidemia reduces glomerular injury in obese Zucker rats. *Kidney Int* 1988;33:667.

Keane WF, et al. Hyperlipidemia and progressive renal disease. *Kidney Int* 1991;39:541.

Klahr S, Levey S, Beck GJ, et al. The effect of dietary protein restriction and blood pressure control on the progression of chronic renal disease. *N Engl J Med* 1994;330:877–884.

Kluthe R, et al. Protein requirements in maintenance hemodialysis. *Am J Clin Nutr* 1978;31:1812.

Kontessis P, et al. Renal metabolic, and hormonal responses to proteins of different origin in normotensive, nonproteinuria type I diabetic patients. *Diabetes Care* 1995;18:1233–1240.

Krediet RT, et al. Peritoneal permeability to proteins in diabetic and non-diabetic continuous ambulatory peritoneal dialysis patients. *Nephron* 1986;42:133.

KROC Collaborative Study Group. Blood glucose control and the evolution of diabetic retinopathy and albuminuria: a preliminary multicenter trial. *N Engl J Med* 1984;311:365.

Krumlovsky FA. Disorders of protein and lipid metabolism associated with chronic renal failure and chronic dialysis. *Ann Clin Lab Sci* 1981;11:350.

Legrain M, Rottembourg J. Peritoneal dialysis in diabetics. In Nolph KD, ed. *Peritoneal dialysis.* Boston: M. Nijhoff; 1985:506.

Levine SF, et al. Protein-restricted diets in diabetic nephropathy. *Nephron* 1989;52:55.

Lindholm B, et al. Hormonal and metabolic adaptation to the glucose load of CAPD in non-diabetic patients. In: Keen H, Legrain M, eds. *Prevention and treatment of diabetic nephropathy.* Boston: MTP; 1983:353.

Löfberg F, et al. Ribosome and free amino acid content in muscle during hemodialysis. *Kidney Int* 1991;39:984.

Mak RHK. Intravenous 1,25 dihydroxycholecalciferol corrects glucose intolerance in hemodialysis patients. *Kidney Int* 1992;41: 1049.

May RC, et al. Specific defects in insulin-mediated muscle metabolism in acute uremia. *Kidney Int* 1985;28:490.

May RC, Kelly RA, Mitch WE. Metabolic acidosis stimulates protein degradation in rat muscle by a glucocorticoid-dependent mechanism *J Clin Invest* 1986;77:614.

May RC, Kelly RA, Mitch WE. Mechanisms for defects in muscle protein turnover in rats with chronic uremia: the influence of metabolic acidosis. *J Clin Invest* 1987;79:1099.

McCaleb ML, et al. Induction of insulin resistance in normal adipose tissue by uremic human serum. *Kidney Int* 1984;25:416.

Mitch WE, Goldberg A. Mechanisms of muscle wasting. *N Engl J Med* 1996;335:1897–1905.

Mitch WE, Medina R, Greiber S, et al. Metabolic acidosis stimulates muscle protein degradation by activating the adenosine-triphosphate-dependent pathway involving ubiquitin and proteasomes. *J Clin Invest* 1994;93:2127-2133.

Mitch WF, et al. The effect of a keto acid-amino acid supplement to a restricted diet on the progression of chronic renal failure. *N Engl J Med* 1984;311:623.

Mogensen CE, Christensen CK. Predicting diabetic nephropathy in insulin-dependent patients. *N Engl J Med* 1984;311:89.

Moller DE, Flier JS. Insulin resistance mechanisms, syndromes, and implications. *N Engl J Med* 1991;325:939.

Morel DW, Chisolm GM. Antioxidant treatment of diabetic rats inhibits lipoprotein oxidation and cytotoxicity. *J Lipid Res* 1989; 30:1827.

Mulec H, Johnson SA, Bjorek S. Relation between serum cholesterol and diabetic nephropathy. *Lancet* 1990;1:1537.

Munoz JM. Fiber and diabetes. *Diabetes Care* 1984;7:2.

Nair KS, et al. Effect of poor diabetic control and obesity on whole body protein metabolism in man. *Diabetologia* 1985;25:400.

Nath KA, Hostetter MK, Hostetter TH. Pathophysiology of chronic tubulointerstitial disease in rats: interactions of dietary acid load, ammonia, and complement component C3. *J Clin Invest* 1985;76:667.

Nath KA, Kren SM, Hostetter TH. Dietary protein restriction in established renal injury in the rat: selective role of glomerular capillary pressure in progressive glomerular dysfunction. *J Clin Invest* 1986;78:1199.

Nath KA, Salahudeen AK. Induction of renal growth and injury in the intact rat kidney by dietary deficiency of antioxidants. *J Clin Invest* 1990;86:1179.

Nikkila EA. High density lipoproteins in diabetes. *Diabetes* 1981; 30(Suppl 2):82.

Ohlson LO, Larsson B, Svärdsudd K, et al. The influence of body fat distribution on the incidence of diabetes mellitus 13.5 years of follow-up of the participants in the study of men born in 1913. *Diabetes* 1985;34:1055–1058.

Okubo M, et al. Deranged fat metabolism and the lowering effect of carbohydrate poor diet on serum triglycerides in patients with chronic renal failure. *Nephron* 1980;25:8.

Oldrizzi L, et al. Progression of renal failure in patients with renal disease of diverse etiology on protein-restricted diet. *Kidney Int* 1985;27:553.

Olefsky JM, Kolterman OG. Mechanisms of insulin resistance in obesity and noninsulin-dependent (type II) diabetes. *Am J Med* 1981;70:151.

Papadoyannakis NJ, Stefanidis CJ, McGeown M. The effect of the correction of metabolic acidosis on nitrogen and potassium balance of patients with chronic renal failure. *Am J Clin Nutr* 1984; 40:623.

Parillo M, et al. Metabolic consequences of feeding a high-carbohydrate, high-fiber diet to diabetic patients with chronic kidney failure. *Am J Clin Nutr* 1988;48:255.

Parthasarathy S. Novel atherogenic, oxidative modification of low-density lipoprotein. *Diabetes Metab Rev* 1991;7:163.

Pedersen O, et al. Postbinding defects of insulin action in human adipocytes from uremic patients. *Kidney Int* 1985;27:780.

Pedrini M. et al. The effect of dietary protein restriction on the progression of diabetic and non-diabetic renal diseases: a meta-analysis. *Ann Intern Med* 1996;124:627.

Pitts RF. Acid–base regulation by the kidneys. *Am J Med* 1950;9:356.

Price SR, Baily JL, Wang X, et al. Muscle wasting in insulinopenic rats results from activation of the ATP dependent ubiquitin-proteasome pathway by a mechanism including gene transcription. *J Clin Invest* 1996;307:369.

Randle PJ, et al. The glucose fatty-acid cycle: its role in insulin sensitivity and the metabolic disturbances of diabetes mellitus. *Lancet* 1963;2:785.

Reaven GM. How high the carbohydrate? *Diabetologia* 1980;19:409.

Reaven GM. Effect of dietary carbohydrate on the metabolism of patients with non-insulin dependent diabetes mellitus. *Nutr Rev* 1986;44:65.

Reaven GM. Banting Lecture 1988: the role of insulin resistance in human disease. *Diabetes* 1988;37:1595.

Reichley KB, Mueller WH, Hanis CL, et al. Centralized obesity and cardiovascular disease risk in Mexican Americans. *Am J Epidemiol* 1987;125:373.

Rivellese A, et al. A fibre rich diet for the treatment of diabetic patients with chronic renal failure. *Diabetes Care* 1985;8:620.

Rizza RA, et al. Production of insulin resistance by hyperinsulinemia in man. *Diabetologia* 1985;28:70.

Robbins DL, Howard BV. Lipoprotein(a) and diabetes. *Diabetes Care* 1991;14:347.

Rosman JB, et al. Prospective randomized trial of early dietary protein restriction in chronic renal failure. *Lancet* 1984;2:1291.

Rubenstein AH, Mako ME, Horowitz DL. Insulin and the kidney. *Nephron* 1975;150:306.

Rylance PB, et al. Fish oil modifies lipids and reduces platelet aggregability in haemodialysis patients. *Nephron* 1986;43:196.

Salahudeen AK, Clark EC, Nath KA. Hydrogen peroxide-induced renal injury. *J Clin Invest* 1991;88:186.

Sanfelippo ML, Swenson RS, Reaven GM. Reduction of plasma triglycerides by diet in subjects with chronic renal failure. *Kidney Int* 1977;11:54.

Sanfelippo ML, Swenson RS, Reaven GM. Response of plasma triglycerides to dietary change in patients on hemodialysis. *Kidney Int* 1978;14:180.

Santeusanio F, et al. Evidence for a role of endogenous insulin and glucagon in the regulation of potassium homeostasis. *J Lab Clin Med* 1973;81:809.

Schade DS, et al. Normalization of plasma insulin profiles with intraperitoneal insulin infusion in diabetic man. *Diabetologia* 1980;19:35.

Schmitz O. Insulin-mediated glucose uptake in nondialyzed and dialyzed uremic insulin-dependent diabetic subjects. *Diabetes* 1985; 34:1152.

Scrimshaw NW. An analysis of past and present recommended daily allowances for protein in health and disease. *N Engl J Med* 1976; 294:136.

Sherwin RS, et al. Influence of uremia and hemodialysis on the turnover and metabolic effects of glucagon. *J Clin Invest* 1976;62:722.

Shimada M, Ishibashi S, Gotodec T, et al. Overexpression of human lipoprotein lipase protects diabetic transgenic mice from diabetic hypertriglyceridemia and hypercholesteremia. *Arterioscler Thromb Vasc Biol* 1995;15:1688.

Shimada M, et al. Overexpression of human lipoprotein lipase in transgenic mice: resistance to diet-induced hypertriglyceridemia and hypercholesteremia. *J Biol Chem* 1993;268:17924.

Simpson HCR, et al. A high carbohydrate leguminous fibre diet improves all aspects of diabetic control. *Lancet* 1981;1:1.

Slomowitz LA, et al. Effect of energy intake on nutritional status in maintenance hemodialysis patients. *Kidney Int* 1989;35:704.

Smith D, DeFronzo RA. Insulin resistance in uremia mediated by post-binding defects. *Kidney Int* 1982;22:54.

Snyder D, Pulido LB, Kagan A. Dietary reversal of the carbohydrate intolerance in uremia. *Proceedings of the European Dialysis and Transplantation Association* 1968;5:205.

Tamborlane WV, et al. Restoration of normal lipid and amino acid metabolism in diabetic patients treated with a portable insulin-infusion pump. *Lancet* 1979;1:1258.

Taskinen MR, Nikkila EA. Lipoprotein lipase activity of adipose tissue and skeletal muscle in insulin deficient human diabetes: relation to high density and very low density lipoproteins and response to treatment. *Diabetologia* 1979;17:351.

Tepper T, et al. Loss of amino acids during hemodialysis: effect of oral essential amino acid supplementation. *Nephron* 1981;29:25.

Tessari P, et al. Defective suppression by insulin of leucine-carbon appearance and oxidation in type I insulin-dependent diabetes mellitus. *J Clin Invest* 1986;77:1797.

Tolins JP, Hostetter MK, Hostetter TH. Hypokalemic nephropathy: role of ammonia in chronic tubular injury. *J Clin Invest* 1987;79:1447.

Tsukamoto Y, et al. Effects of a polyunsaturated fatty acid-rich diet on serum lipids in patients with chronic renal failure. *Nephron* 1982;31:236.

Unger RH, Orei L. Glucagon and the A cell: physiology and pathophysiology. *N Engl J Med* 1981;304:1575.

Vaag A, et al. Effect of the antilipolytic nicotinic acid analogue acipimox on whole-body and skeletal muscle glucose metabolism in patients with noninsulin-dependent diabetes mellitus. *J Clin Invest* 1991;88:1282.

Vannini P, et al. Lipid abnormalities in insulin-dependent diabetic patients with albuminuria. *Diabetes Care* 1984;7:151.

Viberti GC, et al. Long term correction of hyperglycaemia and progression of renal failure in insulin dependent diabetes. *Br Med J* 1983;286:598.

Wahren J, Felig P, Hagenfeldt J. Effect of protein ingestion on splanchnic and leg metabolism in normal man and in patients with diabetes mellitus. *J Clin Invest* 1976;57:987.

Walker JD, et al. Restriction of dietary protein and progression of renal failure in diabetic nephropathy. *Lancet* 1989;2:1411.

Wassner SJ, et al. Protein metabolism in renal failure: abnormalities and possible mechanisms. *Am J Kidney Dis* 1986;7:285.

Wen SF, Huang TP, Moorthy AY. Effect of a low protein diet on experimental diabetic nephropathy in the rat. *J Lab Clin Med* 1985;106:589.

Williams B, et al. Metabolic acidosis and skeletal muscle adaptation to low protein diets in chronic uremia. *Kidney Int* 1991;40:779.

Williamson JR, et al. Glucose-induced microvascular functional changes in non-diabetic rats are stereospecific and are prevented by an aldose reductase inhibitor. *J Clin Invest* 1990;85:1167.

Wilson PW, McGee DL, Kannel WB. Obesity, very low density lipoproteins, and glucose intolerance over fourteen years: the Framingham Study. *Am J Epidemiol* 1981;114:697.

Wing SS, Goldberg AL. Glucocorticoid activate the ATP ubiquitin dependent proteolytic system in skeletal muscle during fasting. *Am J Physiol* 1994;264:E688.

Wiseman MJ, et al. Effect of blood glucose control on increased glomerular filtration rate and kidney size in insulin-dependent diabetes. *N Engl J Med* 1985;312:617.

Wiseman MJ, et al. Glycemia and dietary protein in the modulation of glomerular filtration rate and albuminuria in insulin-dependent diabetes. *Kidney Int* 1986;29:389.

Wolf BA, et al. Diacylglycerol accumulation and microvascular abnormalities induced by elevated glucose levels. *J Clin Invest* 1991;87:31.

Working Group on Management of Patients with Hypertension and High Blood Cholesterol. National Education Programs Working Group report on the management of patients with hypertension and high blood cholesterol. *Ann Intern Med* 1991;114:224.

Young GA, Parsons FM. Impairment of phenylalanine hydroxylation in chronic renal insufficiency. *Clin Sci* 1973;45:89.

Zatz R, et al. Predominance of hemodynamic rather than metabolic factors in the pathogenesis of diabetic glomerulopathy. *Proc Natl Acad Sci U S A* 1985;82:5963.

Zeller K, et al. Effect of restricting dietary protein on the progression of renal failure in patients with insulin-dependent diabetes mellitus. *N Engl J Med* 1991;324:79.

The Nephrotic Syndrome: Nutritional Consequences and Dietary Management

George A. Kaysen

The nephrotic syndrome results from urinary loss of albumin and other plasma proteins of similar size and is characterized by hypoalbuminemia, hyperlipidemia, and edema formation. It is more difficult to quantitate the losses of tissue protein; however, marked muscle wasting (sometimes obscured by edema) has been described in patients with continuous, massive proteinuria. Micronutrients such as vitamin D, iron, and zinc are bound to proteins in plasma and are lost into the urine in the nephrotic syndrome, making it possible for depletion syndromes to occur when proteinuria is massive and continuous.

The major rationales for changing a patient's diet are to blunt manifestations of the syndrome (e.g., edema), to replace nutrients lost in the urine, and to reduce risks either of progression of renal disease or of atherosclerosis. The latter two could be a consequence of altered lipid metabolism. It might also be possible that specific allergens contained in food may cause renal disease in some patients. In this rare instance, dietary modification might prove curative.

DIETARY PROTEIN

Metabolic abnormalities in the nephrotic syndrome include depletion of plasma and tissue protein pools. In superficial ways, the nephrotic syndrome is similar to protein-calorie malnutrition (i.e., kwashiorkor). In both cases, the plasma albumin concentration is reduced, plasma volume is expanded, and albumin pools shift from the extravascular to the vascular compartment. In the case of protein malnutrition, it is possible to correct all of the manifestations by providing the needed protein and calories, whereas this is not the case in the nephrotic syndrome. Although average values for proteinuria (grams of protein lost into the urine per day) are approximately 6 to 8 g/day (the amount contained in a hen's egg), simply increasing dietary protein is of little demonstrable benefit. In fact, dietary protein supplementation further damages the filtration barrier of the glomerular capillary, resulting in increased urinary protein losses (Fig. 9-1). Dietary protein restriction, in contrast, reduces urinary protein excretion, maintains nitrogen balance, and may have a salutary effect on the rate of progression of the renal disease, especially in proteinuric patients.

There are several reasons why reducing urinary protein excretion is a desirable end. In addition to the consequences of losing proteins from plasma, proteinuria is thought to be directly damaging to the renal interstitium because of a variety of putative mechanisms. Filtered proteins are reabsorbed by the tubule, carrying iron, complement components, and biologically active lipids into the interstitial space. For example, it is proposed that lipids are chemoattractive for monocytes, which promote renal

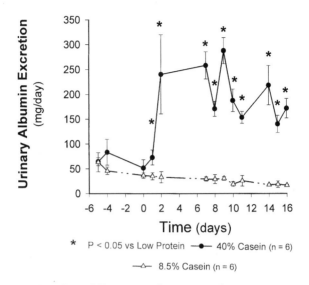

Fig. 9-1. The effect of dietary protein augmentation on urinary albumin excretion in rats with the nephrotic syndrome. The nephrotic syndrome was induced by injection of anti-FX 1A antibody to produce passive Heymann nephritis. Twelve rats were initially fed a diet containing 8.5% protein as sodium caseinate. On day 0, six animals had dietary protein increased to 40% casein. Urinary albumin excretion increased significantly in these animals by the second day after the change in diet, and remained significantly greater thereafter.

injury. Reabsorbed iron from proteinuria is biologically active and may act as an oxidant, injuring the kidney. Diets that are high in protein are also high in acid content, leading to acidosis and obligating the kidney to increase ammoniagenesis. Accelerated rates of renal ammonia production that result from increased dietary acid loads accompanying a high-protein diet may also lead to renal injury. The reduction in urinary protein excretion that follows institution of a low-protein diet potentially can have a salutary effect on progressive renal injury through any or all of these mechanisms (Table 9-1).

The degree of hyperlipidemia also rises as urinary protein losses increase. Thus, reduction in urinary protein excretion reduces blood lipid levels.

Several studies suggest that the composition of proteins in the diet may be as important as its absolute nitrogen content. In experimental studies in rats, dietary augmentation with some amino acids causes a prompt increase in urinary albumin excretion, whereas other amino acids, specifically the branched-chain amino acids, arginine, proline, glutamine, glutamate, aspartate, or asparagine, are devoid of any effect on proteinuria. Specific types of dietary proteins may be of importance in humans with renal disease. When patients with the nephrotic syndrome were fed a vegetarian soy diet, their urinary protein excretion decreased, as did blood lipid levels. The diet was also low in fat

Table 9-1. Adverse renal effects of proteinuria

Processes that may cause interstitial fibrosis by
   macrophage recruitment and increased transforming
   growth factor-β and platelet-derived growth factor
      Tubular exposure to filtered components of the complement
        cascade not normally present in tubular fluid
      Tubular exposure to reabsorbed iron
      Tubular exposure to proinflammatory lipids reabsorbed
        from filtered proteins
Exposure to growth factors, such as insulin-like
   growth factor-1 causing renal hypertrophy
Decreased renal response to atrial natriuretic factor causing
   distal sodium retention and resulting in edema formation

(28% of calories) and the protein content was low (0.71 g/kg ideal body weight), so the benefit of a soy-based diet in nephrotic patients may be a consequence of the amino acid composition in those diets, although differences in lipid composition or in protein absorption may also explain the apparent benefit of these diets as well. Curiously, there was little difference between a diet containing 1.1 or 0.7 g protein/kg on urinary protein excretion.

Recommendations

Because urinary protein excretion varies from day to day in individual patients, we collect three, separate 24-hour specimens and make three measurements of serum albumin and protein to establish a baseline value. Patients are then placed on a 35 kcal/kg diet containing 0.7 to 1.0 g protein/kg and restricted to 2 g of sodium. We then measure the 24-hour urinary urine excretion every 2 to 3 months and monitor the urinary urea excretion to ensure that patients are not eating more (or less) protein than recommended. Our goal is to decrease proteinuria without lowering serum albumin and protein concentration. This is usually possible when dietary protein intake is restricted to these levels (Table 9-2).

**Table 9-2. Dietary recommendations
in the nephrotic syndrome**

Protein
   35kcal/kg energy containing 0.7-1.0g protein per kg
   Soy protein may be less harmful than "high-quality protein"
Fat
   Less than 30% of total calories
   Low cholesterol (less than 200 mg/day)
   High in polyunsaturated fatty acids (10% of energy)
   Fish oil may be useful for IgA nephropathy (12g/day)
Minerals
   Less than 2g Na
   Do not administer iron unless
      there is clear evidence of iron deficiency
   Calcium: patients may have hypovitaminosis D

Dietary protein intake can be estimated because, in the steady state, dietary protein intake is equal to protein catabolic rate (PCR). If total body urea pools do not change during the 24-hour period (blood urea nitrogen and weight neither decrease nor increase), it is possible to estimate the amount of protein that has been eaten by the formula:

PCR = (10.7 + [24-hour urinary urea excretion/0.14])g/day
        + urinary protein excretion

For example, if urinary urea excretion is 6 g/day, then protein intake is equal to protein losses, and is 53.6 g/day + urinary protein excretion.

If there is variance from the prescribed diet, an accurate nutritional history should be obtained and the diet adjusted accordingly.

Although high-quality protein (meat and dairy products) is usually recommended, it has been found that vegetarian diets based on soy protein are more effective in reducing urinary protein loss, increasing serum protein levels, and correcting hyperlipidemia. Consequently, we recommend soy-based protein in the diet.

LIPIDS

One hallmark of the nephrotic syndrome is hyperlipidemia, characterized by high serum levels of total cholesterol and triglycerides, mostly in the low-density lipoprotein (LDL), very–low-density lipoprotein (VLDL), and intermediate-density lipoprotein (IDL) fractions. There also is a lower level of high-density lipoprotein (HDL) cholesterol. There are at least two reasons why reversing these changes in the plasma lipid levels is desirable in nephrotic patients with hyperlipidemia: 1) to reduce the risk of cardiovascular disease, and 2) to retard the progression of renal injury.

The plasma lipoprotein composition in patients with the nephrotic syndrome is a pattern associated with accelerated atherosclerosis in patients without kidney disease. In the nephrotic syndrome, plasma levels of LDL, VLDL, and IDL are increased, whereas HDL levels are either unaffected or are reduced. This leads to an increased ratio of LDL/HDL cholesterol. In addition, the plasma lipoprotein(a) [Lp(a)] is increased in nephrotic patients, and an elevated Lp(a) level is a predictor of accelerated atherosclerosis. The concentration of Lp(a) is genetically determined in patients without kidney disease and largely depends on the specific isoform of the apolipoprotein(a) moiety synthesized by the liver. Plasma Lp(a) levels are increased in nephrotic patients independently of a specific isoform, and the level falls when proteinuria abates.

In the nephrotic syndrome, plasma fibrinogen is also increased as a consequence of a high rate of synthesis in the liver. A high plasma concentration of fibrinogen is another predictor of atherogenesis. Based on these abnormalities, patients with the nephrotic syndrome should be at increased risk of atherogenesis, and this is most likely the case. Consequently, efforts should be made to reduce high plasma lipid levels, both by nutritional and by pharmacologic means, in patients who are anticipated to have the nephrotic syndrome for a prolonged duration. If the underlying condition can be easily treated (e.g., minimal-change nephrotic syndrome), treatment of the underlying disease should be the primary goal.

Regarding the issue of progressive renal damage, there is strong evidence in animals that elevated lipid levels alone can induce severe and progressive renal injury and that reducing plasma lipid levels in animals with established renal disease favorably alters the course of the disease. Even though the impact of hyperlipidemia on the progression of renal disease in humans is less secure, there is evidence that lipids play a role in renal disease; for example, hereditary lecithin cholesterol acyltransferase deficiency may be linked to progressive mesangial and glomerular sclerosis. Second, hypercholesterolemia is an independent risk factor for progression of renal disease in insulin-dependent diabetics and predicts the onset of microalbuminuria. In a 6-week study of a small number of nephrotic patients, simvastatin did not decrease protein losses despite the presence of a significant decrease in serum cholesterol. Over longer periods, simvastatin was associated with a significant decrease in urinary protein excretion plus an increase in serum albumin, but no changes in serum creatinine. Although the study was carried out prospectively, there were no contemporaneously treated control subjects, the study was not randomized, and the investigators were not blinded. Nevertheless, treatment of the hyperlipidemia in nephrotic patients may have a salutary effect on the degree of renal injury. There are fewer data available about how treatment of hyperlipidemia influences the ultimate renal outcome (death or dialysis), although a reduction in urinary protein excretion is a reasonable surrogate for an improved outcome. There is no basis for providing lipid-lowering drugs to nephrotic patients who are not hyperlipidemic. At the same time, it would be unwise to allow patients with elevated LDL cholesterol and low levels of HDL cholesterol to go untreated.

Lipids comprise a group of compounds, including prostaglandins (PG) and leukotrienes, that are important regulators of vascular resistance. These compounds are products of metabolism of polyunsaturated fatty acids (PUFA), but PUFA are not synthesized by mammals and are available only through the diet. Thus, dietary supplementation with specific PUFA could affect the levels of these important vasoactive compounds. Lipids derived from marine sources are enriched with omega-3 PUFA (e.g., eicosapentaenoic acid), whereas those derived from vegetable oils are enriched with omega-6 PUFA (e.g., arachidonic acid). Eicosapentaenoic acid competes with arachidonic acid as a substrate for cyclooxygenase and lipooxygenase, and cyclooxygenase converts arachidonic acid and eicosapentaenoic acid to the diene (e.g., PGI_2, thromboxane [TX] A_2) and triene metabolites (e.g., PGI_3, TXA_3), respectively. TXA_2, an arachidonic acid metabolite, is a potent vasoconstrictor, whereas TXA_3, a metabolite of eicosapentaenoic acid, is biologically inert. In contrast, the vasodilators PGI_2 and PGI_3 are equipotent. Alterations in the generation of both vasodilatory prostaglandins (PGE_2, PGI_2) and vasoconstricting cyclooxygenase metabolites (TXA_2) can occur during renal injury or during physiologic stress, such as plasma volume contraction. Lipooxygenase converts arachidonic acid and eicosapentaenoic acid to the 4 and 5 series of leukotrienes. These compounds can also cause vasoconstriction or vasodilatation. Although changes in eicosanoid metabolism can support the glomerular filtration rate during adaptation to renal injury or plasma volume contraction, they may also play a pathogenic role. Because of the differences in biologic activity of their vaso-constrictive and vasodilatory metabolites, substitution of eicos-apentaenoic acid for arachidonic acid in the diet may alter the expression of renal injury.

The availability of specific PUFA has been demonstrated to alter the course of renal injury in experimental animals and to reduce blood lipid levels. In humans, however, adding as much as 5 g of fish oil per day to the diet of nephrotic patients eating a soy vegetarian diet produced no added beneficial effect on either proteinuria or on blood lipids compared with patients main-tained on the soy diet without fish oil supplements. In contrast, larger doses of fish oil (e.g., 15 g/day) given to subjects eating an unrestricted diet caused a decrease in plasma total triglycerides and in LDL triglycerides and an increase in LDL cholesterol. Donadio and colleagues treated 55 IgA nephropathy patients with 12 g of fish oil per day in a prospective, randomized, placebo-controlled study and found a significant reduction in the rate of progression of renal disease. At the end of the treatment period, the fish oil-treated group had a lower prevalence of hypertension, a slower rise in serum creatinine, and fewer cases of nephrotic-range proteinuria.

Recommendations

Dietary fat restriction has been shown to be partially effec-tive in reducing blood lipid levels in nephrotic patients. Diets low in fat (<30% of total calories) and cholesterol (<200 mg/day) and rich in PUFA and linoleic acid (10% of energy) can reduce blood lipid levels.

If the serum total cholesterol remains elevated (>200 mg/dl) after dietary lipid restriction and attempts to minimize urinary protein excretion, then pharmacologic therapy should be instituted.

Giving fish oil supplements may be beneficial for patients with IgA nephropathy (see Table 9-2).

VITAMIN D

Hypocalcemia, including both a reduced serum ionized as well as total calcium level, is frequent in nephrotic patients. Hypocalcemia does not result entirely from a reduced fraction of calcium bound to albumin. Plasma levels of vitamin D are reduced, and the degree of abnormality inversely correlates with urinary albumin excretion. Hypovitaminosis D is not the result of loss of renal mass because plasma vitamin D levels are also low in nephrotic patients with normal renal function. Synthesis of vitamin D by the proximal nephron has been shown to be impaired in some experimental models of the nephrotic syndrome in the rat; however it is unknown how or whether this applies to nephrotic patients. Vitamin D-binding protein is present in the urine of nephrotic patients, and vita-min D levels normalize when proteinuria resolves. It is unknown whether the synthesis of vitamin D-binding protein rises in response to its urinary loss, or is modulated by changes in dietary protein. Moreover, plasma albumin and vitamin D

concentrations correlate closely. Labeled vitamin D administered to nephrotic subjects appears rapidly in their urine, suggesting that vitamin D loss is the cause of hypovitaminosis D in
these patients.

The clinical significance of hypovitaminosis D is controversial.
Some find that although total 1,25-dihydroxyvitamin D is reduced,
free vitamin D is not, but serum parathyroid hormone levels are
often increased for the level of ionized calcium and vitamin D, suggesting functional hypovitaminosis D. Nephrotic patients malab-
sorb calcium, a defect that can be corrected by exogenously administered vitamin D. Hypovitaminosis D of the nephrotic syndrome
can cause rickets, especially in children. Unlike many of the other
manifestations of the nephrotic syndrome, hypovitaminosis D can
be managed with replacement therapy.

Recommendations

Measure the plasma parathyroid hormone level: if it is high,
then treat with 1,25-dihydroxyvitamin D and calcium supplements. Alternatively, the free 1,25-dihydroxyvitamin D level can
be measured.

IRON

Although urinary iron losses in transferrin rise, the anemia is
more likely to be due to losses of erythropoietin rather than
iron. Unless there is unequivocal evidence of iron deficiency, do
not administer iron, because iron is released from transferrin in
the tubule (especially when the urine pH is < 6) and may be
reabsorbed by renal tubular cells, causing or contributing to
interstitial fibrosis.

Recommendations

Anemia associated with the nephrotic syndrome should not be
assumed to be a consequence of iron deficiency. Iron should not
be administered unless iron deficiency is documented.

SALT AND WATER

Edema formation is one of the most bothersome symptoms of
the nephrotic syndrome and frequently brings the patient to the
attention of the nephrologist. Edema is a consequence of pathologic retention of salt and water.

The classic model of edema formation in the nephrotic syndrome is based on the assumption that a decrease in plasma albumin concentration would lead to a decrease in the difference
between the interstitial and plasma oncotic pressures ($\Delta\pi$) and,
ultimately, to plasma volume contraction. Edema would occur
when the amount of fluid entering the interstitium exceeded maximal lymph flow, leading to a decreased circulatory volume. The
plasma volume contraction would then activate the renin–
angiotensin–aldosterone axis and cause secondary renal sodium
retention—the so-called "underfill" edema. Because plasma volume contraction also causes an increase in vasopressin release,
water should also be retained, leading to hyponatremia (as seen in
other edema-forming states, specifically congestive heart failure
and liver disease). Dietary sodium restriction should, therefore,
play an important role in management of edema in patients with
the nephrotic syndrome.

Edema formation in the nephrotic syndrome results from this and another mechanism. There is a reduced ability of the nephrotic kidney to excrete a sodium load, either in response to plasma volume expansion or to atrial natriuretic factor (ANF). Experimentally, this problem appears to be intrinsic to the nephrotic kidney itself and unrelated to changes in circulating blood volume. For example, the normal increase in urinary cyclic guanosine monophosphate during saline infusion is blunted in nephrotic rats because of increased phosphodiesterase activity in the inner medullary collecting duct cells. The rise in phosphodiesterase activity would accelerate the hydrolysis of cyclic guanosine monophosphate, the effector of ANF, thereby reducing the effectiveness of ANF. The reduced ability to excrete sodium leads to salt retention and edema. The proteinuric kidney avidly reabsorbs filtered salt in the distal nephron and is less responsive to ANF. Consequently, the systemic capillary bed is faced with increased hydrostatic pressure, even though defense mechanisms to counteract edema formation (i.e., increased lymphatic flow and decreased interstitial protein concentration) have already been activated. Thus, unlike in liver disease or congestive heart failure, the measured plasma volume may not be reduced. Diuretics and restriction of dietary sodium chloride are effective in treating edema.

Recommendations

A low sodium diet is recommended.

ZINC AND COPPER

The most important zinc-binding protein is albumin, and urinary zinc losses can be substantial in the nephrotic syndrome. Documented zinc deficiency, however, is probably a consequence of both reduced absorption of zinc plus urinary loss. The effect of proteinuria on zinc metabolism has been largely ignored, and it is not known to what extent zinc depletion plays a role in the clinical manifestations of the nephrotic syndrome.

Copper, like iron, is also bound to a circulating plasma protein, ceruloplasmin. Although the urinary loss of this 151-kDa protein may cause a decrease in blood copper, it results in no clinically recognized manifestations.

In summary, there is reason to believe that the loss of protein in patients with the nephrotic syndrome could result directly or indirectly in excessive losses of several ions and trace elements. The importance of these losses to clinical manifestations of the nephrotic syndrome is not established, and routine administration of a supplement is not recommended. If a specific deficit is documented, replacement therapy is appropriate.

The principal effects of dietary manipulation in the nephrotic syndrome are summarized in Table 9-3.

The following is a list of a suggested 2-day diet using a high-quality protein source and a 2-day diet using a vegetarian (Vegan) soy protein source for a 65-kg man who participates in moderate physical activity. We have made no adjustment for urinary protein losses, and in general have not advised adjustment for urinary protein losses. The amounts of food may be adjusted for patients of different weights.

**Table 9-3. Potential effects of diet
on the expression of the nephrotic syndrome**

Effects on the rate of disease progression
    High-protein diets increase proteinuria and cause hyperfiltration
        Increased proteinuria delivers complement, iron, and
            other potential toxins to the renal interstitium
    High-lipid diets increase blood lipid levels, increasing the risk
      of atherogenesis, and may contribute to loss of renal function
Effects on the signs or symptoms of the nephrotic syndrome
    Dietary sodium restriction reduces edema
        Many patients are volume expanded and tolerate sodium
           restriction and diuretics
    Dietary protein restriction (0.8g/kg/day) and use of soy protein
      reduces proteinuria and may increase serum albumin
      concentration

Nonvegetarian High-Quality Protein
Day 1
Breakfast
    2 waffles, plain (4 tbsp. fat-free cool whip,
      ½ cup frozen strawberries)
    ½ cup low-fat yogurt, plain
    6 oz. apple juice
Lunch
    1 chicken salad sandwich
      (2 oz. chicken salad sprinkled w/salt, 1 tbsp. mayonnaise,
      2 slices whole-wheat bread)
    1 cup romaine lettuce, shredded
      (2 tbsp. oil and vinegar dressing)
    1 blueberry muffin
    1 cup 1% milk
Dinner
    3 oz. lean roast beef (cooked w/1/8 tsp. salt)
    ½ cup mashed potatoes (1 tsp. margarine)
    ½ cup broccoli, seasoned
    2 dinner rolls (2 tsp. margarine)
    1 orange
    1 cup tea/coffee (2 tsp. sugar)
Day 2
Breakfast
    ¼ cup egg beater (1 tsp. vegetable oil)
    1 cup oatmeal (2 tsp. sugar)
    1 slice whole-wheat toast (1 tsp. jelly)
    1 cup 1% milk
Lunch
    1 tuna fish sandwich (2 oz. tuna, 1 tsp. mayonnaise,
      2 slices whole-wheat bread)
    4 carrot sticks
    1 apple
    4 graham crackers
    1 cup tea/coffee (2 tsp. sugar)
Dinner
    3 oz. baked chicken, seasoned (cooked w/¹/₈ tsp. salt)

$^{1}/_{2}$ cup rice
$^{1}/_{2}$ cup boiled cabbage
$^{1}/_{2}$ cup corn
$^{1}/_{12}$ angelfood cake
6 oz. grape juice

SEPARATE DIETS

Strict Vegetarian–Soy Diets
Day 1
Breakfast
    2 oz. tofu scramble
    1 cup oatmeal (2 tsp. sugar)
    $^{1}/_{2}$ English muffin (2 tsp. jelly)
    1 medium orange
    1 cup soy milk
Lunch
    1 tempeh (soy product) burger
        ($^{1}/_{4}$ cup tempeh, 1 hamburger bun, 1 tbsp. mayonnaise)
    $^{1}/_{2}$ cup baked beans, homemade ($^{1}/_{2}$ tsp. salt)
    $^{1}/_{2}$ cup applesauce
    1 cup grape juice
Dinner
    8 oz. soy spaghetti
    2 oz. soy cheese
    4 oz. fruit salad
    1 medium baked potato (1 tbsp. margarine)
    tea/coffee (nondairy creamer, 2 tsp. sugar)
Day 2
Breakfast
    $^{1}/_{2}$ cup soy sausage
    2 pancakes (4 tbsp. syrup)
    $^{1}/_{2}$ cup applesauce
    6 oz. orange juice
Lunch
    3 oz. soy bologna
        (2 slices whole-wheat bread, 1 tbsp. mayonnaise)
    $^{1}/_{2}$ cup corn
    $^{1}/_{2}$ cup carrot– raisin salad
        (2 tsp. mayonnaise, 1 tsp. sour cream substitute)
Dinner
    6 oz. tofu stir-fry
    1 cup mixed vegetables
        ($^{1}/_{2}$ cup broccoli, $^{1}/_{2}$ cup cauliflower, 1 tsp. oil, $^{1}/_{8}$ tsp. salt)
    $^{1}/_{2}$ cup stewed potatoes ($^{1}/_{8}$ tsp. salt)
    1 cup soy milk
    2 oatmeal–raisin cookies

Soy Products
Breakfast
    Soy milk (8 oz.)
        Protein = 7 g
        Fat = 5 g
        Na = 40 mg
        Carbohydrate = 5 g
    Tempeh (soy bacon)
    Soy sausage (per serving):
        Protein = 9 g

        Fat = 0 g
        Na = 240 mg
        Carbohydrate = 8 g
    Soy pancake mix
    Tofu scramble
Lunch
    Soy bologna (per serving)
        Protein = 14 g
        Fat = 0 g
        Na = 335 mg
        Carbohydrate = 8 g
Dinner
    Tofu stir fry (3 oz.)
        Protein = 5 g
        Fat = 1 g
        Na = 70 mg
        Carbohydrate = 19 g
    Brand names of soy products
        Eden
        Pacific
        Yves
        Mori-NV

SELECTED READINGS

Alfrey AC. Role of iron and oxygen radicals in the progression of chronic renal failure. *Am J Kidney Dis* 1994;23:183–187.

D'Amico G, Gentile MG, Manna G, et al. Effect of vegetarian soy diet on hyperlipidemia in nephrotic syndrome. *Lancet* 1992;339: 1131–1134.

D'Amico G, Remuzzi G, Maschio G, et al. Effect of dietary proteins and lipids in patients with membranous nephropathy and nephrotic syndrome. *Clin Nephrol* 1991;35:237–242.

Davies RW, Staprans I, Hutchison FN, et al. Proteinuria, not altered albumin metabolism, affects hyperlipidemia in the nephrotic rat. *J Clin Invest* 1990;86:600–605.

Don BR, Kaysen GA, Hutchison FN, et al. The effect of angiotensin-converting enzyme inhibitors and dietary protein restriction in the treatment of proteinuria. *Am J Kidney Dis* 1991;17:10–17.

Donadio JV Jr, Bergstralh EJ, Offord KP, et al. A controlled trial of fish oil in IgA nephropathy. *N Engl J Med* 1994;331:1194–1199.

Gentile MG, Fellin G, Cofano F, et al. Treatment of proteinuric patients with a vegetarian soy diet and fish oil. *Clin Nephrol* 1993; 40:315–320.

Goldstein DA, Haldimann B, Sherman D, et al. Vitamin D metabolites and calcium metabolism in patients with nephrotic syndrome and normal renal function. *J Clin Endocrinol Metab* 1981;53: 116–121.

Joven J, Villabona C, Vilella E, et al. Abnormalities of lipoprotein metabolism in patients with nephrotic syndrome. *N Engl J Med* 1990;323:579–584.

Kaysen GA, Gambertoglio J, Jiminez I, et al. Effect of dietary protein intake on albumin homeostasis in nephrotic patients. *Kidney Int* 1986;29:572–577.

Kaysen GA, Martin VI, Jones H Jr. Arginine augments neither albuminuria nor albumin synthesis caused by high-protein diets in nephrosis. *Am J Physiol* 1992;263:F907–F917.

Kaysen GA, Myers BD, Couser WG, et al. Mechanisms and consequences of proteinuria. *Lab Invest* 1986;54:479–498.

Paller MS, Hostetter TH. Dietary protein increases plasma renin and reduces pressor reactivity to angiotensin II. *Am J Physiol* 1986; 251:F34–F39.

Peterson C, Madsen B, Perlman A, et al. Atrial natriuretic peptide and the renal response to hypervolemia in nephrotic humans. *Kidney Int* 1988;34:825–831.

Rabelink A, Erkelens D, Hene R, et al. Effects of simvastatin and cholestyramine on lipoprotein profile in hyperlipidemia of nephrotic syndrome. *Lancet* 1988;2:1335–1337.

Rabelink A, Hene R, Erkelens D, et al. Partial remission of the nephrotic syndrome on long-term simvastatin. *Lancet* 1990;335: 1045–1046.

Reichel M, Mauro TM, Ziboh VA, et al. Acrodermatitis enteropathica in a patient with the acquired immune deficiency syndrome. *Arch Dermatol* 1992;128:415–417.

Remuzzi G, Imberti L, Rossini M, et al. Increased glomerular thromboxane synthesis as a possible cause of proteinuria in experimental nephrosis. *J Clin Invest* 1985;75:94–101.

Schmitz PG, Kasiske BL, O'Donnell MP, et al. Lipids and progressive renal injury. *Semin Nephrol* 1989;9:354–369.

Sinclair HM. Essential fatty acids in perspective. *Human Nutrition, Clinical Nutrition* 1984;38:245–260.

Stec J, Podracka L, Pavkovcekova O, et al. Zinc and copper metabolism in nephrotic syndrome. *Nephron* 1990;56:186–187.

Thomas ME, Freestone A, Varghese Z, et al. Lipoprotein(a) in patients with proteinuria. *Nephrol Dial Transplant* 1992;7:597–601.

Wanner C, Rader D, Bartens W, et al. Elevated plasma lipoprotein(a) in patients with the nephrotic syndrome. *Ann Intern Med* 1993; 119:263–269.

Wilhelmsen LK, Svärdsuud K, Korsan-Bengsten B, et al. Fibrinogen as a risk factor for stroke and myocardial infarction. *N Engl J Med* 1984;311:501–505.

Nutritional Support in Acute Renal Failure

Wilfred Druml

In the predialysis era and the early years of hemodialysis, severe or total restriction of nutrient intake was recommended for patients with acute renal failure (ARF). Subsequently, "minimal requirements" were used in analogy to chronic renal failure (CRF) and, later, liberal nutritional support was used with little regard to renal function. Modern nutritional therapy includes a tailored regimen that takes into consideration the complex metabolic alterations and substrate requirements of patients with ARF and various degrees of stress and hypercatabolism. Preexisting or hospital-acquired malnutrition is an important factor contributing to the persistent high mortality in critically ill patients, including those with ARF. The primary goals of nutritional support are similar for patients with ARF or with other catabolic clinical conditions—namely, to maintain protein stores and correct preexisting or disease-related deficits in lean body mass. The objectives differ fundamentally from those for CRF patients because diets or infusions that satisfy minimal requirements in CRF will not necessarily be sufficient for ARF patients. The degree of hypercatabolism caused by the disease associated with ARF, the nutritional state of the patient, and the type and frequency of dialysis therapy are the determinants of nutrient requirements (and outcome) in ARF patients.

Modern nutritional support of ARF patients is directed at supplying the requirements for all nutrients necessary for preservation of lean body mass, immunocompetence, wound healing, and so forth, while preventing specific metabolic alterations and limiting uremic toxicity. The multiple metabolic alterations associated with ARF and the methods for estimating nutrient requirements are discussed, as is experimental and clinical experience and current concepts as to the type and composition of nutritional programs.

THE METABOLIC CONSEQUENCES OF ACUTE RENAL FAILURE

Acute renal failure is often a complication of sepsis, trauma, or multiple organ failure, so it is difficult to ascribe specific metabolic alterations to ARF. Metabolic changes in most patients are determined not only by acute loss of renal function and the underlying disease (infection and organ dysfunction), but by the type and intensity of renal replacement therapy. The acute loss of renal function does not permit the adjustments in water, electrolyte, and acid–base metabolism seen in CRF, and it causes specific and distinct alterations in protein–amino acid, carbohydrate, and lipid metabolism.

Energy Metabolism

Acute renal failure in experimental animals decreases oxygen consumption even when hypothermia and acidosis are corrected.

Impairment of oxidative phosphorylation was implicated as the cause of this "uremic hypometabolism." In contrast, oxygen consumption in patients with ARF is increased by approximately 20%, almost certainly because of the underlying disease rather than the ARF (energy expenditure is increased in septic patients but normal in nonseptic subjects with ARF). Even in the multiple organ failure syndrome, oxygen consumption depends on the injury rather than ARF. Consequently, if uremia is controlled by hemodialysis or hemofiltration, there is little if any change in energy metabolism in ARF.

The pattern of substrate oxidation in ARF is similar to that in other acute disease. The oxidation of fat is increased, whereas carbohydrate oxidation is reduced (at least after an overnight fast). The preferential oxidation of fat may reflect insulin resistance or decreased hepatic glycogen stores in ARF.

Protein and Amino Acid Metabolism

The hallmark of metabolic alterations in ARF is activation of protein catabolism with excessive release of amino acids from skeletal muscle and sustained negative nitrogen balance. Not only is protein breakdown accelerated, but there is defective utilization of amino acids for protein synthesis in muscle, and amino acid transport into skeletal muscle is impaired. This abnormality can be linked both to insulin resistance and to a generalized defect in ion transport in uremia; both the activity and receptor density of the sodium pump are abnormal in adipose cells and muscle tissue. Consequently, amino acids are redistributed from muscle to the liver. Hepatic extraction of amino acids from blood, hepatic gluconeogenesis, and ureagenesis are all increased. Finally, hepatic synthesis and secretion of acute-phase proteins are stimulated.

Amino Acid Pools and Amino Acid Utilization in Acute Renal Failure

These metabolic alterations in ARF lead to imbalances in amino acid pools with a typical plasma amino acid pattern. Plasma concentrations of cystine, taurine, methionine, and phenylalanine are elevated, whereas valine and leucine are decreased in patients with ARF. As expected from the increased hepatic extraction of amino acids observed in animal experiments, overall amino acid clearance and especially that of amino acids used in gluconeogenesis is enhanced. In contrast, the clearance of phenylalanine, proline, and, remarkably, valine is decreased in ARF.

Causes of Protein Catabolism in Acute Renal Failure

The causes of hypercatabolism in ARF are complex (Table 10-1). Accelerated protein breakdown could be a secondary response induced to support the stimulation of hepatic gluconeogenesis from amino acids. In healthy subjects or patients with CRF, hepatic gluconeogenesis from amino acids is readily and completely suppressed by an infusion of glucose. In ARF, however, hepatic glucose formation is decreased but not halted, because during a glucose infusion there is persistent gluconeogenesis from amino acids. These findings have important implications for nutritional support in patients with ARF: 1) it is impossible to achieve a positive nitrogen balance in a patient with ARF; 2)

**Table 10-1. Contributing factors to
protein catabolism in acute renal failure**

Impairment of metabolic functions by uremic toxins

Endocrine factors
  Insulin resistance
  Increased secretion of catabolic hormones (catecholamines,
    glucagon, glucocorticoids)
  Hyperparathyroidism
  Suppression of release of or resistance to growth factors

Acidosis

Systemic inflammatory response syndrome (activation of cytokines)

Release of proteases

Inadequate supply of nutritional substrates

Loss of nutritional substrates (renal replacement therapy)

protein catabolism cannot be suppressed by feeding or infusing nutritional substrates; and 3) future advances will require a method that suppresses protein catabolism. Experimentally, the stimulation of muscle protein catabolism and enhanced hepatic gluconeogenesis is mediated by a glucocorticoid-dependent pathway. Increased protein catabolism in rats with ARF is normalized by treatment with a steroid receptor antagonist.

A major stimulus of muscle protein catabolism in experimental ARF is insulin resistance: the maximal rate of insulin-stimulated protein synthesis is depressed and protein degradation is increased even in the presence of insulin. There may be a link between protein and glucose metabolism; tyrosine release from muscle (as a measure of protein catabolism) is highly correlated with the ratio of lactate release to glucose uptake. This suggests that inefficient energy metabolism stimulates protein breakdown and interrupts the normal control of protein turnover.

A second stimulus of muscle protein breakdown is acidosis. Experimentally, metabolic acidosis activates the catabolism of protein and amino acids independently of azotemia. In patients with CRF, there also is compelling evidence that increased protein and amino acid degradation can be eliminated by correcting metabolic acidosis. It is unknown whether these findings apply to patients with ARF.

Several other catabolic factors are operative in ARF, including release of hormones (catecholamines, glucagon, glucocorticoids), hyperparathyroidism, suppression or decreased sensitivity to growth factors, and the release of proteases from activated leukocytes. The release of inflammatory mediators such as tumor necrosis factor (TNF) and interleukins also could mediate hypercatabolism in acute disease states.

The type and frequency of renal replacement therapy have an important impact on protein balance. Aggravation of protein catabolism during dialysis is in part mediated by the loss of nutritional substrates, but there is also activation of protein breakdown and inhibition of protein synthesis in muscle (see later; see also Chapter 2). Last, but not least, inadequate nutrition contributes to the loss of lean body mass in ARF.

*Metabolic Functions of the Kidney and Protein
and Amino Acid Metabolism in Acute Renal Failure*

Protein and amino acid metabolism are also affected by the impairment of kidney function: various amino acids are synthesized by the kidneys and released into the circulation, including cysteine, methionine (from homocysteine), tyrosine, arginine, and serine. Because of this, certain amino acids, such as arginine or tyrosine, which are termed "nonessential" might become "conditionally indispensable" in ARF patients. The kidney is also an important organ where proteins are degraded; multiple peptides are filtered and then catabolized in the proximal tubule so that the constituent amino acids are recycled into the metabolic pool. In renal failure, catabolism of peptide hormones is retarded (insulin requirements decrease in diabetic patients in whom ARF develops). Although this could impair the efficacy of dipeptides as a source of amino acids, most dipeptides used as nutritional substrates contain alanine or glycine at the *N*-terminus and are rapidly hydrolyzed even when there is renal dysfunction.

Carbohydrate Metabolism

Acute renal failure is commonly associated with hyperglycemia, mainly because of insulin resistance. Experimentally, the plasma insulin concentration is elevated, maximal insulin-stimulated glucose uptake by skeletal muscle is decreased by 50%, and glycogen synthesis is impaired. Because insulin concentrations causing half-maximal stimulation of glucose uptake are normal, a postreceptor defect rather than impaired insulin sensitivity must be causing defective glucose metabolism in ARF. A second feature of abnormal glucose metabolism in ARF is accelerated hepatic gluconeogenesis, mainly from conversion of amino acids released during protein catabolism. Hepatic extraction of amino acids, their conversion to glucose, and urea production are all increased in ARF. As detailed earlier, alterations of glucose and protein metabolism in ARF are interrelated; impaired cellular glucose utilization is associated with accelerated protein catabolism. Metabolic acidosis also contributes to deterioration of glucose tolerance in normal subjects and uremic patients.

Insulin metabolism is grossly abnormal in ARF: endogenous insulin secretion is reduced in the basal state and during glucose infusion. Because the kidney is a major organ of insulin disposal (see earlier), insulin degradation is decreased in ARF. Surprisingly, insulin catabolism by the liver is also consistently reduced in ARF. This results in normal or high plasma insulin concentrations and could explain the normal blood glucose levels in the fasted state in some animal models of ARF.

Lipid Metabolism

Profound alterations of lipid metabolism occur in patients with ARF. The triglyceride content of plasma lipoproteins, especially very–low-density lipoprotein (VLDL) and low-density lipoprotein, is increased, whereas total cholesterol and particularly high-density lipoprotein cholesterol are decreased. In addition, concentrations of apolipoproteins A I, A II, and B become abnormal. The major cause of lipid abnormalities in ARF is impaired lipolysis; the activities of both lipolytic systems, peripheral lipoprotein lipase and hepatic triglyceride lipase, are decreased to less than 50% of normal. Compared with healthy subjects, the decrease in lipolytic activity after heparin is accelerated in ARF patients. Finally, metabolic acidosis may contribute to the impaired lipolysis of ARF by inhibiting lipoprotein lipase.

Whether increased hepatic triglyceride secretion contributes to the hypertriglyceridemia of ARF remains controversial. Fatty acid and VLDL secretion are reportedly increased, normal, or decreased in ARF rats, but in patients with ARF, plasma triglyceride levels are not correlated with triglyceride clearance or postheparin lipolytic activity. This suggests that hepatic triglyceride synthesis might be increased in ARF (in contrast to CRF).

Changes in lipid metabolism develop rapidly; impaired fat elimination becomes apparent within 48 to 96 hours of renal failure and a creatinine clearance of 30 to 50 ml/minute appears to be a critical threshold for the development of these metabolic alterations. Oxidation of fatty acids is not affected by ARF. During infusion of long-chain fatty acids, carbon dioxide production from lipid was found to be comparable between healthy subjects and patients with ARF.

Fat particles in the artificial fat emulsions used in parenteral nutrition are degraded similarly to endogenous VLDL. Thus, there is delayed elimination of intravenously infused lipid emulsions in ARF; the elimination half-life is doubled and the clearance of conventional fat emulsions is reduced by more than 50% (Fig. 10-1). An impairment in lipolysis in ARF cannot be bypassed with medium-chain triglycerides; the elimination of fat emulsions containing long-chain or medium-chain triglycerides is equally retarded in ARF (see Fig. 10-1). Carnitine deficiency does not participate in the development of lipid abnormalities in ARF. In contrast to CRF, plasma carnitine levels are increased in ARF. This is due to both an increased release during muscle catabolism plus an activated hepatic carnitine synthesis.

Electrolytes

Acute renal failure frequently is associated with hyperkalemia and hyperphosphatemia, but as many as 12% of patients have a low serum potassium on admission. Nutritional support, especially a parenteral nutrition regimen with a low electrolyte content, can cause hypophosphatemia and hypokalemia in as many as 50% and 19% of patients, respectively. This is of interest because potassium or phosphate depletion in patients with normal kidney function increases the risk for development of ARF and can retard the recovery of renal function. With modern nutritional support, hyperkalemia is an indication for initiation of extracorporeal therapy in <5% of patients. Because hyperkalemia and hyperphosphatemia result from impaired renal excretion, increased release during catabolism, impaired cellular uptake, and acidosis, the type of underlying disease and degree of hypercatabolism determine the occurrence and severity of electrolyte abnormalities. Hyperphosphatemia can also predispose to the development and maintenance of ARF.

Acute renal failure is frequently associated with hypocalcemia (because of hypoalbuminemia), a high serum phosphate plus

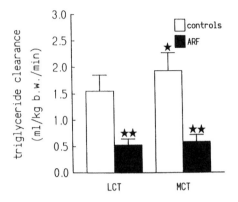

Fig. 10-1. Triglyceride clearance during infusion of lipid emulsions containing long-chain triglycerides (LCT) and long- and medium-chain triglycerides (MCT) in healthy subjects (N = 5) (open bars) and patients with acute renal failure (ARF) (N=7) (closed bars). *p < 0.05 versus LCT, **p<0.001 ARF versus controls. Adapted from W. Druml et al. Fat elimination in acute renal failure: Long chain versus medium chain triglycerides. *Am J Clin Nutr* 1992; 55:468-472.

skeletal resistance to the calcemic effect of parathyroid hormone, and impaired activation of vitamin D. In ARF caused by rhabdomyolysis, a rebound hypercalcemia may develop during the diuretic phase.

Micronutrients

As in CRF, plasma levels of 25(OH) vitamin D_3 and 1,25-$(OH)_2$ vitamin D_3 are severely depressed in ARF despite reduced calcitriol degradation (Fig. 10-2). In contrast to CRF, where vitamin A and retinol-binding protein are elevated, vitamin A serum levels are decreased in patients with ARF. Similarly, the plasma concentration of the antioxidant, vitamin E, is depressed by >50% in patients with ARF. Vitamin K levels are normal or even elevated (see Fig. 10-2).

Micronutrients are part of the defense mechanism against oxygen free radical–induced injury to the cell. There is a reduced antioxidant status in patients with ARF, and in experimental ARF, a low vitamin E or selenium level exacerbates the degree of ischemic renal injury, worsens the course of renal failure, and increases mortality; repletion with antioxidants exerts the opposite effect. These results support a crucial role of reactive oxygen species in ischemia or reperfusion injury.

NUTRIENT REQUIREMENTS IN ACUTE RENAL FAILURE

Energy Substrates

Energy requirements of patients with ARF have been grossly overestimated in the past. Although an energy intake of >50 kcal/kg/day (i.e., 100% above basic energy expenditure [BEE]) has been advocated to promote nitrogen balance, an exaggerated nutrient intake has adverse effects, and energy supply should not exceed the actual energy consumption.

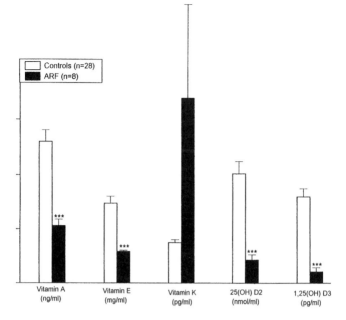

Fig. 10-2. Plasma concentrations of fat soluble vitamins in healthy controls (N=28) (open bars) and patients with acute renal failure (ARF) (N=8) (closed bars). For better comparison, y-axis presents an arbitrary scale. *** p<0.001 ARF versus controls. Adapted from Druml W. Fat soluble vitamins in acute renal failure. *Miner Electrolyte Metals* 1998; 25:220–226.

Direct measurement of the energy requirement of an individual patient is usually not available because few institutions perform indirect calorimetry or measure pulmonary thermodilution. Nevertheless, calculation of energy requirements from a standard formula provides an acceptable estimate of oxygen consumption. This includes the calculation of BEE with multiplication by a "stress factor"; the additional multiplication by 1.3 (or 1.25, as recommended in the past) is unnecessary (Table 10-2). Even in hypermetabolic conditions such as sepsis or multiple organ failure, energy requirements rarely exceed 130% of calculated BEE.

Amino Acid/Protein Requirements in Patients With Acute Renal Failure

In most clinical situations, daily protein or amino acid requirements exceed the minimal intake of 0.6 g protein/kg recommended for stable CRF patients or the recommended allowance of 0.8 g/kg/day for normal subjects. Unfortunately, few studies have attempted to define these requirements in ARF. In nonhypercatabolic patients during the polyuric phase of ARF, a protein intake of 0.97 g/kg/day was required to achieve a positive nitrogen balance. In the polyuric recovery phase of patients with sepsis-induced ARF, a nitrogen intake of 15 g/day

Table 10-2. Estimation of energy requirements

a. *Calculation of basic energy expenditure* (BEE; Harris-Benedict equation):

Men: $66.47 + (13.75 \times BW) + (5 \times height) - (6.76 \times age)$

Women: $655.1 + (9.56 \times BW) + (1.85 \times height) - (4.67 \times age)$

The average BEE is approximately 25 kcal/kg BW/day

b. *Stress factors to correct calculated energy requirement* for hypermetabolism:

Postoperative (no complications)	1.0
Long bone fracture	1.5–1.30
Cancer	1.0–1.30
Peritonitis/sepsis	1.20–1.30
Severe infection/multiple trauma	1.20–1.40
Burns	1.20–2.00*

Corrected energy requirements (kcal/day) = BEE × stress factor

BW, body weight.

*$\approx$ BEE + % burned body surface area.

(averaging an amino acid intake of 1.3 g/kg/day) was superior to 4.4 g/day (about 0.3 g/kg amino acids) in reducing negative nitrogen balance. Positive nitrogen balance was not maintained even with this regimen, however.

In a randomized, double-blinded trial of catabolic ARF patients, infusions of 21 g of essential amino acids (EAA) (averaging 0.25 g/kg/day) were compared with the same amount of EAA plus 21 g of nonessential amino acids (NEAA; a third group received glucose alone). There were no differences in recovery of renal function or survival, and urea appearance tended to be higher with increased amino acid intake when the influence of 21 g of EAA was compared with a mixture of EAA plus NEAA in amounts equaling or slightly exceeding the urea nitrogen appearance (UNA) of the previous day (on average, 76 g amino acids/day). The higher amino acid intake increased urea appearance, but the nitrogen balance was less negative (–3.0 vs. –5.2 g N/day; P not significant).

More recently, hypercatabolic patients, receiving 1.5 or 1.7 g amino acids/kg during continuous hemofiltration therapy, had less nitrogen loss compared with an infusion containing 0.7 g amino acids/kg (-3.4 vs. -8.1 g N/day). Since nitrogen balance is invariably negative in catabolic patients, there is no justification for exceeding a protein intake of 1.5 g/kg/day.

In summary, if the period of renal insufficiency is brief and there is no associated catabolic illness, the intake of protein or amino acids should be 0.8 g/kg/day. Otherwise, the intake should exceed 0.8 g/kg/day. Hypercatabolism *cannot* be overcome by increasing protein or amino acid intake to more than 1.3 to 1.5 g/kg/day, and excessive protein simply stimulates the formation of urea and other nitrogenous waste products, therefore aggravating uremic complications.

For patients treated by hemodialysis, continuous hemofiltration, or peritoneal dialysis, an extra protein/amino acid intake of 0.2 g/kg/day should be provided to compensate for losses occurring during therapy.

Assessment of Protein Catabolism

Because virtually all nitrogen arising from amino acids liberated during protein degradation is converted to urea, the degree of protein catabolism can be judged clinically by calculating the urea nitrogen appearance rate (UNA). When UNA is multiplied by 6.25, it can be converted to protein equivalents. Because muscle contains about 20% protein, multiplying the estimated protein loss by 5 yields an approximation of the loss of muscle mass. Obviously, UNA does not reflect a "true" rate of protein catabolism because it does not take into account the high endogenous rate of protein turnover (3 to 4 g of protein/kg/day in adults).

In patients with renal insufficiency, urea produced is not excreted completely but accumulates in body fluids. Because urea is distributed equally in body water (about 60% of body weight), changes in the urea pool can easily be calculated (Table 10-3). Besides urea in urine, nitrogen losses in other body fluids (e.g., gastrointestinal or choledochal losses) must be added to the net change in urea pool. In addition, nonurea nitrogen must be taken into account. These losses do not vary substantially with the diet and can be estimated to be 0.031 g N/kg/day. If this value is added to the UNA, total waste nitrogen production can be estimated. When nitrogen intake from the diet or parenteral nutrition is known, the nitrogen balance can be calculated.

Amino Acid Solutions for
Parenteral Nutrition in Acute Renal Failure

The most controversial question is what type of amino acid solution should be used: exclusively EAA, solutions of EAA plus NEAA, or specifically designed "nephro" solutions with proportions of EAA and specific NEAA that might become "conditionally essential" in ARF (Table 10-4).

The use of EAA alone is based on principles established for treating CRF patients with low-protein diets plus an EAA supplement. However, the metabolic adaptations to low-protein diets that occur in CRF patients may not occur in ARF patients; in addition, there are fundamental differences in the goals of nutritional therapy.

Table 10-3. Estimating the extent of protein catabolism

Urea nitrogen appearance (UNA; g/day)
    = urinary urea nitrogen excretion + change in urea nitrogen pool
    = $(UUN \times V) + (BUN_2 - BUN_1) \, 0.006 \times BW +$
      $(BW_2 - BW_1) \times BUN_2/100$

If there are substantial gastrointestinal losses, add urea nitrogen in secretions:
    = volume of secretions $\times BUN_2$
    Net protein breakdown (g/day) = UNA $\times$ 6.25
    Muscle loss (g/day) = UNA $\times$ 6.25 $\times$ 5

UUN, urinary urea nitrogen concentration; V, urinary volume; BUN_1 and BUN_2, blood urea nitrogen in mg/dl on days 1 and 2, respectively; BW_1 and BW_2, body weights in kg on days 1 and 2, respectively.

Table 10-4. Amino acid solutions for the treatment of ARF

	Rose requirements**	RenAmin (Clintec)	Aminess (Clintec)	Aminosyn RF (Abbott)	Nephr-Amine (McGaw)	Nephrotect (Fresenius)
Amino acids (g/l)		65	52	52	54	100
(= g/%)		6.5%	5.2%	5.2%	5.4%	10%
Volume (ml)		500	400	1000	1000	500
mOsmol/l		600	416	475	435	908
Nitrogen (g/l)		10	8.3	8.3	6.5	16.3
Essential amino acids (g/l)						
Isoleucine	1.40	5.00	5.25	4.62	5.60	5.80
Leucine	2.20	6.00	8.25	7.26	8.80	12.80
Lysine-Acetate/HCl	1.60	4.50	6.00	5.35	6.40	12.00
Methionine	2.20	5.00	8.25	7.26	8.80	2.00
Phenylalanine	2.20	4.90	8.25	7.26	8.80	3.50
Threonine	1.00	3.80	3.75	3.30	4.00	8.20
Tryptophan	0.50	1.60	1.88	1.60	2.00	3.00
Valine	1.60	8.20	6.00	5.20	6.40	8.70

Nonessential amino acids (g/l)

Alanine	5.60				6.20
Arginine	6.30		6.00		8.20
Glycine	3.00				6.30*
Histidine	4.20	4.12	4.29	2.50	9.80
Proline	3.50				3.00
Serine	3.00				7.60
Tyrosine	0.40				3.00†
Cysteine	0.40			0.20	0.40

Electrolytes (mEq/l)

Acetate	60	50	105	44	71
Sodium				5	
Potassium			5.4		
Chloride	31				3

*Glycine in part is a component of the dipeptide glycyl-L-tyrosine. **"Adequate intake" of essential amino acids.
†Tyrosine is included as a dipeptide (glycyl-L-tyrosine).

Solutions of EAA may be therapeutically suboptimal because:

Amino acid requirements seem to be higher when assessed by isotope turnover techniques, compared with the nitrogen balance methods of the 1940s.

Certain amino acids designated as NEAA for healthy subjects may become conditionally indispensable in sick patients (e.g., histidine, arginine, tyrosine, serine, cysteine), and arginine-free solutions can cause life-threatening hyperammonemia, coma, and acidosis.

Changes in amino acid metabolism caused by ARF (or hypercatabolism) can cause serious imbalances of amino acid pools.

Infusion of more than 0.6 g EAA/kg/day simply increases the production of waste products. A complete amino acid mixture may improve net nitrogen retention more than an EAA solution.

Taken together, solutions including both EAA and NEAA in standard proportions or in special proportions designed to counteract the metabolic changes of renal failure ("nephro" solutions) should be used in nutritional support of ARF patients. Although 0.6 g EAA/kg/day might suffice for noncatabolic patients, a mixture of EAA and NEAA, and especially those amino acids that might become conditionally essential in ARF, should be used if more is required. Unfortunately, the claim that amino acid solutions enriched in branched-chain amino acids exert a clinically significant anticatabolic effect has not been substantiated. Glutamine, traditionally an NEAA, has been found to improve immunologic functions and the integrity of the gastrointestinal barrier. Because glutamine is not stable in aqueous solutions, glutamine dipeptides are used in parenteral nutrition. It must be recognized that the use of dipetides in part depends on intact renal function, and renal failure may impair hydrolysis (see earlier).

Because of the low solubility of tyrosine, dipeptides containing tyrosine (such as glycyl-tyrosine) are included in modern "nephro" solutions as a tyrosine source (see Table 10-4). Note that N-acetyl tyrosine, which has been used as a tyrosine source, cannot be converted into tyrosine in humans, and might stimulate protein catabolism.

Micronutrients

In patients with ARF, balance studies of micronutrients (vitamins, trace elements) are not available. With dialysis, many small molecules, including minerals and several vitamins, are lost and should be replaced. For example, depletion of thiamine (vitamin B_1) by continuous hemofiltration plus an inadequate intake can result in lactic acidosis and heart failure. On the other hand, ascorbic acid (vitamin C) is converted to a toxic product, oxalic acid, so its intake should be <200 mg/day. Fat-soluble vitamins are not lost during hemodialysis, but their requirements may rise in ARF, except for vitamin K, which has a high plasma concentration (see Fig. 10-2).

Most commercial multivitamin preparations for parenteral infusions contain the recommended dietary allowances (RDA) of vitamins and can be safely used in patients with ARF. However, a daily parenteral supply of trace elements should be avoided. Trace element homeostasis depends on both gastrointestinal absorption, which is bypassed by intravenous infusion, and renal excretion, which is impaired in ARF, so the risk of toxicity rises. A possible exception is selenium, the cofactor of glutathione peroxidase, which may be given regularly because its levels are low in hemodialysis patients.

METABOLIC IMPACT OF EXTRACORPOREAL THERAPY

Catabolism during dialysis is caused by substrate losses, activation of protein breakdown from release of leukocyte-derived proteases, and release of interleukins and TNF induced by blood interaction with the dialysis membrane or endotoxin. Dialysis may also inhibit protein synthesis. Because the sieving coefficient of amino acids is within the range of 0.8 to 1.0, amino acids are lost at a rate of approximately 0.2 g/l filtrate (about 5 to 10 g amino acid/day). Membranes used in hemofiltration are more porous, and small proteins are filtered. In view of their short half-life, hormone losses are probably not of pathophysiologic importance. Continuous hemofiltration may be associated with a heat loss accounting for 350 to 700 kcal/day. This is reduced when lactate is added to hemofiltration fluids.

In patients with ARF treated by continuous renal replacement therapies, nutrition must be given during extracorporeal therapy. Because the endogenous clearance of amino acids (i.e., tissue uptake and utilization) is 80 to 1800 ml/minute, it greatly exceeds dialytic clearance, so only a minimal fraction of amino acids infused is removed by dialysis (i.e., only about 10% of the infused amino acids).

IMPACT OF METABOLIC AND NUTRITIONAL INTERVENTIONS ON RENAL FUNCTION AND COURSE OF ACUTE RENAL FAILURE

Starvation accelerates protein breakdown and impairs protein synthesis in the kidney; refeeding has the opposite effects. In experimental ARF, infusion of amino acids or total parenteral nutrition accelerates tissue repair and recovery of renal function, but in patients with ARF a beneficial effect has been much more difficult to prove.

On balance, available evidence suggests that provision of substrates may enhance tissue regeneration and, possibly, renal tubular repair. On the other hand, amino acids infused before or during ischemic or nephrotoxic injury to the rat kidney may enhance tubular damage and accelerate loss of renal function. In part, this is related to the increase in metabolic work for transport processes. During the phase of renal damage, the "ebb phase" immediately after trauma, shock, major operations, and the like, nutritional intake should be avoided (see later). Amino acids may be toxic (e.g., lysine or arginine) or protective, like glycine and to a lesser degree alanine, which limit tubular injury in ischemic and nephrotoxic models of ARF. A high protein intake before an ischemic or nephrotoxic insult accelerated renal damage and increased mortality in ARF rats. Whether a similar response occurs in patients is unknown.

METABOLIC INTERVENTIONS
TO CONTROL CATABOLISM

Excessive mortality in ARF is determined by the extent of hypercatabolism. Potentially, hypercatabolism can be modified at three levels of metabolic intervention:

Substrate level: Unfortunately, it is impossible to halt hypercatabolism and hepatic gluconeogenesis simply by providing conventional nutritional substrates to patients with ARF.

Endocrine level: Therapy with hormones (insulin, insulin-like growth factor, growth hormone) and hormone antagonists (steroid receptor antagonists) seems beneficial in rats. Unfortunately, early clinical trials have yielded less clear-cut results.

Mediator level: Cytokines (interleukins and TNF-α) can stimulate amino acid release from skeletal muscle and activation, so therapies to limit the actions of inflammatory mediators (e.g., cyclooxygenase inhibitors, thromboxane antagonists, and antibodies to TNF-α, platelet-activating factor, interleukins) could prove beneficial.

Early reports attempted to define the effect of nutritional support by comparing it with glucose infusion alone. In one study, a solution including 16 g EAA was compared with infusion of glucose alone in a double-blinded protocol. Survival rate was especially improved in high-risk patients (e.g., those requiring dialysis or with pneumonia, sepsis, or a gastrointestinal hemorrhage). There was also a tendency toward a shorter duration of renal dysfunction. A potential benefit for high-risk patients with ARF was confirmed in uncontrolled studies, but the benefit was either not statistically significant or there were problems in the design of the study. Taken together, the studies suggest that a nutritional strategy of infusing amino acids is superior to glucose alone, especially in high-risk patients, and that hypercatabolic patients should receive both EAA and NEAA. The difficulties with convincingly demonstrating a beneficial effect of nutritional support are not surprising: ARF patients are extremely heterogenous because of varying degrees of renal failure and associated complications.

NUTRITIONAL STRATEGIES
IN ACUTE RENAL FAILURE

General Considerations

What Patient Needs Nutritional Support?

This decision is influenced by the patient's ability to meet nutritional requirements by eating, the nutritional status of the patient, the underlying illness, and the degree of catabolism. In any patient with evidence of malnutrition (based on low serum albumin and transferrin, anthropometric measurements, and, most important, clinical judgment), nutritional therapy should be initiated. However, if a patient is well nourished and will resume a normal diet within 5 days, no specific nutritional support is necessary. In patients with excess protein catabolism, nutritional support should be initiated early.

When Should Nutrition Be Started?

The timing of nutritional support is determined by the nutritional status and the degree of catabolism. The higher the degree of malnutrition and/or the extent of catabolism, the earlier nutritional support should be initiated. The decision should be made early in the course of disease to avoid the development of deficiencies and of hospital-acquired malnutrition. During the acute phase of ARF (within 24 to 48 hours after trauma or surgery), nutritional support should be withheld. Infusions of large quantities of amino acids or glucose during this "ebb phase" increase oxygen requirements and aggravate tubular damage and the degree of renal functional loss.

At What Degree of Renal Dysfunction
Should the Nutritional Regimen Be Adjusted?

Animal experiments have shown that muscle protein synthesis falls when renal function is <30% of normal. In patients with CRF, glucose intolerance and lipid abnormalities occur when creatinine clearance is <40 ml/minute. Thus, at a serum creatinine >3 mg/dl or creatinine clearance <40 ml/minute, a nutritional regimen should be designed to counteract the specific metabolic abnormalities of ARF.

Patient Classification

Ideally, a nutritional program should be designed for each individual ARF patient. Clinically, it is useful to distinguish three groups of ARF patients based on the extent of protein catabolism associated with the underlying disease. This provides guidelines for the dietary requirements (Table 10-5).

Group I includes patients without excessive catabolism and a UNA <6 g N above nitrogen intake/day. ARF is usually caused by nephrotoxins (aminoglycosides, contrast media, or mismatched blood transfusions). In most cases, these patients are fed orally and the prognosis for recovery of renal function and survival is excellent.

Group II consists of patients with moderate hypercatabolism and a UNA exceeding nitrogen intake by 6 to 12 g N/day. These patients frequently have complicating infections, peritonitis, or moderate injury. Tube feeding or intravenous nutritional support is usually required, as is dialysis/hemofiltration (to limit waste product accumulation).

Group III comprises ARF patients with severe trauma, burns, or overwhelming infections. UNA is markedly elevated to >12 g N above nitrogen intake/day. Treatment strategies usually include parenteral nutrition plus blood pressure and ventilatory support. Dialysis or hemofiltration is used to maintain fluid balance and blood urea nitrogen (BUN) below 100 mg/dl (see Table 10-5). Mortality in such patients exceeds 60% to 80%. It is not the loss of renal function that accounts for the poor prognosis but the superimposed hypercatabolism and the severity of underlying illness. Unfortunately, there are no reliable methods for stopping or reducing hypercatabolism, and nutritional therapy should be directed at minimizing the loss of protein mass (see earlier).

Table 10-5. Patient classification and substrate requirements in patients with acute renal failure

	Extent of Catabolism		
	Mild	Moderate	Severe
Excess urea appearance (above N intake)	<5 g	5–10 g	>10 g
Clinical setting (examples)	Drug toxicity	Elective surgery ± infection	Severe injury or sepsis
Mortality	20%	~60%	>60%
Dialysis/hemofiltration frequency	Rare	As needed	Frequent
Route of nutrient administration	Oral	Enteral or parenteral	Enteral or parenteral
Energy recommendations (kcal/kg BW/day)	25	25–30	25–35
Energy substrates	Glucose	Glucose + fat	Glucose + fat
Glucose (g/kg BW/day)	3.0–5.0	3.0–5.0	3.0–5.0 (max. 7.0)
Fat (g/kg BW/day)		0.5–1.0	0.8–1.5
Amino acids/protein (g/kg/day)	0.6–1.0	0.8–1.2	1.0–1.5
	EAA (+NEAA)	EAA + NEAA	EAA + NEAA
Nutrients used			
Oral/enteral	Food	Enteral formulas	Enteral formulas
Parenteral	EAA + specific NEAA solutions (general or "nephro") Multivitamin and multitrace element preparations	Glucose 50–70% + fat emulsions 10% or 20%	Glucose 50–70% + fat emulsions 10% or 20%

BW, body weight; EAA, essential amino acids; NEAA, nonessential amino acids

Nutrient Administration

Oral Feeding

In all patients who can tolerate them, oral feedings should be used. Calories are provided by simple carbohydrates (e.g., sugar, jellies, sweets) at regular intervals. Initially, 40 g of high-quality protein per day is given (0.6 g/kg/day); this is gradually increased to 0.8 g/kg/day as long as the BUN remains <100 mg/dl. For patients treated by hemodialysis, protein intake should be increased to 1.0 to 1.2 g/kg/day to make up for amino acids lost and the catabolism occurring during dialysis. For peritoneal dialysis patients, protein intake should be raised to 1.4 g/kg/day to counteract losses of both amino acids and protein into the dialysate. A supplement of water-soluble vitamins is recommended, but vitamin C intake should be limited to <200 mg/day.

Enteral Nutrition (Tube Feeding)

The gastrointestinal tract should be used whenever possible because nutrients may help to maintain gastrointestinal functions and the mucosal barrier (i.e., prevent the translocation of bacteria and systemic infections). Even small amounts of enterally administered diets exert a protective effect on the intestinal mucosa.

In patients with ARF who are anorectic or unable to eat, enteral nutrition should be provided through small, soft feeding tubes with the tip positioned in the stomach or jejunum. If feeding solutions are given continuously, the stomach should be aspirated every 2 to 4 hours until adequate gastric emptying and intestinal peristalsis are established. This practice prevents vomiting and reduces the risk of bronchopulmonary aspiration. To avoid diarrhea, the formula should be diluted initially and the amount and concentration of the solution gradually increased over several days until nutritional requirements are met. Undesired but potentially treatable side effects include nausea, vomiting, abdominal distention, cramping and diarrhea.

ENTERAL FORMULAS. There are standardized tube feeding formulas for subjects with normal renal function that can also be given to patients with ARF. Alternatively, enteral feeding formulas designed for patients with CRF can be used because they are limited in potassium and phosphates (Table 10-6). The protein content is lower and confined to high-quality proteins (in part as oligopeptides and free amino acids), the electrolyte concentrations are low, and most contain recommended allowances of vitamins and minerals. The diets can be supplemented with electrolytes, protein, lipids, and so forth as required.

Parenteral Nutrition

If nutrient requirements cannot be met by the enteral route, total parenteral nutrition should be used. Because fluids are usually restricted, hyperosmolar solutions are infused through central venous catheters to avoid damage to peripheral veins. Ideally, the dialysis access catheter should not be used for parenteral nutrition.

Table 10-6. Enteral formulas for nutritional support in patients with renal failure

	Amin-Aid (McGaw)	Travasorb renal* (Travenol)	Salvipeptide nephro† (Clintec)	Replena (Abbott)	Survimed Renal‡ (Fresenius)
Volume (ml)	750	1050	500	500	1000
Calories					
kcal	1470	1400	1000	1000	1320
cal/ml	1.96	1.35	2.00	2.00	1.32
Energy distribution (proteins:fat:carbohydrates) (%)	4:21:75	7:12:81	8:22:70	6:43:51	6:10:84
kcal/g N	832:1	389:1	313:1	427:1	398:1
Proteins (g)	14.6	24.0	20.0	15.0	20.8
EAA (%)	100	60	23		
NEAA (%)	0	30	20		
Hydrolysate (%)			23	100	100
Full protein (%)			34	100	
Nitrogen (g)	1.76	3.6	3.2	2.4	3.32
Carbohydrates (g)	274	284	175	128	276
Monodisaccharides (%)	100	100	3	10	
Oligosaccharides (%)			28		
Polysaccharides (%)			69	90	100

Fat (g)	34.6	18.6	24	48	15.2
LCT (%)		30	50	100	70
Essential fatty acids (%)		18	31	22	52
MCT (%)		70	50		30
Nonprotein kcal/g N	800	363	288	393	374
Osmolality (mOsmol/kg)	1095	590	507	615	600
Sodium (mmol/l)	11		7.2	34.0	15.2
Potassium (mmol/l)			1.5	28.5	8
Vitamins	b	a	a	a	a
Minerals	b	b	a	a	a

EAA, essential amino acids; NEAA, nonessential amino acids; LCT, long-chain triglycerides; MCT, medium chain triglycerides; a, 2000 kcal/day meet recommended dietary allowance for most vitamins and minerals; b, must be added.
*3 bags + 810 ml water = 1050 ml.
†1 × component I + 1 × component II + 350 ml water = 500 ml.
‡4 bags + 800 ml water = 1000 ml.

COMPONENTS OF PARENTERAL NUTRITION. **Energy Substrates.** *Carbohydrates.* Glucose is the main energy substrate because it can be used by all organs even under hypoxic conditions, and has the potential to reduce nitrogen requirements. Because ARF impairs glucose tolerance, insulin is frequently needed. Note that a glucose intake >5 g/kg/day promotes lipogenesis and fatty infiltration of the liver, as well as excessive carbon dioxide production and hypercarbia. If energy requirements cannot be met by glucose infusion plus insulin, a portion should be supplied by lipid emulsions. For prolonged therapy, the most suitable means of providing the energy requirements in critically ill patients is not glucose or lipids, but glucose and lipids. Other carbohydrates, including fructose, sorbitol, or xylitol, should be avoided because of potential adverse metabolic effects.

Fat Emulsions. Advantages of intravenous lipids include a high specific energy content, a low osmolality, provision of essential fatty acids to prevent lipid deficiency syndromes, a lower frequency of hepatic side effects, and a reduced carbon dioxide production (especially in patients with respiratory failure). The changes in lipid metabolism induced by ARF should not prevent the use of lipid emulsions. However, the amount of lipid should be adjusted to meet the patient's capacity to use lipids; usually, 1 g fat/kg/day does not increase plasma triglycerides substantially, and about 20% to 25% of energy requirements can be met. Lipids should be avoided in patients with hyperlipidemia (plasma triglycerides >350 mg/dl), intravascular coagulation, acidosis (pH < 7.25), impaired circulation, or hypoxemia.

Parenteral lipid emulsions are usually composed of long-chain triglycerides mostly derived from soybean oil, but emulsions containing a mixture of long- and medium-chain triglycerides are available. Proposed advantages include a faster uptake by tissues because of a higher affinity for the lipoprotein lipase enzyme, a more complete, carnitine-independent metabolism, and a triglyceride-lowering effect. Medium-chain triglycerides alone do not promote faster lipolysis because both types of fat emulsions are equally retarded in ARF (see Fig. 10-1).

Amino Acid Solutions. Potential advantages of specifically designed "nephro" mixtures and recommended daily nitrogen intake have been discussed. Although 0.6 g EAA/kg/day is probably sufficient for noncatabolic patients, those patients who require a higher level should receive a mixture including both EAA and NEAA in standard proportions or in proportions designed to counteract the metabolic changes of renal failure (see Table 10-4).

Electrolytes. Electrolytes should be added to the solution as required. Remember that the infusion of glucose or amino acids causes a shift of potassium and phosphate into cells, producing hypokalemia and hypophosphatemia. If phosphates are added to "all-in-one" solutions, it is preferable to use organic phosphates (e.g., glycerophosphate, glucose-1-phosphate) to avoid incompatibilities with other ions (e.g., calcium, magnesium) in the solution. Divalent ions (calcium, magnesium) can impair the stability of fat emulsions and should be used cautiously in lipid-containing nutrition solutions.

Micronutrients. Multivitamin preparations can safely be added to the nutrition solution, but vitamin C should be kept at

<200 mg/day. Trace elements should be restricted to twice weekly to avoid toxic effects.

PARENTERAL SOLUTIONS. Standard solutions containing amino acids, glucose, and lipids plus vitamins, trace elements, and electrolytes contained in a single infusion bag are available ("all-in-one" solutions; Table 10-7). The stability of fat emulsions in such mixtures should be tested. If hyperglycemia is present, insulin can be added or administered separately. To ensure maximal nutrient use and to avoid metabolic derangements (e.g., mineral unbalance, hyperglycemia, or excessive BUN), the infusion should be started at a low rate (providing about 50% of requirements) and gradually increased over several days. Optimally, the solution should be infused continuously over 24 hours to avoid marked changes in substrate concentrations.

Table 10-7. Renal failure fluid ("all-in-one solution")*

Component	Quantity		Remarks
Glucose	40–70%	500 ml	In the presence of severe insulin resistance switch to D30W
Fat emulsion	10–20%	500 ml	Start with 10%, switch to 20% if triglycerides are <350 mg/dl
Amino acids	6.5–10%	500 ml	General or special "nephro" amino acid solutions including essential and nonessential amino acids
Water-soluble vitamins†	Daily		Limit vitamin C intake to <200 mg/day
Fat-soluble vitamins†	Daily		
Trace elements†	Twice weekly		Beware of toxic effects
Electrolytes	As required		Beware of hypophosphatemia or hypokalemia after initiation of total parenteral nutrition
Insulin	As required		Added directly to the solution or given separately

*"All-in-one solution" with all components contained in a single bag. Infusion rate initially 50% of requirements, to be increased over a period of 3 days to satisfy requirements.
†Combination products containing the recommended dietary allowances.

**Table 10-8. Minimal suggested schedule
for monitoring parenteral nutrition**

Variables	Patient's Metabolic Status	
	Unstable	Stable
Blood glucose	$1–6 \times$ Daily	Daily
Osmolality	Daily	$2 \times$ Weekly
Electrolytes (Na^+, K^+, Cl^+)	Daily	Daily
Calcium, phosphate, magnesium	Daily	$3 \times$ Weekly
BUN/BUN rise/day	Daily	Daily
Urinary nitrogen appearance	Daily	$2 \times$ Weekly
Triglycerides	Daily	$2 \times$ Weekly
Blood gas analysis/pH	Daily	$1 \times$ Weekly
Ammonia	$2 \times$ Weekly	$1 \times$ Weekly
Transaminases + bilirubin	$2 \times$ Weekly	$1 \times$ Weekly

BUN, blood urea nitrogen.

COMPLICATIONS. Technical problems and infectious complications originating from the central venous catheter, and chemical and metabolic complications of parenteral nutrition are similar in patients with ARF and in nonuremic subjects. Obviously, the tolerance to fluid is limited and electrolyte derangements may develop rapidly, whereas an exaggerated protein or amino acid intake results in excessive BUN (and waste product) accumulation; glucose intolerance and decreased fat clearance can cause hyperglycemia and hypertriglyceridemia. Thus, nutritional therapy in patients with ARF requires more frequent monitoring. Most complications are related to an excess intake of substrates (e.g., hyperglycemia, fatty infiltration of the liver, increased carbon dioxide production, hypertriglyceridemia, hyperkalemia, accelerated BUN increase) or development of deficiencies (e.g., of minerals, vitamins, essential fatty acids). By gradually increasing the infusion rate, by limiting the infusion to supply requirements, and by combining glucose with lipids, many of these side effects can be minimized.

MONITORING PARENTERAL NUTRITION. Table 10-8 summarizes laboratory tests required to monitor patients treated with parenteral nutrition. The frequency of testing depends on the patient's metabolic stability; plasma glucose, potassium, and phosphate should be monitored repeatedly after the start of parenteral nutrition.

CONCLUSIONS

All patients require adequate nutritional support to maintain protein stores and to correct preexisting or disease-related deficits in lean body mass. In patients with ARF, it is not the impairment of renal function per se that determines the decision to start nutritional support, but the nutritional status, type and severity of underlying disease, and the degree of associated hypercatabolism.

An increased understanding of the pathophysiologic mechanisms underlying the metabolic changes induced by ARF, better definitions of nutritional requirements, and advances in the techniques of parenteral and enteral nutritional support have greatly improved the success of nutritional therapy. Nevertheless, the optimal nutritional regimen for ARF has not been defined, nor has nutritional support convincingly reduced morbidity and mortality in ARF patients. The poor prognosis in patients with ARF is related to the severity of the underlying illness and to hypercatabolism, and nutritional therapy, like dialysis, should be viewed as a means of supporting the patient until the underlying illness is controlled and hypermetabolism is reversed. Future advances will require metabolic interventions that control accelerated catabolism.

SELECTED READINGS

Abel RM, Beck CH, Abbott WM, et al. Improved survival from acute renal failure after treatment with intravenous essential amino acids and glucose: results of a prospective double-blind study. *N Engl J Med* 1973;288:695–699.

Chima CS, Meyer L, Hummell AC, et al. Protein catabolic rate in patients with acute renal failure on continuous arteriovenous hemofiltration and total parenteral nutrition. *J Am Soc Nephrol* 1993;3:1516–1521.

Clark AS, Mitch WE. Muscle protein turnover and glucose uptake in acutely uremic rats. *J Clin Invest* 1983;72:836–845.

Druml W, Lochs H, Roth E, et al. Utilization of tyrosine dipeptides and acetyl-tyrosine in normal and uremic humans. *Am J Physiol* 1991;260:E280–E285.

Druml W, Fischer M, Sertl S, et al. Fat elimination in acute renal failure: long chain versus medium chain triglycerides. *Am J Clin Nutr* 1992;55:468–472.

Druml W, Fischer M, Liebisch B, et al. Elimination of amino acids in renal failure. *Am J Clin Nutr* 1994;60:418–423.

Druml W, Mitch WE. Metabolism in acute renal failure. *Semin Dial* 1996;9:484–490.

Druml W, Mitch WE. Enteral nutrition in renal disease. In: Rombeau JL, Rolandelli RH, eds. *Enteral and tube feeding*. Philadelphia: WB Saunders; 1997:439–461.

England BK, Mitch WE. Acid-base, fluid and electrolyte aspects of parenteral nutrition. In: Kokko JP, Tannen R, eds. *Fluid and electrolytes*. Philadelphia: WB Saunders; 1990:1024–1042.

Feinstein EI, Blumenkrantz MJ, Healy M, et al. Clinical and metabolic response to parenteral nutrition in acute renal failure: a controlled double blind study. *Medicine* 1981;60:124–135.

Fürst P, Stehle P. The potential use of dipeptides in clinical nutrition. *Nutr Clin Pract* 1993;8:106–114.

Hübl W, Druml W, Roth E, et al. Importance of liver and kidney for the utilization of glutamine-containing dipeptides in man. *Metabolism* 1994;43:1104–1107.

Macias WL, Alaka KJ, Murphy MH, et al. Impact of nutritional regimen on protein catabolism and nitrogen balance in patients with acute renal failure. *J Parenter Enteral Nutr* 1996;20:56–62.

Maroni BJ, Steinman T, Mitch WE. A method for estimating nitrogen intake of patients with chronic renal failure. *Kidney Int* 1986;27:58–63.

May RC, Clark AS, Goheer MA, et al. Specific defects in insulin-mediated muscle metabolism in acute uremia. *Kidney Int* 1985;28:490–497.

May RC, Kelly RA, Mitch WE. Mechanisms for defects in muscle protein metabolism in rats with chronic uremia: the influence of metabolic acidosis. *J Clin Invest* 1987;79:1099–1103.

Mitch WE. Amino acid release from the hindquater and urea appearance in acute uremia. *Am J Physiol* 1981;241:E415–E419.

Mitch WE, Chesney RW. Amino acid metabolism by the kidney. *Miner Electrolyte Metab* 1983;9:190–202.

Schneeweiss B, Graninger W, Stockenhuber F, et al. Energy metabolism in acute and chronic renal failure. *Am J Clin Nutr* 1990;52:596–601.

Toback FG. Regeneration after acute tubular necrosis. *Kidney Int* 1992;41:226–246.

Nutritional Therapy and the Progression of Renal Disease

William E. Mitch

Protein-restricted diets can improve many uremic symptoms because most uremic toxins result from the metabolism of protein. These diets also ameliorate specific complications of chronic renal failure (CRF), including metabolic acidosis, renal osteodystrophy, and hypertension, because a low-protein diet invariably results in restriction of the intake of acid phosphates, sodium, and potassium. Although controversial, evidence suggests that low-protein diets can also slow the progressive loss of renal function.

An unexplained complication of CRF is that renal function continues to decline even when the disease that initially damaged the kidney is no longer active. This means that CRF in general progresses toward end-stage renal disease (ESRD), but each patient seems to progress at different rates even though he or she has the same type of kidney disease. There is reason to believe that progression of renal disease is connected to the amount of protein in the diet. It has been recognized for more than 50 years that a high-protein diet fed to rats with experimental CRF leads to increasing proteinuria, renal damage, and mortality. Conversely, dietary protein restriction protects the kidney from further damage. Investigators have also examined whether restricting dietary protein can delay the loss of residual renal function in patients with CRF. Two facts should be emphasized: first, despite intensive investigation, the mechanism(s) causing the progressive loss of renal function have not been identified. Suggested mechanisms include: 1) a lower level of an unidentified nephrotoxin produced from the metabolism of protein or amino acids; 2) a decrease in proteinuria (proteinuria is proposed as a nephrotoxin and is a sign of more severe kidney damage); and 3) better control of hypertension with a restricted diet. The second fact is that multicenter trials testing the influence of a low-protein diet on progression have not yielded a statistically significant benefit, at least when an intention-to-treat analysis was used (i.e., whether patients did or did not ingest the prescribed diet is ignored). On the other hand, several studies of small groups of patients with CRF have shown that low-protein diets can slow the loss of renal function. Results of studies of experimental animals are not reviewed in this chapter because the mechanism(s) causing progression have not been identified.

When evaluating reports that any type of dietary manipulation slows the loss of renal function in patients with CRF, at least three questions should be addressed: first, does the diet maintain an adequate nutritional status? Second, has dietary compliance been achieved? Third, does the restricted diet change the rate of loss of renal function?

DO LOW-PROTEIN DIETS CAUSE MALNUTRITION?

For many years it has been suggested that low-protein diets be used cautiously in patients with CRF to prevent loss of body protein stores. The concern arises from two observations: 1) there is evidence that patients with CRF experience a spontaneous decrease in protein intake; and 2) there is a statistical association between the presence of hypoalbuminemia and increased mortality in hemodialysis patients. Signs of malnutrition are common in dialysis patients; it is assumed that hypoalbuminemia arises from an inadequate diet or a catabolic influence of uremia. Concern about both of these issues is misplaced. First, with proper counseling and management, a low-protein diet is associated with neutral nitrogen balance, normal levels of serum proteins, and normal anthropometric indices during long-term therapy. Second, the mechanism causing hypoalbuminemia in hemodialysis patients appears to be more closely related to signs of inflammation rather than an inadequate diet. Perhaps most important, the proper implementation of a low-protein diet was found to be associated with an improved survival of patients with CRF who subsequently began dialysis therapy.

As noted in Chapter 7, the successful use of a protein-restricted diet depends on two factors: 1) ensuring that the requirements of different nutrients are included in the diet, and 2) a regular assessment of nutritional adequacy. Most reports indicate that long-term therapy with low-protein diets is nutritionally sound. For example, patients treated with a very–low-protein diet (VLPD; ~0.3 g protein/kg/day) supplemented with a mixture of ketoacids and amino acids (ketoacids), were in neutral nitrogen balance and sustained stable anthropometric values as well as serum albumin and transferrin levels (indices of visceral protein stores) for > 1 year of therapy. The same diet plus a supplement of either ketoacids or a mixture of essential amino acids (EAA) was associated with an increase in serum protein concentrations in patients who had subnormal values before dietary therapy. On the other hand, if the diet is inadequate or there is insufficient monitoring of compliance, patients are at risk of losing lean body mass.

MONITORING CHANGES IN RENAL FUNCTION

The functional mass of the human kidney is best assessed by the glomerular filtration rate (GFR). It follows that measuring the rate of decrease in GFR provides an estimate of the loss of renal mass. In Table 11-1, the methods for measuring the rate of loss of renal function are listed. Changes in GFR are most often estimated from serial measurements of the renal clearance of ^{125}I-iothalamate or ^{99m}Tc-DTPA, the plasma clearance of a compound largely cleared by glomerular filtration, or indirect estimates of GFR such as the serum creatinine (Scr) or creatinine clearance (Ccr). Because a low-protein diet can reduce creatinine production, the impact of this fact on the use of Scr or Ccr to monitor renal function is worth noting.

Serum Creatinine and Creatinine Clearance

A single value of Scr is a crude estimate of either the Ccr or GFR because Scr depends on the rate of creatinine production, the volume of distribution of creatinine, the degree of renal tubular creatinine secretion, and the rate of extrarenal creatinine clearance. On the other hand, Scr is an inexpensive test, and in patients with renal disease, the day-to-day coefficient of variation is only 6.5% (this is far below the variability in Ccr, which

Table 11-1. Methods of assessing progression of chronic renal failure

Method	Benefits	Drawbacks
Change in Scr	Inexpensive	Influenced by diet and changes in renal function Difficult to analyze the rate of change
Change in Scr^{-1}	Inexpensive Simple to analyze rate of progression	Influenced by diet and changes in renal function
Creatinine clearance	Relatively inexpensive compared with GFR markers	High degree of day-to-day variability
Renal clearance of compounds cleared by the kidney (e.g., ^{125}I-iothalamate)	Best estimate of GFR	Expense of personnel and marker Requires 4 hr by the patient Potential hazards of radioactive compound
Plasma clearance of compounds cleared by the kidney (e.g., iohexol)	Good estimate of GFR	Expense of personnel and marker Requires > 4 hr by the patient if there is renal insufficiency

Scr, serum creatinine; Scr^{-1}, the reciprocal of serum creatinine; GFR, glomerular filtration rate.

has been estimated to be $\geq 25\%$). Obviously, a change in Scr reflects a change in GFR because creatinine is largely cleared by the kidney. In fact, the reciprocal of Scr (Scr^{-1}) declines linearly with time in most patients with CRF, indicating that Ccr and GFR decline at a constant rate, and this has been verified. The decline in Scr^{-1} in individual patients varies: in the initial report of 34 patients, the rate of decline in Scr^{-1} varied from 0.0011 to 0.0152 dl/mg/month and was linear in all but 3 subjects (in other reports, the decline in Scr^{-1} was found to be linear in 60% to 80% of patients). All reports emphasize that the decline in Scr^{-1} varies widely in individual patients with CRF; in patients with diabetic nephropathy, there is as much as a 40-fold difference in the rates of progression, even though they have the same disease.

There are problems in using Scr to assess the rate of progression of renal disease: 1) creatinine excretion varies with the amount of well cooked meat in the diet, 2) creatinine production may be low in patients with CRF, and 3) creatinine is metabolized to a limited extent. If this extrarenal creatinine clearance changes, it would make interpretation difficult, but the amount of extrarenal clearance is small. In assessing the importance of these factors, the following considerations are important: prolonged adherence to a meat-restricted diet leads to a lower Scr because the contribution of creatinine arising from creatine in meat decreases. However, a false decrease in Scr persists only as long as renal function remains stable. If renal function continues to decline, then Scr will rise.

Creatinine is nonenzymatically formed from the dehydration of creatine and creatine phosphate. Consequently, the half-life of the creatine pool determines the rate of creatinine production. More important, the half-life of creatinine is ~41 days. Therefore, judgments about whether a low-protein diet has slowed the progression of CRF based on changes in Scr require a minimum wait of 4 months (i.e., > 3 half-lives). After this period, if Scr rises (or Scr^{-1} declines), the explanation must be that renal insufficiency has progressed, but if Scr and Scr^{-1} do not change, then the loss of kidney function has slowed. These considerations depend on the assumption that CRF does not slow creatinine production, and this seems to be correct. Rates of creatinine production in patients with CRF were indistinguishable from the value predicted for normal subjects of the same age, weight, and sex. Moreover, the creatine concentration in muscle of patients with CRF is normal (this is important because the conversion of creatine to creatinine is a nonenzymatic process). This leaves the concern about extrarenal creatinine clearance, but the critical issue is whether extrarenal clearance changes over time or with the severity of renal insufficiency. These questions have not been tested. In summary, measures of Scr or Scr^{-1} are useful for assessing changes in renal function but not very precise as an estimate of the GFR. A persistent increase in Scr means that renal function has declined, whereas prolonged stabilization of Scr (i.e., > 4 months) means that renal function is stable. A more precise estimate of GFR (e.g., the renal clearance of inulin, ^{125}I-iothalamate, or [99m] Tc-DTPA) has been used in several intervention trials to assess how the diet changes in renal function. First, these methods provide a more precise estimate of the remaining functioning mass of the kidney. Second, they are time consuming; a high urine flow is required to improve the accuracy, and there should be at least three urine collection periods of 20 to 30 minutes each. They are also expensive because of the personnel required and the costs of using radioisotopically labeled compounds. Even when an unlabeled compound (e.g., iohexol) is used to measure the plasma clearance and avoid timed urine collections, patients with GFR values < 30 ml/minute require more than 6 hours for the measurement. The tools and methods used to measure progression must be understood, just like instruments for measuring the nutritional adequacy of the diet.

NUTRITIONAL ADEQUACY OF LOW-PROTEIN DIETS

Three types of dietary regimens have been used in studies examining whether the progression of CRF can be slowed: 1) a low-protein diet providing 0.6 g protein/kg ideal body weight/day; 2) a VLPD containing 0.3 g protein/kg/day of predominantly vegetable protein supplemented with a mixture of EAA; or 3) a VLPD supplemented with a mixture of EAA and the nitrogen-free analogs of amino acids (ketoacids). Because restricting dietary protein also limits the intake of phosphates, sulfates, acid, and the like, any positive impact on progression may be due to restriction of some other component of the diet (see Chapter 7). The diets are based on the requirements for EAA and protein of normal adults plus measurements of the nitrogen balance of patients with CRF. Kopple and Coburn demonstrated that the minimal protein requirement of normal subjects (i.e., 0.6 g protein/kg/day), also maintains neutral nitrogen balance in patients with CRF. With the more restrictive VLPD regimens, nitrogen balance also is neutral and, importantly, serum albumin and transferrin are maintained during long-term therapy.

MONITORING DIETARY ADEQUACY AND COMPLIANCE

Successful therapy with a low-protein diet requires regular assessment of nutritional status and compliance with such a diet. Fortunately, the protein intake of patients with CRF can be estimated easily. The method depends on the fact that waste nitrogen derived from degraded protein is converted principally into urea, so the urea nitrogen appearance rate (i.e., the sum of urea excretion plus accumulation) closely parallels protein intake. In contrast, nonurea nitrogen excretion (i.e., the nitrogen in urinary creatinine, uric acid, ammonia, and feces) does not vary significantly with protein intake and averages 0.031 g nitrogen/kg body weight/day. The estimate of nitrogen (and hence, protein) in the diet is based on the assumption that the patient is in neutral nitrogen balance (B_N). In this case, nitrogen intake (I_N) equals urea nitrogen appearance (U) plus nonurea nitrogen (NUN) excretion (i.e., if $B_N = 0$, then $I_N = U + NUN$). Assuming the patient is in the steady state (i.e., serum urea nitrogen and weight are constant), then urea nitrogen appearance (U) will equal the 24-hour urinary urea nitrogen excretion (UUN). When the estimated protein intake is similar to the amount prescribed, it can be concluded that the patient is compliant with the protein prescription (Table 11-2). If the estimated nitrogen (and hence, protein) intake is less than the amount of prescribed dietary protein, the patient should be

**Table 11-2. Estimating dietary protein intake
from the 24-hour urinary urea nitrogen excretion**

Example: A 45-year-old man has received instruction in a diet
   providing 0.6 protein/kg/day (i.e., 42 g protein). Weight: 70 kg;
   UUN = 4.5 g/day; NUN = 0.031 g N × 70 kg = 2.2 g N/day
if B_N = 0, then I_N = UUN + NUN
$$= 4.5 + 2.2 = 6.7 \text{ g N}$$
$$= 6.7 \text{ g N} \times 6.25 \text{ g protein/g N}$$
$$= 42 \text{ g protein/day}$$

N, nitrogen; UUN, 24-hour urinary urea nitrogen excretion (g N/day); NUN,
nonurea nitrogen (g N/day); B_N, nitrogen balance (g N/day) I_N, nitrogen intake
(g N/day).

instructed to increase protein intake; if the estimated protein
intake exceeds the amount prescribed by more than 25%, there
are three possible explanations: 1) there is a catabolic stimulus
(e.g., metabolic acidosis) causing degradation of body protein
with increased waste nitrogen production; 2) there is gastrointestinal bleeding; or 3) the patient is noncompliant with the
diet. The patient must be examined and, if no clinical abnormality is found, referred to the dietitian for assistance in
achieving dietary compliance.

An adequate energy intake is critical for the proper use of a
low protein diet; patients with CRF should eat ~35 kcal/kg/day
to utilize the diet protein maximally. In contrast to estimating
protein intake, dietary diaries or diet recall are the only available methods for assessing energy intake (see Chapters 3 and
15). Nutritional status can be monitored by serial measurements
of anthropometric indices, serum albumin, and transferrin. Once
a patient understands the goals and the use of a dietary regimen, he or she can be followed as an outpatient every 3 months,
but at each visit there should be an estimate of 1) protein intake
from the 24-hour UUN excretion plus an estimate of NUN losses
as 0.031 g N/kg/day; 2) caloric intake from 3-day food diaries;
and 3) serum albumin, transferrin, and anthropometric measurements. These indices are used to provide the patient with
feedback to achieve compliance.

**LOW-PROTEIN DIETS AND
THE PROGRESSION OF RENAL INSUFFICIENCY**

**Conventional Low-Protein Diets
and Nondiabetic Nephropathy**

Early trials examining how a low-protein diet influences the
progression of CRF were based on changes in Scr (Table 11-3). In
one study of 390 patients treated with a low-protein diet (0.6 g pro-
tein/kg ideal body weight/day) for 54 ± 28 months, more than half
of the patients had stable Scr values, 11% had slower deterioration (defined as a lower rate of decline of Scr^{-1} with time), and 32%
had more rapid loss of kidney function. Patients who began the
low-protein diet early seemed to benefit, and patients with interstitial nephritis fared better than those with chronic glomerulonephritis or polycystic kidney disease. The initial level of Scr, the

Table 11-3. Trials of conventional low-protein diets in patients with nondiabetic progressive renal failure

Diet	Assessment of Progression	Patients	Reference
0.6 g protein/kg/day vs. unrestricted diet	Change in Scr^{-1}	390	*Kidney Int* 1989;36:S103
0.6 g protein/kg/day vs. unrestricted diet	Change in Scr^{-1}	149	*Lancet* 1984;2:1291
0.4 g protein/kg/day vs. unrestricted diet	Change in plasma clearance of GFR marker	64	*N Engl J Med* 1989;321:1773
0.6 g protein/kg/day and 0.8 g phosphate/day vs. 0.8 g protein/kg/day and 1 g phosphate/day vs. 0.8 g protein/kg/day and no phosphate restriction	Change in Ccr	95	*Q J Med* 1991;81:837
0.6 vs. 1 g protein/kg/day	Doubling of Scr	456	*Lancet* 1991;357:1299

Scr^{-1}, the reciprocal of serum creatinine; Scr, serum creatinine; Ccr, creatinine clearance.

severity of proteinuria, and hypertension were independent risk factors associated with a more rapid increase in Scr. Importantly, indices of protein nutrition including weight, anthropometric measurements, and serum proteins were maintained. However, after 5 years of the dietary therapy there were problems in a subgroup of eight patients: the serum albumin and transferrin and the protein concentration in muscle biopsy samples decreased significantly, despite stable anthropometric measurements.

In a prospective, randomized trial involving 149 patients followed for an average of 24 months, the average difference in protein intake between the low-protein diet and control groups was 18 g/day. From an analysis of changes in Scr^{-1}, Rosman and colleagues concluded that the low-protein diet reduced the rate of progression by three- to fivefold. There were no adverse changes in nutritional status. After 4 years, the slowing of the loss of renal function was largely restricted to patients with more advanced renal insufficiency or with glomerulonephritis. There was a more beneficial effect in men; the response was minimal in women, and patients with polycystic kidney disease benefited only if blood pressure control was successful.

Ihle and colleagues conducted an 18-month, prospective, randomized trial of the influence of a low-protein diet on changes in GFR. The treatment group was given a low-protein diet of 0.4 g protein/kg/day, whereas the control group consumed an isocaloric diet providing at least 0.75 g protein/kg/day. Progression was assessed as changes in GFR calculated from the plasma disappearance of ^{51}Cr-EDTA; dietary compliance and nutritional adequacy were monitored every 3 months. Eight of the 72 patients were excluded from the analysis (3 withdrew voluntarily, and 5 were excluded for noncompliance with their diet or medications). Thus, the analysis was restricted to the 64 patients who were compliant with therapy. The results were impressive: ESRD developed in 9 of 33 patients (27%) who were eating an unrestricted diet compared with only 2 of 31 (6%) who were compliant with the protein-restricted diet ($P < 0.05$). In the control group, the mean GFR decreased from 15 to 6 ml/min (60% reduction; $P < 0.01$); in the low protein diet group, it fell from 14 to 12 ml/min (13% reduction; P = NS; Fig. 11-1). The average protein intake (calculated from urea excretion using the method described) was about 0.7 g/kg day in the low-protein diet group. Over the 18 months, serum albumin and anthropometric measurements remained stable, but there was a small, significant decrease in weight, serum transferrin, and total lymphocyte count during the first 6 to 9 months only. These results indicate that dietary protein restriction can slow the rate of progression of renal failure in some patients and delay the onset of ESRD.

In contrast, others have found no benefit of a low-protein diet on progression. Ninety-five patients with CRF were followed for 19 ± 3 months after random assignment to three groups: one group was given a diet containing 0.6 g protein/kg/day and 800 mg phosphorus; another group, > 0.8 protein/kg/day and 1 g phosphorus/day (a minimal phosphorus restriction); and for a third group, the diet had 0.8 g protein/kg/day and no phosphorus restriction (control group). After randomization, the rate of decline in Ccr in the low-protein and low-phosphorus groups slowed, but only by 2.2 ml/minute/1.73 m^2/year; it accelerated by

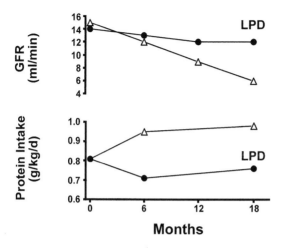

**Fig. 11-1. Changes in glomerular filtration rate (GFR)
measured from the plasma clearance of iothalamate in patients
with chronic renal failure prescribed a protein-restricted or
unrestricted diet. The calculated level of dietary protein based
on urea excretion is also shown. The low-protein regimen
significantly reduced the decline in GFR ($P < 0.01$).** (Modified from
Ihle BU, Becker GJ, Whitworth JA, et al. The effect of protein restriction on
the progression of renal insufficiency. *N Engl J Med* 1989;321:1773–1777.)

1.0 ml/minute/1.73 m²/year in the control group (P = NS).
Changes in body weight, midarm muscle circumference, and
serum transferrin, albumin, and immunoglobulins did not differ
between groups, so assignment to a protein-restricted diet did
not adversely affect nutritional status.

Another study showing no benefit of prescribing a low-protein
diet was the Northern Italian multicenter trial of 456 patients.
The patients were assigned to a low-protein diet of 0.6 g/kg/day (N
= 226) or a control diet containing 1.0 g/kg/day (N = 230). Patients
were stratified according to the severity of their renal insufficiency and progression was evaluated by analyzing the time to
dialysis or doubling of Scr ("renal survival"). Although there was
a trend for fewer patients to reach ESRD, in the low-protein diet
group (27 vs. 42 endpoints in the control group; $P < 0.06$), Locatelli
and colleagues reported that there was no difference in the number experiencing a doubling of Scr in the control and low-protein
diets. There was a minimal difference in dietary protein (i.e.,
about 9.5 g protein/day) suggesting that compliance was poor.
Another problem is that the rates of renal progression were very
slow in both groups, so that the study lacked sufficient statistical
power to detect any difference. Regarding nutritional status, only
weights were recorded, and they did not change significantly.

Conventional Low-Protein Diets and Diabetic Nephropathy

In the United States, diabetes mellitus is the most common
cause of ESRD, and the number of these patients on dialysis

continues to rise. Strategies that slow the rate of progression of diabetic nephropathy are clearly needed. In an early study, 19 patients with type I insulin-dependent diabetes mellitus and persistent proteinuria were evaluated while they consumed an unrestricted diet (1.13 g protein/kg/day). When the diet was restricted to 0.67 g protein/kg/day, the rate of decrease in GFR and the severity of albuminuria decreased significantly (GFR slowed from a loss of 0.61 to 0.14 ml/minute per month). This beneficial response was significant even after the results were adjusted for differences in blood pressure, energy intake, and blood glucose control (i.e., glycosylated hemoglobin levels).

In another study, 32 type I diabetic patients were given diets containing 0.8 or $\geq$ 1.6 g protein/kg/day and compared over a 6-month period. Those given the low-protein diet exhibited no decline in GFR, and their proteinuria significantly decreased. Patients consuming the high-protein diet lost GFR at an average rate of 1.3 ml/minute/1.73 m^2, and their proteinuria increased. These differences could not be attributed to blood pressure or glycemic control.

Zeller and associates studied type I diabetic patients for a longer period using a randomized, prospective, controlled trial design (average initial GFR was 48 ml/minute and there was 3.7 g/d of proteinuria). The groups were assigned to a control (1.0 g protein/kg/day) or a low-protein diet (0.6 g protein/kg/day) and followed for at least 12 months (average, 35 months). Blood pressure was well controlled and the degree of glycemic control was comparable in both groups. The calculated dietary protein was 1.08 in the control group and 0.72 g protein/kg/day in the low-protein diet group (after excluding two patients whose intakes persistently exceeded 0.8 g protein/kg/day). In patients consuming the low-protein diet, the rate of decline in GFR was fourfold slower (12.1 vs. 3.1 ml/year, respectively; $P < 0.02$). The beneficial effect of the low-protein diet could not be attributed to better glycemic control or more frequent visits to the clinic. There was no decrease in weight, midarm circumference, or serum albumin, indicating that this degree of protein restriction did not have adverse nutritional consequences over the 3 years of the study.

Very–Low-Protein Diets With Supplements of Essential Amino Acids or Ketoacids

Evidence that a diet containing only 0.3 g protein/kg/day (VLPD) supplemented with a mixture of EAA slows progression is tenuous but has not been studied extensively. When a VLPD is supplemented with a mixture of the nitrogen-free analogs of EAA (i.e., ketoacids), there appears to be slowing of progression. Early studies (Table 11-4) compared rates of decline in Ccr or Scr^{-1} before and after beginning the ketoacid regimen. Likewise, when changes in GFR were measured, there appeared to be a benefit from the ketoacid regimen.

THE MODIFICATION OF DIET IN RENAL DISEASE STUDY

The largest study designed to test whether a low-protein diet can slow the progression of renal failure was the National Institutes of Health-sponsored Modification of Diet in Renal Disease Trial (MDRD Study). It was a multicenter, randomized,

Table 11-4. Trials of conventional low-protein diets in diabetic patients with progressive renal failure

Diet	Assessment of Program	Patients	Reference
1.1 to 0.6 g protein/kg/day	Change in GFR	19	*Lancet* 1989;2:1411
0.8 vs. 1.6 g protein/kg/day	Change in GFR and proteinuria	32	*Am J Clin Nutr* 1994;60:579
0.6 vs. 1 g protein/kg/day	Change in GFR, Ccr, and proteinuria	35	*N Engl J Med* 1991;324:78

GFR, glomerular filtration rate; Ccr, creatinine clearance.

prospective trial in which patients were assigned to one of two levels of blood pressure control (usual mean arterial pressure = 107 mm Hg [~140/90] or low mean arterial pressure = 92 mm Hg [~125/75] and different levels of dietary protein. In Study A, 585 patients with GFR between 25 to 55 ml/minute were randomly assigned to a standard or a low-protein diet (1.3 vs. 0.58 g protein/kg/day). In Study B, 255 patients with GFR between 13 to 24 ml/minute were assigned to a low-protein diet or a VLPD (0.58 vs. 0.28 g protein/kg/day); the VLPD was supplemented with a ketoacid–amino acid mixture. There was no control diet in Study B because both groups of patients were treated with a low-protein diet, and in both Study A and B insulin-requiring diabetics were excluded and GFR was measured every 4 months as the renal clearance of ^{125}I-iothalamate. During the initial 4 months, renal function declined *more* rapidly in Study A patients assigned to the low-protein and

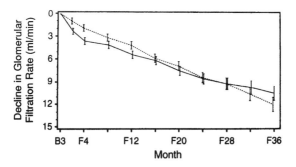

Fig. 11-2. Changes in glomerular filtration rate (GFR) in patients with moderately severe renal insufficiency (Study A) extrapolated to 3 years (mean follow-up, 2.2 years) in the Modification of Diet in Renal Disease (MDRD) Study. Note the initial more rapid decline in patients assigned to the low-protein diet (solid line), followed by a slower decline in GFR. (From Klahr S, Levey AS, Beck GJ, et al. The effects of dietary protein restriction and blood-pressure control on the progression of chronic renal failure. *N Engl J Med* 1994;330:878–884.)

low–blood-pressure groups (P = 0.004 and 0.01, respectively; Fig. 11-2). Thereafter, the rate of decline in GFR was 28% less in the low-protein (P = 0.009) and 29% less in the low–blood-pressure group (P = 0.006). However, when the change in GFR was examined from the initial randomization to the end of the trial (average, 2.2 years) using an intention-to-treat analysis, the projected decline in GFR at 3 years did not differ significantly between the diet or blood pressure groups. In those with more advanced CRF (Study B), the rate of decline in GFR was 19% slower in the very–low-protein compared with the low-protein group (P = 0.065), but the cumulative incidence of ESRD or death did not differ between the diet groups. Interestingly, there was no beneficial effect of low blood pressure control compared with the usual blood pressure level in either Study A or Study B, with the exception that progression was slower in patients with proteinuria (> 1 g/day) assigned to the low–blood-pressure group. In summary, there were no statistically significant benefits of prescribing a low-protein diet or more vigorous blood pressure control.

The interpretation of these conclusions are complicated by several factors. First, there was no requirement that patients enrolling in this trial must have evidence for loss of renal func-

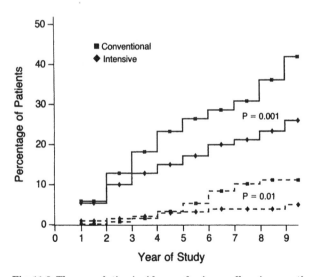

Fig. 11-3. The cumulative incidence of urinary albumin excretion > 300 mg/day (dashed lines) and > 40 mg/day (solid lines) in diabetic patients receiving standard insulin therapy or intensive insulin therapy to control blood glucose in the Diabetes Control and Complications Trial (DCCT). Note that the benefit of intensive insulin therapy was not detectable until 3 to 4 years of therapy. (From Anonymous. The effect of intensive treatment of diabetes on the development and progression of long-term complications in insulin-dependent diabetes mellitus: the Diabetes Control and Complications Trial. *N Engl J Med* 1993;329:977–986.)

tion (i.e., progression). Approximately 15% of the Study A control group had no evidence of decline in GFR during the trial. Whether the same is true for other groups is unknown. Second, there was a disproportionate number of patients (~20%) with polycystic kidney disease, and these patients did not benefit from either a low-protein diet or aggressive treatment of hypertension. Both of these problems increase the number of patients needed to detect any slowing of progression. Third, the sample size requirements were calculated based on a projected decline in GFR of 6 ml/minute/year, but overall, the rates of progression were ~30% slower than expected, again increasing the number of patients needed to detect a benefit of the interventions. Fourth, the intention-to-treat analysis does not take into account whether patients were compliant with the diet. In fact, when the results were analyzed according to the amount of protein actually consumed, a benefit of dietary protein restriction was demonstrated: a 0.2 g/kg/d reduction in protein intake was associated with a 29% slower rate of decline in GFR and a 41% prolongation in the time to dialysis ($P < 0.01$). In this analysis, no independent influence of the ketoacid regimen could be detected. Fifth, the more rapid initial decline in renal function in Study A patients assigned to the low-protein and low–blood-pressure groups was unexpected and presumably a hemodynamic rather than pathologic response to therapy. Unfortunately, this pattern complicates interpretation of the results because the study lasted only 2.2 years. For example, during the initial 2 years of the Diabetes Control and Complications Trial, strict glycemic control appeared to worsen diabetic retinopathy; the positive response on retinal vessels and kidney disease (i.e., albuminuria; Fig. 11-3) was not detected until about 4 years after beginning the trial.

META-ANALYSES OF LOW-PROTEIN DIETS IN CHRONIC RENAL INSUFFICIENCY

Why do conclusions from these studies differ? One answer is that dietary protein restriction does not slow progression. However, in those patients consistently eating a low-protein diet, there was slowing of the loss of kidney function. Another possibility is that the number of patients in each study may have been insufficient to detect a benefit on progression. To address the latter question, there have been meta-analyses of the effectiveness of low-protein diets on the progression of CRF. This technique is based on combining results from several studies and is valid as long as the outcome being examined in each trial is similar.

Fouque and coworkers examined results of six clinical trials including 890 randomly assigned, nondiabetic patients with CRF who were followed for at least 1 year. The results were based on an intention-to-treat analysis and the outcome measure was the odds ratio for the initiation of dialysis or death. The meta-analysis revealed that five of the six trials showed a reduction in the number of patients with renal failure or death (61 for patients assigned to the low-protein diet vs. 95 for the control diets). The odds ratio was calculated to be 0.54 in patients prescribed a low-protein diet ($P < 0.002$), corresponding to a 46%

decrease in the likelihood of kidney failure. It was concluded that the results strongly support the hypothesis that a low-protein diet delays the onset of ESRD.

Pedrini and colleagues examined the course of renal failure of 1413 patients participating in five studies of patients with nondiabetic renal disease (including the MDRD Study) and five studies including 108 patients with type I diabetic nephropathy. In nondiabetic patients, the low-protein diet was associated with a 33% reduction in the risk of renal failure or death ($P < 0.007$). In diabetic patients, a low-protein diet reduced the risk of further kidney damage (a decrease in Ccr or GFR or an increase in proteinuria by 46%; $P < 0.001$). In this analysis, the beneficial effect of a low-protein diet could not be explained by differences in blood pressure or glycemic control. Moreover, angiotensin-converting enzyme inhibitors were used in only 9 of the 108 diabetic patients, so the results were not confounded by this drug. Based on these calculations, it can be estimated that at least 1000 patients would have to be studied to detect a 33% reduction in the risk of renal failure. Neither the MDRD study nor any other clinical trial has included this many patients. Finally, two items should be noted. First, a low-protein diet could reduce the risk of renal failure by slowing the progression of renal disease or by ameliorating uremic symptoms. The secondary analysis of the MDRD study reveals a correlation between achieved protein intake and both the rate of decline in GFR as well as the incidence of renal failure in patients with advanced renal disease. This finding makes it likely that both mechanisms contribute to the beneficial effect of a low-protein diet. Second, a meta-analysis cannot prove or disprove a hypothesis, so the effectiveness of low-protein diets on progression has not been established.

CONCLUSIONS

Randomized trials enrolling nondiabetic patients yield results that have not consistently demonstrated that dietary protein restriction slows progression when analyzed according to diet assignment (rather than achieved intake). Two meta-analyses indicate there can be a 33% to 46% reduction in the risk of renal failure for patients with nondiabetic renal disease. Based on smaller numbers of patients, evidence that a low-protein diet slows the loss of renal function or worsening proteinuria (a predictor of progressive renal failure) in patients with type I insulin-dependent diabetes mellitus appears more secure.

For the CRF patient, the initial focus should be on blood pressure control, aiming for a goal of < 125/75 mm Hg, especially in patients with proteinuria exceeding 1 g/day (angiotensin-converting enzyme inhibitors are the preferred drug). For diabetic patients, blood pressure control may be even more important, and strict glycemic control can slow the development of diabetic complications, including nephropathy. However, if the Scr of a patient with CRF continues to rise in spite of these measures, dietary protein restriction is warranted. From a practical point of view, compliance with low-protein diets can be assessed reliably, and the dietary regimens do not cause malnutrition if patients are monitored for nutritional adequacy.

Finally, the suggestion that a spontaneous decrease in dietary intake in patients with progressive CRF is a sign to avoid low-protein diets must be discarded. Evidence suggests just the opposite, and that low-protein diets will maintain an adequate nutritional status and limit uremic symptoms. There is the added possibility that the course of CRF to ESRD can be slowed.

ACKNOWLEDGMENT

This work was supported in part by National Institutes of Health grants DK40907, DK49243, DK45215, and DK37175.

SELECTED READINGS

Anonymous. The effect of intensive treatment of diabetes on the development and progression of long-term complications in insulin-dependent diabetes mellitus: the Diabetes Control and Complications Trial. *N Engl J Med* 1993;329:977–986.

Bingham SA. The dietary assessment of individuals: methods, accuracy, new techniques and recommendations. *Nutrition Abstracts Reviews* 1987;57:705–742.

Coresh J, Walser M, Hill S. Survival on dialysis among chronic renal failure patients treated with a supplemented low-protein diet before dialysis. *J Am Soc Nephrol* 1995;6:1379–1385.

Dullart RP, Bdusekamp BJ, Meiger S, et al. Long-term effects of protein-restricted diet on albuminuria and renal function in IDDM patients without clinical nephropathy and hypertension. *Diabetes Care* 1993;16:483–492.

Ihle BU, Becker GJ, Whitworth JA, et al. The effect of protein restriction on the progression of renal insufficiency. *N Engl J Med* 1989; 321:1773–1777.

Klahr S, Levey AS, Beck GJ, et al. The effects of dietary protein restriction and blood-pressure control on the progression of chronic renal failure. *N Engl J Med* 1994;330:878–884.

Levey AS, Adler S, Caggiula AW, et al. Effects of dietary protein restriction on the progression of advanced renal disease in the Modification of Diet in Renal Disease Study. *Am J Kidney Dis* 1996;27:652–663.

Locatelli F, Alberti D, Graziani G, et al. Prospective, randomized, multicentre trial of effect of protein restriction on progression of chronic renal insufficiency. *Lancet* 1991;337:1299–1304.

Maroni BJ, Steinman T, Mitch WE. A method for estimating nitrogen intake of patients with chronic renal failure. *Kidney Int* 1985; 27:58–65.

Mitch WE. Measuring the rate of progression of renal insufficiency. In: Mitch WE, ed. *The progressive nature of renal disease*. New York: Churchill Livingstone; 1992:203–222.

Oldrizzi L, Rugiu C, Maschio G. The Verona experience on the effect of diet on progression of renal failure. *Kidney Int* 1989;36: S103–S105.

Pedrini MT, Levey AS, Lau J, et al. The effect of dietary protein restriction on the progression of diabetic and nondiabetic renal diseases: a meta-analysis. *Ann Intern Med* 1996;124:627–632.

Rosman JB, Meijer S, Sluiter WJ, et al. Prospective randomized trial of early dietary protein restriction in chronic renal failure. *Lancet* 1984;2:1291–1295.

Walser M. Does prolonged protein restriction preceding dialysis lead to protein malnutrition at the onset of dialysis? *Kidney Int* 1993; 44:1139–1144.

Zeller KR, Whittaker E, Sullivan L, et al. Effect of restricting dietary protein on the progression of renal failure in patients with insulin-dependent diabetes mellitus. *N Engl J Med* 1991;324:78–83.

Nutritional Requirements of Hemodialysis Patients

T. Alp Ikizler and Raymond M. Hakim

Despite substantial improvements in the science and technology of renal replacement therapy, the morbidity and mortality of patients on chronic hemodialysis (CHD) remains excessively high, approaching 24% per year in the United States. Among the many factors that adversely affect patient outcome, protein-calorie malnutrition plays a major role. In this chapter, we will attempt to define the importance of nutrition in the outcome of CHD patients, and explore the possible mechanisms that cause or promote poor nutritional status in these patients, with a specific emphasis on their special dietary requirements. We also discuss measures to prevent malnutrition in stable CHD patients, as well as several treatment options in CHD patients who are already malnourished.

THE ASSOCIATION OF MALNUTRITION WITH MORBIDITY AND MORTALITY IN CHRONIC HEMODIALYSIS PATIENTS

Goal: To identify the relationship between poor nutritional status and increased morbidity and mortality in CHD patients

A number of studies have documented the increased mortality and morbidity in CHD patients with malnutrition. In the patient with end-stage renal disease (ESRD), malnutrition is rarely documented as a cause of death. It is most likely that malnourished patients are at increased risk for other comorbid illnesses such as infections, which are usually the cause of morbid events. An early indication of the relationship between suboptimal nutrition and poor outcome in CHD patients came from the analysis of the National Dialysis Cooperative Study (NCDS) results. In this comprehensive study of 262 CHD patients divided into four groups, the patient group with the lowest protein catabolic rate (PCR), which presumably reflects the dietary protein intake (DPI) in stable CHD patients, had the highest treatment failure and dropout rate. In addition, the same group of patients had the highest death rate in the 12 months after the termination of the study. More recently, Lowrie and colleagues, in their cross-sectional analysis of more than 12,000 CHD patients, identified serum albumin concentration as the most powerful indicator of mortality. Specifically, the risk of death in patients with serum albumin concentration below 2.5 g/dl was close to 20-fold that of patients with a serum albumin of 4.0 to 4.5 g/dl (the normal range). More important, when compared with this reference range, even serum albumin values of 3.5 to 4.0 g/dl resulted in a twofold increase in the relative risk of death. This latter level of albumin is in the range of "normal" for many laboratories, confirming that a small difference in serum albumin concentrations, even when they are in the "normal" range, may adversely affect the relative mortality risk in CHD patients. In addition to serum albumin, Lowrie and colleagues uncovered a close relationship between mortality and other biochemical markers of nutrition such as low blood urea nitrogen (BUN) and low serum cholesterol concentrations (indicators of low protein and energy intake), as well as a low serum creatinine (an indicator of decreased muscle mass in CHD patients) and percentage of ideal body weight. Several more complex nutritional parameters also have been associated with increased risk of death, including serum transferrin, prealbumin, and insulin-like growth factor-1 (IGF-1), as well as total lymphocyte counts and abnormal plasma amino acid profiles. However, their validity, or relationship to serum albumin, remains to be determined. Finally, body composition may be associated with mortality in CHD patients because it has been suggested that decreased total body nitrogen (a marker of low lean body mass) is also associated with a worse outcome in CHD patients.

In summary, several lines of evidence suggest that a poor nutritional status as determined by a number of nutritional markers is associated with worse outcome in CHD patients. However, whether malnutrition per se is a comorbid condition or one that predisposes the CHD patient to other comorbidities remains to be determined.

INDICES OF NUTRITIONAL STATUS

Goal: To discuss nutritional indices and determine the most appropriate method(s) for use in CHD patients

The appropriate interpretation of tests for nutritional assessment in CHD patients remains a challenge. The nutritional state of patients with different diseases can be monitored by using various anthropometric and biochemical indices. Although significant relationships have been established between the nutritional state of the patients and the various markers, the variance of these associations is quite large. In part, this is because nutritional indices are influenced by many nonnutritional factors, especially in CHD patients. The assessment of nutritional status in renal failure is discussed in detail in Chapter 3 of this book. However, we briefly mention the important clinical aspects of several nutritional indices (Table 12-1).

Biochemical Markers

In CHD patients, biochemical measures reflecting the visceral protein stores, such as serum albumin, creatinine, and BUN, as well as more complex parameters such as transferrin, prealbumin, and IGF-1, have been proposed as nutritional indices. Among these parameters, serum albumin is probably the most extensively examined nutritional index, probably because of its easy availability and strong association with outcome, especially in patients with ESRD. Studies have shown that the serum albumin concentration is closely affected by the level of protein intake. In fact, low serum albumin concentrations are usually accompanied by other markers of malnutrition in different patient populations, including patients with ESRD, and have been accepted as one of the most consistent markers of chronic protein-calorie malnutrition. These observations have led to the general concept that an abnormally low serum albumin concentration by itself is sufficient to diagnose protein-energy malnutrition in patients with ESRD. However, serum albumin may also be affected by coexisting problems besides malnutrition. Specifically, serum albumin is

Table 12-1. Indices of malnutrition in chronic hemodialysis patients

Biochemical Parameters and Limitations

Simple

Serum albumin < 4.0 g/dl

Negative acute-phase reactant, long (20 days) half-life

Lower-than-expected serum creatinine concentrations or low creatinine kinetics

Dependent on renal function and muscle mass

Low BUN

Dependent on degree of renal failure or intensity of dialysis; BUN can increase in catabolic states or with renal obstruction or gastrointestinal bleeding

Complex

Serum transferrin concentrations < 200 mg/dl

Dependent on iron stores, half-life of 8–9 days

Serum prealbumin concentrations < 30 mg/dl

Excreted by the kidney and falsely elevated in renal failure; good predictor of outcome in chronic dialysis patients

Serum insulin-like growth factor-1 concentrations < 200 ng/ml

Good association with other nutritional markers; not readily available; not validated in large-scale studies

Body Composition Techniques and Limitations

Anthropometric measures

Continuous decline in body weight or low percentage of ideal body weight (<85%)

Crude marker; late manifestation

Abnormal skinfold thickness, midarm muscle circumference, or muscle strength

Operator dependent; large variations in measurements; useful if measured repeatedly for a longer time (months to years)

Body composition analysis

Abnormally low percentage of lean body mass (or body cell mass) by bioelectrical impedance analysis or dual-energy x-ray absorptiometry

No gold standard to evaluate the results; both are affected by fluid status

Low total body nitrogen or nitrogen index (observed nitrogen/predicted nitrogen)

Not clinically validated in large studies; equipment hard to obtain

Dietary Assessment

Low spontaneous dietary protein intake by protein catabolic rate (< 1.0 g/kg/d)

Related to short-term dietary intake; not well established association with other nutritional markers

BUN, blood urea nitrogen.

a negative, acute-phase reactant and its serum concentration decreases sharply in response to stress or inflammation, and may not reflect the nutritional status of acutely ill patients. Further, the 20-day half-life of serum albumin is relatively long, and therefore a change in its concentration after a decrease in protein intake occurs rather late, but conditions that promote an acute-phase response such as infection or trauma can induce a prompt and significant decrease in serum albumin concentration. In this context, the decrease in serum albumin concentration closely reflects the degree of illness and inflammation, as well as the overall nutritional status. Finally, hypoalbuminemia in CHD patients may also reflect nonnutritional factors, such as external losses and decreased albumin synthesis.

In addition to serum albumin, BUN and serum creatinine concentrations are also considered simple biochemical markers of nutritional status. Urea is the end-product of the metabolism of dietary protein, and serum creatinine reflects muscle mass. The advantages of these simple markers are that they are easily available and cheap to measure. They also accurately reflect the recent protein and calorie intake of most CHD patients. However, the concentrations of both BUN and serum creatinine are altered because of renal failure and the dose of dialysis, which makes their interpretation as nutritional indices more complicated. They primarily reflect short-term DPI, but there is no established association of BUN or serum creatinine with the other nutritional indices in patients with ESRD.

Estimation of DPI by different methods can be used as a simple marker of overall nutritional status in the stable patient with ESRD. Although dietary recall is a direct and simple measure of DPI, several studies have shown that this method lacks accuracy in estimating the actual intake of patients, even in well controlled settings. Other means of measuring DPI, such as the PCR calculations in dialysis patients, have been used to estimate protein intake, but these indirect estimations of DPI are valid only in stable patients, and may easily overestimate the actual protein intake in a catabolic patient with endogenous protein breakdown leading to a high urea nitrogen appearance. There is an active debate over whether PCR is mathematically linked to Kt/V or is an independent nutritional parameter, because both are calculated using the postdialysis BUN value. The lack of a correlation between PCR and other nutritional markers such as serum albumin suggests that there is mathematical linkage, so an indirect estimation of DPI and nutritional status should be evaluated with caution.

More complex biochemical markers are also used to assess the nutritional status of patients with ESRD. Serum transferrin is a transport protein with a small body pool, and its concentration is affected by DPI. It has a shorter half-life (8 to 9 days) than serum albumin, which makes it more advantageous as an early indicator of visceral protein status. A serum concentration < 200 mg/dl is suggested as an indicator of poor nutrition. However, the transferrin concentration is also affected by iron stores and liver disease, and does not necessarily correlate with other short–half-life proteins (e.g., prealbumin).

Serum prealbumin is a promising nutritional marker because of its short half-life (1 to 2 days) and its measurable increase with nutritional supplementation. It is also a serum transport protein (it transports thyroxine and retinol-binding protein) and has a small body pool. The prealbumin concentration is closely and rapidly affected by nutrient (especially energy) intake and changes in body protein stores. It is a powerful predictor of mortality in patients with ESRD, and the serum concentration correlates well with other nutritional indices. However, its main route of excretion is by the kidneys, so serum concentrations of prealbumin may be falsely elevated in patients with chronic renal failure. Although the prealbumin concentration is not particularly useful in patients with progressive chronic renal failure, it is useful in CHD patients with stable, albeit markedly reduced renal function. Unfortunately, the lower limit of prealbumin that is associated with nutritional depletion has not been established in patients with ESRD. Nevertheless, a decline in serum transferrin or prealbumin concentrations suggests an inadequate nutrient intake.

The serum concentration of IGF-1 has also been suggested as a nutritional marker in patients with ESRD because of its response to nutrients and its short half-life (12 to 15 hours). IGF-1 is a growth factor that is structurally related to insulin and is produced and released primarily by the liver. It is 95% bound to IGF-1–binding proteins, so daily variations in the serum concentration are small. For these reasons, the serum IGF-1 concentration is more informative than the traditional markers of an inadequate diet, such as serum albumin and transferrin, showing a better correlation with a simultaneously evaluated body composition measurement and reflecting changes in dietary protein and calorie intake more precisely. IGF-1 is also a reliable nutritional marker in patients with renal failure. As with serum prealbumin, the concentration of IGF-1 signifying malnutrition is not established in patients with chronic renal failure. Our experience is that serum IGF-1 concentrations < 200 ng/ml are usually associated with other signs of poor nutrition. Longitudinal changes in serum IGF-1 concentrations can prospectively predict the changes that will occur in other nutritional parameters, specifically the serum albumin concentration in CHD patients. The IGF-1 concentration is altered by renal failure and liver disease, however, and depends on changes in release of binding proteins and growth hormone. Finally, its diagnostic accuracy as well as its association with outcome in patients with ESRD have not been validated in large-scale studies.

Body Composition Analysis

The analysis of body composition is another important tool for assessment of nutritional status in patients with ESRD. A list of these methods and their relationship to the presence of malnutrition is provided in Table 12-1. The simplest, but unfortunately the least reliable technique is anthropometric measurement. These largely subjective measurements are readily available and may be used as a confirmatory analysis in any patient with suspected protein-energy malnutrition. There are more reliable and accurate methods of analyzing body composition, such as prompt neutron activation analysis, which measures total body nitrogen content, and dual-energy x-ray absorptiometry. These measurements require expensive equipment and are available only in specialized centers, and their validity needs to be confirmed. A new, promising method is bioelectrical impedance analysis (BIA), which has been proposed as an accurate and reproducible measure of body composition in various populations, including patients with ESRD. Although it provides a good correlation between total body water and lean body mass in normal subjects, the variance of the estimates in patients with ESRD may be large. This is partly because BIA does not detect acute changes in body composition, so for improved consistency and accuracy, the measurements should be done predialysis or 30 minutes postdialysis. Several other issues with the BIA technique are its validity in moderately or severely malnourished patients with ESRD and its usefulness in prospective studies. Finally, body composition can be estimated by creatinine kinetics, a method that correlates well with other lean body mass measurements.

In summary, an assessment of malnutrition should rely on multiple indices of nutritional status measured simultaneously. These indices should include biochemical measures, such as serum albumin, as well as an analysis of body composition, if available. Multiple markers yield estimates of somatic tissue status from body composition analysis and visceral protein status from serum proteins.

EXTENT OF MALNUTRITION IN PATIENTS WITH END-STAGE RENAL DISEASE

Virtually every study that has evaluated the nutritional status of patients with ESRD has reported some degree of malnutrition. The prevalence of malnutrition has been estimated to range from approximately 20% to 50% in different populations of patients with ESRD.

Lowrie and colleagues reported serum albumin concentrations of < 3.7 g/dl in 25% of their population, which included more than 12,000 CHD patients. Similar findings are in a report by the Health Care Financing Administration; in a sample analysis from all ESRD Networks in the United States, 53% of the CHD patients had a serum albumin concentration between 3.5 and 3.9 g/dl, and 22% of the patients had a serum albumin concentration of ≤3.4 g/dl. An analysis of the NCDS population revealed an insufficient protein and energy intake in approximately 23% of patients, as well as low body fat and muscle stores in up to 40% of the population. Of note, serum albumin concentrations were within normal ranges in this population.

Analysis of body composition has also provided evidence of malnutrition in CHD patients. Body protein depletion was detected by dual-energy x-ray absorptiometry in up to 26% of CHD patients who were considered to be nutritionally normal based on other indices of nutrition, including other methods of body composition analysis. Others suggest that 76% of CHD patients have a nitrogen index lower than the predicted value (observed nitrogen/predicted normal nitrogen) when assessed by prompt neutron activation analysis, indicating a subnormal lean body mass.

FACTORS AFFECTING THE NUTRITIONAL STATUS OF PATIENTS WITH END-STAGE RENAL DISEASE

Goal: To identify the factors that promote malnutrition in CHD patients, with a specific emphasis on altered requirements

Multiple factors play important roles in the evolution of malnutrition in patients with ESRD (Table 12-2). Many of these factors act simultaneously during the progression from suboptimal nutrition to apparent malnutrition. The nutritional requirements also are substantially altered in CHD patients compared with predialysis patients.

Nutritional Requirements of Chronic Hemodialysis Patients

Protein Requirements

In general, the "minimal" daily protein requirement is that necessary to maintain a neutral nitrogen balance and prevent malnutrition. It is estimated to be a daily protein intake of approximately 0.6 g/kg in healthy people, with a "safe level" of protein intake equivalent to the minimal requirement plus two standard deviations, or approximately 0.75 g/kg/day. CHD patients require a protein intake of 1.0 g/kg/day to maintain a positive or neutral nitrogen balance during nondialysis days, and even this intake may not be adequate for dialysis days. Therefore, a minimum of 1.2 g/kg/day is probably a safe level of DPI for CHD based on several metabolic balance studies. This higher (almost twofold) level compared with normal adults results from a number of identified factors that actually increase the required protein intake of dialysis patients (see later).

Energy Requirements

The minimum energy requirement of CHD patients is less well defined. It depends on the resting energy expenditure (REE), the activity level of the patient, and the presence of other illnesses. Earlier studies concluded that the REE was not different between normal, healthy control subjects and patients with

Table 12-2. Factors affecting the nutritional status of chronic hemodialysis patients

Non-Dialysis Related

Decreased protein and calorie intake

Hormonal derangements
  Insulin resistance
  Hyperparathyroidism

Metabolic acidosis

Comorbidities
  Diabetes mellitus
  Gastrointestinal diseases

Hospitalizations

Medications

Dialysis Related

Inadequate dose of dialysis

Bioincompatibility of hemodialysis membranes

Increased resting energy expenditure

Losses of nutrients (amino acids or proteins)

chronic renal failure both before and after initiation of renal replacement therapy, but more recent studies conclude that the REE is higher in CHD patients, especially after adjusting the REE for fat-free mass where most of the energy expenditure occurs. Interestingly, the higher level of REE increased further during the hemodialysis procedure, when the nutrient losses and catabolic stress are at maximum. The additional increase in REE during nondialysis days as well as during hemodialysis increases the overall REE by 10% to 20% compared with normal people. The cause of this increase in REE in CHD patients is not well defined.

A minimum of 30 to 35 kcal/kg/day of energy intake is usually suggested for stable CHD patients. This level of energy intake rises with concurrent illnesses, especially if they require hospitalization.

Vitamin and Trace Element Requirements

A more detailed discussion of trace elements and vitamins in different stages of renal failure can be found in Chapter 5. Because of the influence of hemodialysis, we briefly review the important clinical aspects of these requirements.

VITAMINS. The level and response to many vitamins are altered in CHD patients, and both decreased as well as increased concentrations can be found. The vitamin A concentration is usually elevated in CHD patients, and even small amounts can lead to excessive accumulation and vitamin A toxicity. Therefore, vitamin A should not be supplemented. Vitamin E level in CHD patients is not well defined, and there are reports of increased, decreased, or unchanged concentrations, but in addition; no reports of adverse effects of vitamin E supplementation; there may be improved lipid peroxidation. At present, vitamin E supplements are not routinely given. Vitamin K supplements are usually not recommended in CHD patients unless there is a high risk for development of deficiency, such as in prolonged hospitalization with poor dietary intake. Vitamin D is discussed in detail in Chapter 4. The serum concentration of any of the water-soluble vitamins is reported to be low in CHD patients mainly because of decreased intake and increased clearance during hemodialysis. The use of daily multivitamin prescriptions that are specifically designed for patients with renal failure usually alleviates this problem. The daily requirements of vitamin B_6, folic acid, and ascorbic acid are higher than normal in CHD patients, and their levels should be followed with prolonged hospitalization. The influence of high-flux and high-efficiency dialyzers on water-soluble vitamins is not clearly defined.

TRACE ELEMENTS. The serum concentrations of most trace elements depend mainly on the degree of renal failure, but only a few of these elements are thought to be important in CHD patients. Among these, the serum aluminum concentration is important because high levels are associated with dialysis dementia as well as aluminum-related bone disease. The first reports of aluminum intoxication were recognized in patients who were dialyzed with untreated water in the dialysate. This problem is mostly eliminated in developed countries, but the risk persists in many developing countries. Another source of aluminum is phosphate binders that contain aluminum hydroxide. In CHD patients with poor control of phosphate intake, prolonged use of these phosphate binders may cause aluminum intoxication, and the patient's serum aluminum concentration should be monitored frequently. A serum aluminum concentration <10 µg/l is the desired level in CHD patients. Finally, concomitant use of aluminum-based phosphate binders and citrate-containing preparations is contraindicated because citrate increases aluminum absorption and predisposes a patient to acute aluminum intoxication.

Selenium deficiency has been associated with cardiovascular disease because there is increased peroxidative damage to cells. A low concentration of selenium has been observed in CHD patients probably secondary to inadequate dietary intake, but whether selenium supplements are beneficial is not defined. Similarly, low serum concentrations of zinc have been reported in CHD patients. Zinc deficiency is associated with impotence and anorexia, but the beneficial effects of supplemental zinc therapy have not been confirmed in CHD patients.

Nondialysis Factors Promoting Malnutrition in Chronic Hemodialysis Patients

Decreased Dietary Nutrient Intake

One of the most significant clinical indicators of advanced uremia is a decrease in appetite. Although not studied in detail, anorexia seems to worsen as renal failure progresses. It has been suggested that accumulation of a low–molecular-weight (< 5 kDa) compound may be a potential marker of this decreased food intake in uremia because it induces a dose-dependent suppression of appetite in normal rats. This compound has been isolated from uremic plasma ultrafiltrate and normal urine.

Decreased nutrient intake may also be related to other illnesses because the actual daily protein and energy intake of CHD patients admitted to the hospital is at perilously low levels (0.55 ± 0.33 g/kg/day). The urea kinetics of such patients revealed a negative nitrogen balance in 80%, and the serum albumin concentration was significantly decreased. Therefore, frequent hospital admissions may cause an insidious poor dietary intake in CHD patients.

Metabolic and Hormonal Derangements

Multiple metabolic and hormonal abnormalities related to the loss of renal tissue as well as renal function are apparent in CHD patients. Metabolic acidosis, which commonly accompanies progressive renal failure, promotes malnutrition by stimulating protein catabolism. Detailed experimental studies suggest that muscle proteolysis is stimulated by an adenosine triphosphate-dependent pathway involving ubiquitin and proteasomes during metabolic acidosis. In normal adults, induction of metabolic acidosis over 7 days with high doses of NH_4Cl (4.2 mmol/kg) significantly reduced albumin synthesis and caused negative nitrogen balance. Correction of metabolic acidosis improves muscle protein turnover in CHD patients. Thus, available evidence suggests that correction of metabolic acidosis may be nutritionally beneficial in CHD patients.

Several hormonal derangements, including insulin resistance, increased glucagon concentrations, and secondary hyperparathyroidism, could also cause malnutrition in chronic renal failure. A postreceptor defect in tissue insulin responsiveness causes insulin resistance and glucose intolerance in uremia, but it is not clear to what extent insulin resistance affects protein metabolism in CHD patients. Secondary hyperparathyroidism is responsible at least in part for inhibition of insulin secretion by pancreatic β cells. Increased parathyroid hormone has also been implicated as a catabolic factor that promotes protein metabolism in uremia by enhancing amino acid release from muscle. Finally, there are several abnormalities in the thyroid hormone profile of uremic patients, characterized by low serum thyroxine and triiodothyronine concentrations. This profile resembles the changes seen in prolonged malnutrition, and it has been suggested that the thyroid hormone profile is a response to decreased energy intake activated to preserve overall energy balance.

Abnormalities in growth hormone and the IGF-1 axis have also been suggested as important factors in the development of malnutrition in uremic patients. Growth hormone is the major promoter of growth in children and exerts anabolic actions in adults, including enhanced protein synthesis and increased fat mobilization and gluconeogenesis; IGF-1 is the major mediator of these actions. Although plasma concentrations of growth hormone actually rise as renal failure progresses, probably because of its reduced clearance, uremia per se can be associated with the development of cellular resistance to growth hormone action. Uremia in rats is characterized by reduced hepatic growth hormone receptor mRNA as well as hepatic IGF-1 mRNA expression. This blunted response attenuates the anabolic actions of these hormones. Interestingly, these abnormalities can also be observed with decreased food intake, as well as in experimental metabolic acidosis. Clinically, metabolic acidosis and decreased dietary protein and energy intake are also associated with decreased IGF-1, although it is not clear which is the primary response and which is a secondary effect. Thus, the current evidence suggests an interesting, as yet ill-defined interrelationship between hormonal, metabolic, and nutritional factors in the evolution of malnutrition in CHD patients.

Other Non–Dialysis-Related Factors

Specific comorbid conditions facilitate the development of malnutrition in CHD patients. Patients with renal failure secondary to diabetes mellitus have a higher incidence of malnutrition compared with patients who are not diabetic. Diabetic patients are more prone to malnutrition because of gastrointestinal disorders such as gastroparesis, nausea and vomiting, bacterial overgrowth in the gut, and pancreatic insufficiency, as well as a high frequency of the nephrotic syndrome and related complications.

Depression, which is common in patients with ESRD, is associated with anorexia, and chronic renal failure patients are usually prescribed a large number of medications, particularly sedatives, phosphate binders, and iron supplements. Each of these is associated with gastrointestinal complications. Finally, the socioeconomic status of the kidney failure patients with decreased mobility, age, and dietary restrictions are factors that greatly enhance the potential for malnutrition in CHD patients.

Hemodialysis-Related Factors Promoting Malnutrition in Chronic Hemodialysis Patients

Loss of nutrients during a dialysis treatment is an important component of dialysis-related catabolism. There is a loss of 5 to 8 g of free amino acids during each hemodialysis session using low-flux dialyzers. With the use of membranes with larger pore sizes (so-called "high-flux membranes") and higher blood flows, these losses increase by 30%. Simultaneous changes in plasma amino acid concentrations suggest that patients catabolize approximately 25 to 30 g of body protein to compensate for these losses.

Another well defined, at least experimentally, cause of protein catabolism in dialysis patients is the contact between blood and foreign material during hemodialysis (i.e., the effects of bioincompatibility). It is now well established that the type of dialysis membrane affects protein metabolism in CHD patients; bioincompatible membranes that vigorously activate the complement system induce much greater net protein catabolism compared with dialysis membranes that do not activate this inflammatory response. Although both types of membranes induce net protein catabolism, the amino acid losses during hemodialysis make protein catabolism more intense when bioincompatible membranes are used. Protein catabolism in normal adults can be observed at 6 hours after initiation of dialysis. On the other hand, some investigators find no adverse effects of dialysis with bioincompatible membranes on protein metabolism, but amino acids in the postdialysis period were not evaluated.

The mechanism by which membrane biocompatibility and activation of the complement pathway enhance protein catabolism is not clear. Production of cytokines (e.g., interleukin-1 and tumor necrosis factor-α [TNF-α]) may cause muscle protein degradation with amino acid release. In experimental studies, the release of amino acids during dialysis with bioincompatible membranes was most prominent at 6 hours after the initiation of hemodialysis, a time consistent with activation of monocytes and release of cytokines, followed by their action on muscle cells. Complement activation increases the transcription of TNF-α, and serum TNF-α concentration is high in CHD patients dialyzed with a complement-activating membrane.

One of the most important factors affecting the nutritional status of dialysis patients is the dose of dialysis. The results of the NCDS suggested a relationship between underdialysis and anorexia. However, there is no clear cause-and-effect relationship between the dose of dialysis and nutrition, and it is possible that the relationship between the dose of dialysis, as measured by Kt/V and the value of PCR, is actually a mathematical artifact rather than a metabolic response reflecting better nutrition. For example, no significant relationship between serum albumin and the dose of dialysis was observed in one large study. Nevertheless, it is quite clear that an inadequate clearance of uremic substances causes progressive anorexia at all stages of renal failure.

Hormonal and metabolic derangements found in the predialysis stage may persist or even worsen at the CHD stage, regardless of the modality of dialysis. Furthermore, placement of permanent or temporary vascular access in a CHD patient can induce additional medical problems and hospitalization, and an increased frequency of hospitalization can adversely affect the nutritional status of dialysis patients.

In summary, multiple factors predispose patients with ESRD to malnutrition. Although some of these factors, such as anorexia and hormonal and metabolic abnormalities, are encountered at all stages of chronic kidney disease, some are specific to the modality of CHD.

PREVENTION AND TREATMENT OF MALNUTRITION IN ESRD PATIENTS WITH END-STAGE RENAL DISEASE

Goal: To discuss the potential measures of preventing malnutrition in CHD patients and propose treatment methods for CHD patients who are already malnourished

A list of measures to prevent or treat malnutrition at different stages of kidney failure is presented in Table 12-3, and an algorithm for assessment of the nutritional status and dietary interventions in CHD patients is shown in Fig. 12-1.

Dose of Dialysis

An adequate dose of dialysis is required to prevent the development of malnutrition in CHD patients. In a prospective cohort analysis of the effects of increasing the dialysis dose in a group of patients with PCR values < 1 g/kg/day, it was shown that PCR increased significantly in the group of patients whose Kt/V values were increased, whereas there was no change in PCR values in the group of patients whose Kt/V values remained the same. In smaller studies, a significant increase in the serum albumin occurs in CHD patients when their dose of dialysis is increased from inadequate to adequate levels. Thus, in a prospective, observational, 4-year study where the dose of dialysis was increased to 1.33 (measured by delivered Kt/V) in 130 CHD patients, the standardized mortality rates of the patients declined from 22.8% to 9.1%. When nutritional parameters of patients with yearly average Kt/V values < 0.86 and > 1.21 were compared, statistically significant differences were found between serum albumin, transferrin, and PCR measurements. Thus, available evidence points to a close association between dialysis dose and nutrition.

Table 12-3. Interventions to prevent or treat malnutrition

Appropriate amount of dietary protein intake (> 1.2 g/kg/d) along with nutritional counseling to encourage an increased intake

Optimal dose of dialysis (Kt/V > 1.4 or Urea reduction ratio >70%)

Use of biocompatible dialysis membranes

Enteral or intradialytic parenteral nutritional supplements (hemodialysis) and amino acid dialysate (peritoneal dialysis) if oral intake is not sufficient

Growth factors (experimental)
  Recombinant human growth hormone
  Recombinant human insulin-like growth factor-1

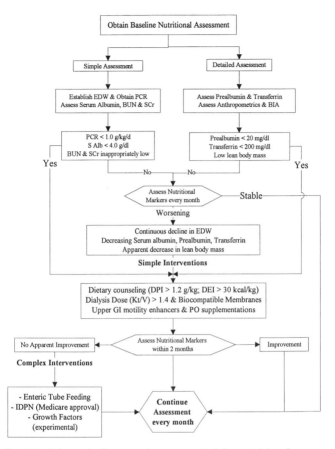

Fig. 12-1. Schematic diagram of assessment of the nutritional status and dietary interventions in patients with end-stage renal disease. EDW, estimated dry weight; PCR, protein catabolic rate; SCr, serum creatinine; BIA, bioelectrical impedance analysis; DPI, dietary protein intake; DEI, dietary energy intake; GI, gastrointestinal; IDPN, intradialytic parenteral nutrition.

Dialysis Membrane

Experimental and cross-sectional studies of patients have highlighted the catabolic and anorectic effects of bioincompatible dialysis membranes. Moreover, there is evidence that biocompatible hemodialysis membranes favorably affect the nutritional status of CHD patients. In a prospective, randomized study of 159 new hemodialysis patients randomized to treatment with a low-flux, biocompatible membrane or a low-flux, bioincompatible membrane, nutritional measurements were taken over 18 months. Treatment with the biocompatible membrane resulted in a mean increase in dry weight of 4.36 ± 8.57 kg, whereas on average no change in weight was observed during treatment with bioincompatible dialysis membranes. In addition, the biocompatible group had an earlier (6 vs. 12 months) and more marked increase in serum albumin concentration than the bioincompatible group, as well as consistently higher IGF-1 values. Reports from the United States Renal Data System (USRDS) also suggest that use of bioincompatible membranes is associated with an increased risk of death compared with biocompatible membranes. Whether a difference in nutritional status plays a role in this increased risk is not clear, but there appears to be a significant increase of infection-related deaths in patients treated with bioincompatible dialysis membrane. It is possible that a poor nutritional status may increase the prevalence of infectious episodes in these patients and eventually increase the risk of death. Further studies are required to evaluate the cause-and-effect relationship between these factors.

Nutrient Intake

Considering the catabolic nature of dialysis, it is clear that patients must maintain an adequate protein and calorie intake. Many patients continue their predialysis diets after beginning dialysis, and it is the nephrologist's and the dietitian's responsibility to ensure that the protein and calorie intake is sufficient for the increased requirements imposed by dialysis. Repetitive, comprehensive counseling by an experienced dietitian is an important step, as well as efforts to detect early signs of malnutrition. Similar efforts should be made during a hospitalization, when these patients often have even lower levels of protein and calorie intake.

Enteral and Intradialytic Parenteral Nutrition

Aggressive dietary counseling to improve nutritional status is usually unsuccessful in optimizing the diet of most malnourished dialysis patients. For these patients, other forms of supplementation such as enteral (including protein and amino acid tablets, protein and energy supplements by mouth, nasogastric tubes, and percutaneous endoscopic gastroscopy or jejunostomy tubes) and intradialytic parenteral nutrition (IDPN) are suggested. Only a limited number of studies evaluating the effects of enteral supplementation in malnourished patients with ESRD are available, and most are not controlled and are small in scope. The degree of success is variable. Nevertheless, it is logical and financially feasible to initiate enteral nutrition in malnourished CHD patients.

There are multiple formulas available as oral supplements for CHD patients. Most of these formulas provide calories in the range of 250 to 375 per box or can. The protein content of these supplements is approximately 15%, and they contain most of the vitamins and trace elements that CHD patients require. The major issues in choosing a supplement is the patient's taste preference and the price and availability of the supplement. When prescribing an enteral supplement, the goal should be to achieve a minimum intake of 1.4 g/kg/day of protein and 30 to 35 kcal/kg/day of energy.

If enteral supplementation fails, IDPN may be considered to treat malnutrition. This mode of treatment should be advocated after a trial of enteral nutritional supplementation. Usually, there are positive nutritional benefits of intradialytic infusions of nutrients, but some investigators were not able to show any benefit of IDPN. Importantly, all studies have drawbacks in their designs and patient populations, so no definitive conclusions can be made. However, in a retrospective analysis of more than 1500 CHD patients treated with IDPN, there was a decreasing risk of death with the use of IDPN, particularly in patients with serum albumin concentrations < 3.5 g/dl and serum creatinine concentrations < 8 mg/dl. There also were substantial improvements in these nutritional parameters with IDPN, suggesting that this mode of treatment is probably most useful in patients with moderate to severe malnutrition.

The prescription of IDPN should be tailored according to the patient's needs; the goals for a minimum daily protein and energy intake should be 1.4 g/kg and 30 to 35 kcal/kg, respectively. When treating a patient with IDPN, side effects such as excessive fluid gain and hyperglycemia should also be monitored closely.

In summary, the available evidence suggests that IDPN may be useful in the treatment of malnourished CHD patients and offers an alternative method of nutritional intervention in patients in whom an inadequate oral or enteral intake cannot be maintained. Most of the evaluations of IDPN are retrospective, uncontrolled, and short term, and there are no clear data to prove that aggressive nutritional supplementation through the gastrointestinal tract is inferior to parenteral supplementation in dialysis patients. Until a controlled study comparing various forms of nutritional supplementation in similar patient groups is completed, the nutritionist should be cautious in choosing highly costly nutritional interventions.

Growth Factors

Growth hormone and its major mediator of growth and metabolic responses, IGF-1, have several anabolic properties. Recombinant human growth hormone (rhGH) has been used in several populations to promote net anabolism. With the recognition that there are defects as well as alterations in growth hormone-IGF-1 axis in CHD patients, rhGH has been proposed as a potential anabolic agent (see Table 12-3). Animal studies suggest administration of rhGH induces a net anabolic action in uremic rats and improves food utilization. In a preliminary, short-term study of CHD patients, a decrease in the predialysis BUN concentration by approximately 25% plus a significant reduction in the net urea generation and PCR during rhGH administration was demonstrated. When rhGH was given to seven malnourished hemodialysis patients in association with IDPN, there were significant improvements in serum albumin, transferrin, and IGF-1 concentrations; IDPN alone did not improve these nutritional parameters. In continuous ambulatory peritoneal dialysis patients, rhGH treatment was associated with a significant decrease in net urea generation and serum potassium and phosphorus concentrations, plus an increase in serum creatinine concentrations, suggesting net anabolism in muscle. Analysis of the amino acid profiles suggested that rhGH shifted amino acid metabolism toward muscle tissues.

Because IGF-1 is the major mediator of growth hormone action, recombinant human IGF-1 has also been proposed to produce anabolism. Although results of nitrogen balance studies in continuous ambulatory peritoneal dialysis patients are consistent with this hypothesis, side effects of this agent may impede its widespread use. Interestingly, the combined use of growth hormone and IGF-1 in healthy subjects seems to provide the most efficient anabolic action with the least number of side effects. It is not known whether the long-term use of these agents in malnourished CHD patients would improve nutritional parameters and outcome.

CONCLUSIONS

Malnutrition is highly prevalent in CHD patients. This is clearly related to multiple factors that begin during the predialysis stage, and continue during CHD. There is an important relationship between malnutrition and a poor outcome in CHD patients. Interventions that improve the poor nutritional status of patients with ESRD may actually improve their morbidity and mortality rates.

ACKNOWLEDGMENTS

This work is partly supported by National Institutes of Health grants nos. DK-45604-05 and HL-36015-10, and Food and Drug Administration grant no. FD-R-000943-03.

SELECTED READINGS

Bergstrom J. Nutrition and mortality in hemodialysis. *J Am Soc Nephrol* 1995;6:1329–1341.

Chertow GM, Ling J, Lew NL, et al. The association of intradialytic parenteral nutrition with survival in hemodialysis patients. *Am J Kidney Dis* 1994;24:912–920.

Hakim RM, Breyer J, Ismail N, et al. Effects of dose of dialysis on morbidity and mortality. *Am J Kidney Dis* 1994;23:661–669.

Ikizler TA, Hakim RM. Nutrition in end-stage renal disease. *Kidney Int* 1996;50:343–357.

Krieg JRJ, Santos F, Chan JCM. Growth hormone, insulin-like growth factor and the kidney. *Kidney Int* 1995;48:321–336.

Lowrie EG, Huang WH, Lew NL, et al. The relative contribution of measured variables to death risk among hemodialysis patients. In: Friedman EA, ed. *Death on hemodialysis*. Amsterdam: Kluwer Academic Publishers; 1994:121–141.

Mitch WE, Medina R, Grieber S, et al. Metabolic acidosis stimulates muscle protein degradation by activating the adenosine triphosphate-dependent pathway involving ubiquitin and proteasomes. *J Clin Invest* 1994;93:2127–2133.

Owen WF Jr, Lew NL, Liu Y, et al. The urea reduction ratio and serum albumin concentrations as predictors of mortality in patients undergoing hemodialysis. *N Engl J Med* 1993;329:1001–1006.

Parker TF III, Wingard RL, Husni L, et al. The effect of the membrane biocompatibility on nutritional parameters in chronic hemodialysis patients. *Kidney Int* 1996;49:551–556.

Schulman G, Wingard RL, Hutchinson RL, et al. The effects of recombinant human growth hormone and intradialytic parenteral nutrition in malnourished hemodialysis patients. *Am J Kidney Dis* 1993;21:527–534.

Nutrition and Peritoneal Dialysis

Ram Gokal and John Harty

Nutrition has a major impact on the outcome of patients on dialysis. To maintain well-being, prevention of malnutrition or reversing any malnourished state must remain major goals in managing peritoneal dialysis patients.

ASSESSMENT OF NUTRITIONAL STATE

The Prevalence of Protein-Calorie Malnutrition in the Peritoneal Dialysis Population

Conventionally, nutritional state is defined in relation to either reference standards or in relation to the clinician's subjective opinion of what constitutes a poor nutritional state. Table 13-1 lists conventional indices of malnutrition.

This approach is complicated by the lack of a specific nutritional gold standard. Protein-calorie malnutrition represents a continuum between marasmus and kwashiorkor. In the former, muscle and fat stores are deficient relative to visceral protein (albumin). In the later state, visceral protein reserves are severely depleted with an apparent preservation of body composition—in part due to edema. In addition, single measures, especially serum albumin, are not specific for nutrition, being influenced by hydration, hepatic synthesis, and inflammatory states. Finally, any single measure, especially anthropometry, is subject to considerable

Table 13-1. Indices of malnutrition in dialysis patients

Anthropometry

A decrease of 10–15% or more in dry weight
   (15–35% dry weight = severe)

Reduction in anthropometric measurements (< 15th percentile = moderate; < 5th percentile = severe malnutrition), body mass index < 20% (severe < 18 kg/m^2)

Low percentage of ideal body weight (< 85%)

Dietary intake

Dietary protein intake < 0.8 g/kg/IBW

Total calorie intake of < 35 g/kg/IBW

Subjective global assessment (B or C)

Nitrogen index < 80%

Serum markers

Serum albumin < 4.0 g/dl

Low insulin-like growth factor-1 (< 300 μg/l), transferrin (< 200 mg/dl), prealbumin (< 30 mg/dl), and cholesterol (< 150 mg/dl)

IBW, ideal body weight; B, mild to moderate malnutrition; C, severe malnutrition (see Table 13-3).

observational error. Reliance on a single marker, such as albumin or estimates of lean body mass, may under- or overrepresent the prevalence of malnutrition in the population. If malnutrition is diagnosed by the presence of only one parameter, up to 25% of the normal population would be regarded as abnormal.

Dietary Protein and Calorie Intake as Nutritional Measures

These are indirect measures and only valid in combination with other assessments (see Nutritional Profiles).

Dietary protein intake (DPI) may be measured using dietary recall. This requires a food diary—collected preferably for 3 days by a skilled dietitian—but there is a tendency to overestimate actual intake. Nevertheless, this is the only technique for estimating calorie intake.

Protein intake can be estimated from urea kinetics. In a patient who is in nitrogen balance, the amount of urea excreted daily is proportional to ingested protein. Furthermore, daily urea removal constitutes 85% of the total daily nitrogen excretion in the urine and peritoneal dialysis effluent. Formulas have been devised to permit calculation of both the urea and, hence, the protein nitrogen appearance rate (PNA), also called the protein catabolic rate (PCR). The PNA can, with caution, be used as a measure of DPI (Table 13-2).

Protein Nitrogen Appearance

A measure of protein intake PNA has many limitations and exhibits only a weak correlation with DPI (0.44 to 0.88). This reflects both considerable variability in the percentage of protein nitrogen converted to urea between low and high protein intake and the excretion of nitrogen in the form of protein, amino acids, and other forms of nonurea nitrogen. Importantly, with catabolic illnesses, the PNA is increased out of proportion to protein intake.

A fundamental problem in using either the dietary recall or PNA as a measure of nutrition is the practice of standardizing such values to body size—expressing protein intake as grams per kilogram of body weight. For smaller and potentially malnourished patients (who have a smaller denominator), use of the patient's actual weight as the denominator often yields sig-

---

Table 13-2. Formula for calculating estimated protein intake based on urea appearance

UNA (g/day) = Vd (dl) × Cd (mg/dl) + Vu (dl) + Cu (mg/dl)

UNA (mmol/day) = Vd (ml) × Cd (mmol/L) + Vu (ml) × Cu (mmol/L)

PNPNA (g/day) = 13 + 7.31 UNA (g/day)

or

13 + 0.261 UA (mmol/d)

Estimated DPI = PNPNA + dialysate and urinary protein loss

Vd, 24-hour drained dialysate volume; Vu, 24-hour urine volume; Cd, dialysate urea concentration; Cu, urinary urea concentration; UNA, urea nitrogen appearance (g/day); UA, urea appearance (mmol/day); PNPNA, protein equivalent of the nonprotein nitrogen appearance (i.e., protein nitrogen appearance – protein losses); DPI, dietary protein intake.

nificantly greater values for protein intake than for larger, well nourished patients. Furthermore, as patients lose weight, the denominator will "shrink," resulting in an apparent preservation of the calculated protein intake. Current recommendations are to standardize PNA to ideal body weight obtained from standard reference tables.

Nutritional Profiles

Many groups have used a nutritional profile or index that incorporates anthropometric measures of fat and muscle mass, serum proteins, and protein intake. Individual nutritional parameters are allocated a score in accordance with established criteria for malnutrition. The patient's nutritional state is then defined in relation to the total score obtained for all nutritional markers. This approach has two significant limitations: the final decision on nutritional state is ultimately based on an arbitrary score, and, more important, such a profile is laborious to perform and relatively insensitive to changes in nutritional state.

Subjective Global Assessment

Such difficulties have led to the development of a clinical scoring technique, the subjective global assessment (SGA), which relies on the clinical appraisal of eight nutritional features (Table 13-3). On the basis of this subjective analysis, the clinician allocates a score to each feature and summarizes the nutritional status of the patient into categories of normal nutrition, mild to moderate malnutrition, or severe malnutrition. Such a technique is easy to perform, has been extensively used in continuous ambulatory peritoneal dialysis (CAPD) patients, and is the currently accepted technique for defining the nutritional state in CAPD and hemodialysis patients. However, being a categorical measure, it is an insensitive technique to monitor change in nutrition over time.

Table 13-3. Subjective global assessment

Historical factors	
1. Weight change	Loss in past 6 mo: 0, <5%, >10%
	Change in past 2 wk: unchanged (recent weight gain negates past losses)
2. Dietary intake	No change or suboptimal intake
	Liquid diet, hypocaloric fluids, starvation
3. Gastrointestinal symptoms	More than 2 wk
	Anorexia, nausea, vomiting, diarrhea
	More than 6 wk
4. Functional capacity	Normal, suboptimal work, ambulatory, bedridden
5. Nutritional stress	None, minimum, high
Physical examination	
1. Loss of subcutaneous fat	Triceps and or mid-axillary line of lateral chest wall
2. Loss of muscle mass	Deltoids, temporals, or quadriceps
3. Edema	

Monitoring Nutritional Status Over Time

This involves the measurement of continuous nutritional variables.

Body Composition

Table 13-4 lists the most commonly used measures of body composition, highlighting their uses and limitations. Most measures are influenced by tissue hydration. In addition, measures of muscle and fat obtained by one technique cannot be directly compared with those quantified by another method.

Biochemical Assays

Biochemical assays include serum proteins, urea, creatinine, and cholesterol. Important serum proteins include albumin, prealbumin, and the insulin-like growth factors (IGF).

Serum albumin is not a particularly sensitive nutritional index. Hypoalbuminemia is often a late manifestation of malnutrition, reflecting a large hepatic reserve in respect to albumin synthesis, so that many months of malnutrition pass before the pool is depleted. Albumin also exhibits poor and often contradictory correlations with other nutritional markers, especially muscle mass and DPI. This is in part due to the many other non-

Table 13-4. Techniques for measurement of body composition in continuous ambulatory peritoneal dialysis patients

Measure	Pros	Cons
Anthropometry	Easy to perform Noninvasive Reproducible to 90% confidence level	Interobserver error Less sensitive
Bioelectrical impedance	Noninvasive Quick	Indirect method Influenced by hydration and electrode site
Total body potassium	Noninvasive Accurate Reproducible	Cost Relatively insensitive to change over time
Total body nitrogen	Very accurate Reveals subtle changes	Cost Lack of availability Does not distinguish inert nitrogen from muscle nitrogen
Dual-energy x-ray absorptiometry	Direct measures of bone mineral, lean body mass, and compartments	Influenced by hydration Cost and availability
Creatinine kinetics	Low cost Ease of calculation	Influenced by catabolism, residual renal function, and hydration

nutritional influences that affect its value, in particular the distribution of albumin between extravascular and intravascular compartments. In fact, normal values of total albumin mass have been found in CAPD patients despite low serum levels, reflecting in part an increase in plasma volume.

Serum prealbumin has a shorter half-life (2 to 3 days) and in some studies has been shown to be a more sensitive nutritional marker than serum albumin. However, because it is excreted through the kidney, higher levels may simply reflect loss of residual renal function.

The plasma IGF-1 level in nonuremic patients is more sensitive and more specific than other nutrition-related serum proteins. IGF-1 has also been shown to be a sensitive marker of wasting in both the hemodialysis and CAPD populations. However, IGF-1 concentrations have wide confidence limits in normal people, making it difficult to identify malnourished patients, and, in renal failure, levels may be either artificially lowered or raised because of alterations in IGF-binding proteins.

PREVALENCE OF MALNUTRITION

Cross-Sectional Analysis

Protein-calorie malnutrition is common in CAPD patients and may be more prevalent than in hemodialysis patients. In a study comparing 224 CAPD patients with 263 patients on maintenance hemodialysis using a clinical scoring technique (SGA), CAPD patients were found to be more malnourished (42.3%) than the maintenance hemodialysis group (30.8%). In particular, CAPD patients had greater muscle wasting and hypoalbuminemia with greater preservation of fat stores. However, diabetes mellitus and ischemic heart disease were more common in the CAPD patients, emphasizing the importance of comorbidity and casemix differences that could influence differences between these two dialysis modalities.

Using a wide range of nutritional techniques, many studies have demonstrated a significant prevalence of malnutrition in CAPD populations; mild to moderate malnutrition is present in 30% to 35% and severe malnutrition in 8% to 10% (Table 13-5). Furthermore, there is often subclinical evidence for protein depletion, including a reduction in both muscle energy and protein stores and abnormalities in plasma and intracellular amino acid patterns.

Nutritional Status on Dialysis: "Nutritional Tracking"

Many CAPD patients remain well nourished, and it is unfair to attribute the majority of the malnutrition solely to the dialysis process. During the first year of CAPD, many patients gain between 5 and 7 kg in weight. Although this is compatible with anabolism, Williams and colleagues have reported that the gain is mainly due to an increase in body water. Body fat has been shown to increase with time, and studies using neutron activation analysis to quantify body protein demonstrate both anabolism and catabolism. Earlier work showed slight reductions in body nitrogen content in the first year of dialysis (especially in larger patients) followed by equilibration at lower levels. More recently, the nitrogen index was found to increase in

**Table 13-5. Studies of nutritional status
in continuous ambulatory peritoneal dialysis patients**

Study	Method	Results
Young et al.	SGA	Mild to moderate malnutrition in 30–35%, severe malnutrition in 8–10%
Fenton et al.	SGA	
Cianciaruso et al.	SGA	
Enia et al.	SGA	
Nelson et al.	Anthropometry	59% MUAC < 25th of NHANES II percentiles
Markman	Nutritional score	Nutritional abnormalities in 50%
Harty et al.	Nutritional score	31% well nourished, 52% mildly to moderately malnourished, 17% severely malnourished
Heide et al.	TBN	20% decrease in TBN over 24 mo
Pollock et al.	TBN	TBN 88% of normal

SGA, subjective global assessment; MUAC, mid-upper arm circumference; NHANES, National Health and Nutrition Examination Survey; TBN, total body nitrogen.

5% to 6% of patients followed from the onset of dialysis for an average of 23 months. Although these gains in body protein were statistically significant, their magnitude suggests that in the absence of peritonitis or significant illness, there is no dramatic change in the nutritional state of these patients. It is possible that the high prevalence of malnutrition in CAPD patients simply reflects the nutritional status of these patients before commencement of dialysis—in effect, a form of "nutritional tracking"

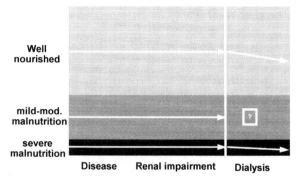

**Fig. 13-1. Nutritional tracking. Evolution of nutritional status
related to progression of renal failure and subsequent dialysis.**

(Fig. 13-1). Nutritional status has been shown to be more influenced by comorbidity than by the dialysis process, and many believe that the nutritional state at the start of dialysis determines the outcome during dialysis. This suggests that patients beginning dialysis in a malnourished state remain so, incurring a poor outcome compared with well nourished patients commencing CAPD. This makes it important to optimize the nutritional milieu in the predialysis period.

MALNUTRITION AND MORTALITY

Malnutrition is closely linked with mortality in dialysis patients. However, it remains to be proven whether the relationship between nutrition and mortality is one of cause and effect, or simply an association.

Biochemical Indices of Nutrition and Mortality

Hypoalbuminemia (<3.5 g/l) has been linked to increased morbidity and mortality, but albumin is influenced by hydration and acute illness and is not a specific nutritional marker in CAPD patients. Accepting these constraints, serum albumin still demonstrates a particularly strong association with survival. CAPD patients with serum albumin levels < 3.5 g/l have a risk of death 3.5 to 4 times that of patients with an albumin level of 4.0 g/l. In the results from the CANUSA (Canadian-USA) study, a decrease of 1 g/l in serum albumin was associated with a 6% increase in the relative risk of death.

A similar association with mortality has been demonstrated for serum prealbumin. Patients with baseline values < 30 mg/dl had a 50% survival of 15 months, in contrast to a 50% survival of 38 months in those with prealbumin levels > 30 mg/dl.

Patients commencing CAPD with low levels of serum creatinine (< 5 mg/dl, reflecting a reduction in muscle mass) have a 2.5- to 5-fold increased risk of death compared with those patients with a baseline creatinine of 12 to 15 mg/dl.

Body Composition and Mortality

Malnutrition as defined by the SGA technique is linked to an increased risk of mortality. In the results from the CANUSA prospective cohort study of 680 patients, a 1 unit lower score was associated with a 25% increase in the relative risk of death.

Low initial values for body protein as measured by total body nitrogen < 80% of the predicted value are associated with a significantly greater risk of mortality or morbidity. By a prospective evaluation, body nitrogen (expressed as grams per kilogram lean body mass) was significantly lower (30.6 vs. 34) in CAPD patients who died compared with those who remained alive.

Although the nutritional state has been linked to survival in dialysis patients, no study has adequately determined whether this is a causal relationship, and a large number of dialysis patients have other medical illnesses that, as in the case of cardiovascular and peripheral vascular disease, are linked to malnutrition and death. Coexisting diseases may result in impaired nutrition and survival, with death occurring in the context of, but not as a consequence of, malnutrition.

PROTEIN AND ENERGY REQUIREMENTS

Nitrogen Balance

Dietary protein and calorie requirements are traditionally derived from nitrogen balance studies. Studies in CAPD patients have demonstrated that nitrogen balance is consistently positive when patients ingest at least 1.2 g protein/kg body weight/day. Anabolism, as demonstrated by an increase in body weight, upper arm muscle circumference, and fat measurements, occurs with the higher-protein diet. There is a curvilinear relationship between nitrogen balance and dietary protein, with a negative nitrogen balance occurring below a protein intake of 1.2 g/kg/day. In contrast, Bergstrom and associates have demonstrated that some CAPD patients can maintain a neutral or positive nitrogen balance with a protein intake as low as 0.7 g/kg/day.

Energy intake is crucial in determining the effectiveness of dietary protein utilization and, hence, the protein requirement, especially in patients ingesting a marginal level of protein. In CAPD patients, energy intake is a major determinant of nitrogen balance; the lowest nitrogen balance is in patients with a total energy intake of less than 35 kcal/kg/day. In peritoneal dialysis patients there is a close correlation between the amount of glucose absorbed and the quantity of glucose instilled in the peritoneum. Energy intake from this source averages 7.4 kcal/kg/day or approximately 20% of the daily total energy intake. Despite this additional energy source, up to 90% of CAPD patients fail to achieve the recommended target of 35 kcal/kg/day.

Based on nitrogen balance studies, a daily target of protein intake of 1.2 g/kg body weight has been recommended, together with a total (diet + dialysate) calorie intake of 35 kcal/kg/day.

Nutritional Adaptation

Protein intake is extremely variable in CAPD patients; most fail to achieve the aforementioned targets and protein-calorie intake diminishes by up to 30% with time. Nevertheless, many patients appear to remain reasonably well nourished. A low-protein diet in nonuremic subjects induces short-term adaptive changes and long-term accommodative changes in both nitrogen metabolism and protein turnover. These responses act to maintain nitrogen balance. Patients with chronic renal failure have been shown to maintain nitrogen balance with protein ingestion as low as 0.67 g/kg/day by activating similar short-term adaptive changes to decrease amino acid oxidation and protein degradation. It seems logical to assume that a suboptimal diet renders the CAPD patient vulnerable to malnutrition during periods of catabolic stress.

ETIOLOGY OF PROTEIN-CALORIE MALNUTRITION

Although the etiology of protein-calorie malnutrition is multifactorial (Table 13-6), the mechanism by which such diverse causes have an adverse impact on nutritional state can be understood in terms of factors that either decrease nutritional intake or enhance protein and energy catabolism.

Table 13-6. Etiology of protein-calorie malnutrition in continuous ambulatory peritoneal dialysis

Inadequate dietary intake

Uremia (inadequate dialysis)

Impact of peritoneal dialysis
  Abdominal bloating
  Absorption of glucose and amino acids
  Peritonitis and exit site infections

Poor diet

Coexisting gastrointestinal disease
  (gastroparesis, peptic ulcer disease)

Comorbid illness (congestive heart failure, atherosclerosis, infection, chronic obstructive pulmonary disease, amyloid)

Medication (calcium binders, antihypertensive agents, iron)

Psychosocial and economic factors
  Isolation and depression
  Ignorance
  Poverty

Poor dentition

Catabolic factors

Comorbid illness (cardiac failure, inflammation, sepsis)

Physical inactivity

Catabolic effect of dialysis procedure
  Peritonitis
  Dialysate protein loss (5–15 g/day)
  Dialysis glucose absorption

Metabolic acidosis

Abnormal energy metabolism

Decreased Intake

Psychosocial and Socioeconomic Factors

Depression, social isolation, and a poor quality of life are common in dialysis patients and are linked to poor appetite. Side effects associated with the use of anxiolytic or antidepressant drugs can further reduce appetite. Financial hardship is common in dialysis patients, and many simply cannot afford either the recommended protein intake or supplements. Many elderly patients are unable to ingest the calories needed to maintain nitrogen balance at protein intakes less than 0.8 g/kg/day.

Comorbid Illness

Coexisting illness is an important determinant of nutritional status and anorexia. In particular, severe malnutrition occurs with atherosclerosis and left ventricular dysfunction. Diabetes with associated gastroparesis is common in dialysis patients and exerts a detrimental influence on appetite, but there are other causes. A prospective study of 97 CAPD patients found that severe comorbidity suppressed appetite over and above the impact of dialysis dose. Those patients with severe comorbidity had a 26% lower protein and a 15% lower calorie intake.

Dialysis-Specific Influences

Eating behavior differs in CAPD patients because of a lower average total food intake plus a lower eating velocity compared with healthy control subjects or hemodialysis patients. Most studies also show that CAPD patients ingest less protein intake than their hemodialysis counterparts. In a cross-sectional study of 147 "stable" patients, only 12% achieved a protein intake of 1.2 g/kg/day and only 8% had a total calorie intake of 35 kcal/kg/day.

DIALYSATE VOLUME. Large infusions of dialysate are associated with symptoms of abdominal bloating and anorexia. An increase in dialysis volume from 2 to 2.5 l was accompanied in some patients by a mean reduction in DPI of 10 g/day. A study of eating behavior has shown that there was a tendency for CAPD patients to be less hungry and have less desire to eat before lunch when their abdominal cavity was full in contrast to periods when there was no dialysate fluid.

OSMOTIC AGENTS. The absorption of glucose from the dialysis fluid provides between 5 to 20 kcal/kg/day, and this continuous glucose absorption can inhibit hunger. Animal studies have shown appetite suppression induced by either glucose or amino acid dialysate solutions, suggesting that the mechanism reducing appetite is more complex than a simple provision of calories.

Dialysis Dose and Nutrition

Anorexia is a characteristic symptom of uremia, and in predialysis patients with chronic renal failure there is evidence for reduced protein intake during progression of renal failure. Amelioration of anorexia with an increase in appetite is characteristic of patients commencing CAPD. This has led to attempts to define an "adequate" amount of dialysis that would be sufficient to facilitate protein intake and prevent or treat protein-calorie malnutrition.

KT/V AND THE NORMALIZED PROTEIN CATABOLIC RATE. Initial enthusiasm for a link between dialysis dose and nutrition stemmed from the observed cross-sectional correlation between dialysis dose (expressed as Kt/V, fractional urea clearance) and protein intake (extrapolated from the normalized PNA, formally referred to as the nPCR). The strength of this correlation (r = 0.5 to 0.6) led to the conclusion that urea clearance was one of the most important determinants of dietary intake, and that in patients with a nPNA <1.0 g/kg/day the dialysis dose should be increased. This approach has since been shown to be seriously flawed.

MATHEMATICAL COUPLING. Because both Kt/V and nPCR share a common numerator (change in blood urea nitrogen) and a common denominator (body weight), their correlation is in part due to the phenomenon of mathematical coupling—namely, that some portion of the relationship between two variables is due to a common component present in both variables. For example, the correlation between Kt/V and nPCR can be recreated using randomly generated numbers for the individual variables in each formula (Fig. 13-2). These findings do not negate a physiologically relevant relationship between dialysis dose and protein

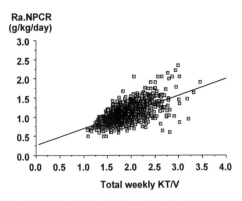

Fig. 13-2. Correlation between fractional urea clearance (Kt/V) and Randerson normalized protein catabolic rate (nPCR) using randomly generated numbers for the variables in each formula. N = 2000. Y = 0.43X + 0.22; r = 0.62; P < 0.0001.

intake, but they do point out the problems with the use of cross-sectional analysis to demonstrate a potential link.

PROSPECTIVE STUDIES: KT/V AND NUTRITION. Five published studies have investigated the impact of increasing dialysis dose on nutritional state. Most were short term and used only nPCR and albumin as nutritional markers (Table 13-7). In a prospective study of 33 patients followed for 1 year, increasing the dialysis dose resulted in an increase in Kt/V from 1.6 to 1.9, but there was a decrease in protein intake by a mean of 2 g/day (possibly because of more problems with abdominal fullness). Importantly, a reduction in the total clearance from a Kt/V of 1.8 to 1.5 (due to loss of residual renal function) was accompanied by a significant fall in protein intake (mean decrease of 8.5 g/day). This reflects the limited ability to augment clearance by increasing the dialysis volume used by CAPD patients, plus the negative impact of larger dialysate volumes and osmotic load on appetite.

Table 13-7. Impact of increasing dialysis dose on nutrition*

Study	Kt/V		nPNA (g/kg/d)		Albumin (g/L)	
	Pre	Post	Pre	Post	Pre	Post
Lindsay and Spanner	1.74	2.70	0.65	0.93	—	—
Tzamaloukas et al.	1.40	2.10	0.74	0.96	33.9	33.3
Heimburger et al.	1.53	1.89	0.81	0.87	29.1	30.5
Williams et al.	1.37	1.65	0.88	0.88	35.4	35.5
	1.70	2.74	1.26	1.42	31	31
Harty et al.	1.50	1.80	0.92	0.94	37	36

Kt/V, fractional urea clearance; nPNA, normalized protein nitrogen appearance.
*Values before (pre) and after (post) increase in dialysis dose.

Residual Renal Function and Nutrition

The importance of residual renal function to nitrogen metabolism and nutrition has been noted since the conception of CAPD. A residual renal creatine clearance of 1 ml/minute is equivalent to 10 l/week and is not inconsequential, given the average creatinine clearance of 40 to 50 l/week achieved by CAPD. During nitrogen balance measurements, residual renal function has a greater influence on the protein intake than CAPD clearance, and in an international cross-sectional study of 224 CAPD patients, Young and colleagues found that anuria was present in 94% of severely malnourished patients. The CANUSA study also showed an association between a decrease in nutritional state and loss of residual renal function.

Increased Catabolism

Table 13-6 lists important catabolic factors that can influence the nutritional status of CAPD patients. Very few catabolic stimuli have been definitely identified as causes of CAPD malnutrition, but it is reasonable to suppose that in a vulnerable, maximally adapted patient, even trivial metabolic insults will result in a profound nutritional deficit.

Peritonitis

Peritonitis results in a negative nitrogen balance, a reduction in serum albumin, and a decrease in lean body mass. The mechanism includes a reduction in protein and energy intake, increased protein catabolism, and increased protein losses into the dialysate. Even with mild peritonitis, the daily dialysate protein loss is about 15 g and it often remains elevated for weeks. Patients who are in nitrogen balance because they have adapted to an inadequate protein and calorie intake will be most vulnerable to such a nutritional insult.

Protein Losses Into the Dialysate

Even in the absence of peritonitis, the daily loss of protein into the peritoneal effluent ranges from 5 to 12 g, in addition to a free amino acid loss of 2 to 4 g. Albumin represents the major type of protein lost, and the increase in albumin clearance is directly related to the peritoneal transport status. Those in the high-transport group have both a greater daily amount of albumin lost and a lower serum albumin. It is still uncertain whether the lower levels of serum albumin seen in this subgroup represent a lower serum albumin mass or a dilutional phenomenon due to overhydration, because overhydration is also common in high transporters. Moreover, it is unclear whether the transport status with differences in dialysis protein loss is deleterious to the nutritional state of CAPD patients.

Metabolic Acidosis

Metabolic acidosis is a potent stimulus increasing protein catabolism. There is some evidence that increasing serum bicarbonate in CAPD patients is associated with anabolism as measured by a decrease in leucine turnover and a disproportionate reduction in urea production compared with the amount of DPI. On the other hand, only 6% of CAPD patients have a serum bicarbonate < 22 mEq/l, and nutritional surveys do not suggest that this subgroup is at special risk for nutritional problems. Oral supplementation with sodium bicarbonate should be used with caution in view of the risk of inducing chronic salt and water overload.

Abnormal Energy State

Energy requirements may be increased in CAPD patients. Although resting energy expenditure has been found to be similar in CAPD patients and nonuremic control subjects, malnourished patients have levels of resting energy expenditure similar to those of well nourished nonuremic control subjects. The continuous peritoneal absorption and subsequent oxidation of glucose elicit a thermogenic response that could interfere with energy conservation in CAPD patients. Thus, dialysate glucose may paradoxically turn out to be detrimental to patients who have a suboptimal protein and energy intake.

PREVENTION OF MALNUTRITION

The various causes leading to protein-energy malnutrition are shown in Table 13-6.

Although uremia and inadequate dialysis are important, there are specific factors related to peritoneal dialysis such as glucose absorption from the peritoneal cavity, a sensation of abdominal fullness, and gastroparesis and diarrhea in diabetics that are additional causes. A preventative strategy consists of eradicating or minimizing these factors, and it is important to identify patients who are at risk for development of malnutrition (Table 13-8). The strongest predictors of a low serum albumin include diabetes and advanced age; there is debate whether a high dialysate/plasma creatinine ratio (hyperpermeable membrane) is a risk factor in addition to a dilution of serum albumin. Other vulnerable groups include socially isolated, depressed patients and those who have recurrent peritonitis.

Table 13-8. Patients at risk for development of malnutrition

Elderly

Socially isolated

Diabetes mellitus

Recurrent peritonitis

Active comorbid conditions

Loss of residual renal function

Inadequate solute removal

Malnutrition risk	
Dietary protein intake	< 0.8 g/kg IBW/day
Calories	< 30 kcal/kg IBW/day
Mid-upper arm circumference	< 15th percentile = mild to moderate < 5th percentile = severe
Weight	< 80% IBW (NHANES)
Serum albumin	< 30 g/l

IBW, ideal body weight; NHANES, National Health and Nutrition Examination Survey.

The first step in the prevention of malnutrition is a careful assessment of the patient's nutritional status at the beginning of dialysis and every 3 to 6 months thereafter. Early diagnosis and a correction strategy can avoid the clinical deterioration that makes the patient more difficult to treat, because malnutrition may cause anorexia. This relationship is suggested because an improved nutritional status is associated with improved food intake, at least in hemodialysis patients who received parenteral nutrition. They showed an increase in food intake before any change in nutritional status. Regular monitoring includes SGA and serum albumin, the best parameters to use, but the clinician needs to be aware of the shortcomings of these parameters (see Table 13-3).

Nutritional Tracking

The predialysis nutritional status may have a major impact on nutritional status after dialysis. This tracking phenomenon (see Fig. 13-1) suggests that dialysis therapy should begin before malnutrition sets in. Although there is no strong evidence for this suggestion, longitudinal studies are suggestive.

Strategy for Maintaining an Adequate Nutritional Status

Sufficient protein, calories, and other nutrients are required to maintain adequate nutritional status. There must be regular assessments of patients at risk. Optimum intakes of protein and calories may not be possible to achieve, but must be the nutritional goals for CAPD patients.

MONITORING NUTRITIONAL STATUS

The methods for monitoring nutritional status are outlined in Tables 13-3 and 13-4. The goal in monitoring the nutritional status of CAPD patients is to identify malnutrition early to make optimal use of dietary and dialysis manipulation, thus improving patient's the nutritional status and outcome.

Reliable estimates of lean body mass are limited and the methods are expensive and not widely available. Creatinine kinetics based on a 24-hour dialysate and urine collection should give a reasonable approximation of the lean body mass in patients who are in steady state, but the creatinine generation rate has a wide standard deviation and is influenced by meat intake. Another parameter is DPI by diet diary, but this is time consuming. The indirect method (PNA) only indirectly relates to protein uptake and then only in the steady state.

Practical Approach to Monitoring

Surveillance needs to be built into the routine clinical care of all patients. The important parameters are:

1. Body weight (<80% of desired level)
2. PNA (normalized to ideal body weight; <0.8 g/kg)
3. Serum albumin (limit of <35 g/l)

None of these is necessarily specific, but if they are below the minimum target (given in parenthesis above) it should alert the physician to impending nutritional deficit and to make other assessments (e.g., SGA, measurement of lean body mass, protein intake) at every clinic visit. Dietary instructions should be

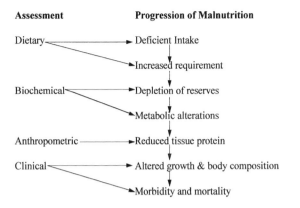

Assessment   **Progression of Malnutrition**

Dietary ——————→ Deficient Intake

→ Increased requirement

Biochemical ————→ Depletion of reserves

→ Metabolic alterations

Anthropometric ——————→ Reduced tissue protein

Clinical ——————→ Altered growth & body composition

→ Morbidity and mortality

Fig. 13-3. The four major criteria used to assess the progression of malnutrition.

reviewed at least quarterly, or more often if clinically indicated. The need to monitor dialysis dose, residual renal function, and fluid status cannot be overemphasized, and patients with a low plasma albumin concentration should be evaluated for malnutrition. It is important to exclude or treat any overt or occult comorbid disease or psychosocial problems that could impair nutritional status, and give advice to increase protein and calorie intake. Failure to do this will lead to progressive malnutrition (Fig. 13-3).

NUTRITIONAL REQUIREMENTS FOR PERITONEAL DIALYSIS PATIENTS

Energy

An adequate energy intake is a prerequisite for efficient utilization of dietary protein and maintenance or repletion of body nutrient stores. Energy requirements do not appear to be different in patients undergoing maintenance dialysis therapy and normal adults (Table 13-9). The recommended calorie intake for sedentary, nonuremic people of ideal body weight averages 30 kcal/kg/day; because dialysis patients have impaired energy metabolism and negative energy balance, sedentary, stable, nonobese dialysis patients should ingest 35 kcal/kg/day from all sources (including glucose absorption from the dialysate). A higher calorie intake is required for patients who perform strenuous labor, who are below their desired body weight, and who are catabolic (e.g., those with peritonitis). Patients older than 60 years of age may be prescribed about 30 kcal/kg/day because normal adults of the same age seem to require less energy.

Calories Gained From Dialysis Solutions

Peritoneal dialysis regimens (primarily 1.36 g/dl glucose, with one or two at 3.86 g/dl glucose) provide about 400 to 600 kcal/day. For nightly intermittent peritoneal dialysis (NIPD) regimens containing 15 l of dialysis solution, the calorie uptake would be between 390 and 860 kcal. The amount of glucose

**Table 13-9. Recommended dietary
nutrient intakes for peritoneal dialysis patients**

Protein	1.0–1.2 g/kg/day; for severe malnutrition > 1.2 g/kg/day
Calories	> 35 kcal/kg/day
Fat (% of total energy)	30–40
Carbohydrate	Rest of calories
Fiber intake	20–25 g/day
Sodium	1–2 g/day
Potassium	40–70 mEq/day
Calcium	800–1000 mg/day
Magnesium	200–300 mg/day
Phosphorus	8–15 mg/kg/day
Zinc	15 mg/day
Thiamin	1.5 mg/day
Riboflavin	1.8 mg/day
Pantothenic acid	5 mg/day
Niacin	20 mg/day
Pyridoxine	10 mg/day
Vitamin B_{12}	3 µg/day
Vitamin C	60 mg/day
Folic Acid	1 mg/day
Vitamins A E K	No addition
Vitamin D	See text

absorbed can be easily calculated from the volume and glucose concentration of a 24-hour collection of dialysate. A rough, but clinically accurate estimate of the amount of glucose absorbed from the dialysate by a CAPD patient with normal peritoneal transport characteristics can be made by multiplying the 24-hour glucose infused by 0.6. A patient using four exchanges of anhydrous glucose, 2.27% (or 2.5% in the United States) will absorb about 110 g of glucose, corresponding to about 440 kcal in 24 hours.

Proportion of Various Components

The protein, carbohydrate, and fat distribution of calories ingested is not clearly defined, but in dialysis patients about 40% to 50% of calories should be carbohydrates. A further reduction of carbohydrate intake is difficult to achieve except by restricting concentrated sweets and alcohol. Cholesterol restriction should be practiced with restraint because many cholesterol-containing foods such as meat and eggs are excellent sources of high–biologic-value protein. Patients can gain much of the advantage of the high protein value of eggs by consuming the egg whites only. Ingestion of fish or white meat is preferable to consumption of red meat.

Protein

The recommended protein allowance for healthy adults is 0.8 g/kg/day, but most Americans eat a much greater amount (1 to 1.5 g/kg/day). Most nitrogen balance studies suggest that dialysis patients require a protein intake of at least 1 g/kg/day, at least 50% of which should be of high biologic value (i.e., from meat, fish, and egg white). There is a curvilinear relationship between DPI and nitrogen balance in CAPD patients, and a protein intake of 1.2 g/kg/day ensures neutral to positive nitrogen balance in all clinically stable CAPD patients. This recommendation is based on achieving the maximum nutritional status for the largest number of CAPD patients, but patients who consume 0.9 to 1 g/kg do not necessarily put themselves at risk of malnutrition, assuming that they are stable.

One problem with dietary recommendations for dialysis patients, who are often malnourished, is the weight used in the calculation. To base a patient's requirements on the actual weight will only serve to maintain the present malnourished state, but the amount of food will not necessarily correct malnutrition. Kinetically modeled estimates of protein intakes (nPCR for dialysis) predict protein intake normalized to actual weight. For such patients, protein and calorie recommendations should be based on the average body weight of healthy subjects of the same sex, height, and age as the patient.

Lipids

There is a high incidence of lipid abnormalities in CAPD patients, including low serum high-density lipoprotein cholesterol, high very–low-density and low-density lipoprotein cholesterol, and elevated total triglycerides. High serum apolipoprotein concentrations have also been reported, as well as elevation of lipoprotein(a). These are all pathogenic markers of atherosclerosis and their correction should be part of the dietary management of these patients. The American Heart Association diet is usually recommended; it provides for 30% of total calories from fat, with saturated fat below 20% of total calories and cholesterol intake 300 mg or less. The polyunsaturated/saturated fat ratio in the normal American diet is 0.3 : 1. The provision of greater amounts of polyunsaturated fats can lower the plasma triglycerides and cholesterol concentration. Therefore, the advocated ratio is 1 : 1 or 1.5 : 1.

Sodium and Water

A normal sodium intake averages 100 to 300 mmol/day (2.5 to 7 g/day). In CAPD patients, the amount of dietary sodium depends on the amount lost in residual urinary output and peritoneal losses, and the state of hydration. A high sodium intake and dialysate sodium concentration plus certain psychogenic disorders will increase thirst and fluid intake. It is well recognized that CAPD patients are overhydrated (high pulmonary artery wedge pressures), especially those who have a hyperpermeable membrane. For these reasons, fluid restriction is wise and, in general, water intake should equal the urine output plus approximately 500 ml to replace insoluble and peritoneal dialysis losses over a 24-hour period. Patients who are hypertensive (mainly related to salt and water overload) require fluid and salt restriction, but most patients can have a sodium intake of about 2 to 3 g a day and a water intake of 750 to 1000 ml/day.

In patients who are anuric, it is usually not too difficult to remove up to 2 l of fluid per day by ultrafiltration, but frequent use of dialysis solutions containing a high concentration of dextrose is required, especially for patients with a hyperpermeable membrane. There is some concern about the excessive use of hypertonic dialysis solutions because in the long term, there may be damage to the peritoneal membrane integrity, inducing a hyperpermeable membrane. Such a change can also be related to increased glycosylation end products in the peritoneum and is exacerbated by peritonitis.

Potassium

Peritoneal dialysis patients usually do not become hyperkalemic because of increased fecal excretion of potassium. CAPD patients should be prescribed a dietary potassium intake of roughly 70 mmol/day, but hypokalemia may develop in some patients, especially if they are given diuretics or have a low protein intake.

Magnesium, Phosphorus, and Calcium

The requirements for these minerals depend on the dialysate concentration of magnesium and calcium, the state of bone disease and phosphate accumulation, the ingestion of oral phosphate-binding agents, and the use of vitamin D analogs.

Vitamins and Trace Elements

Dialysis patients are prone to deficiencies of water-soluble vitamins, and supplements are needed. Vitamin deficiencies are caused by a poor intake, interference with absorption by drugs, altered metabolism, and losses into the dialysate. Daily requirements of most vitamins are not clearly defined, but supplementation can prevent or correct vitamin deficiencies in CAPD patients.

Water-Soluble Vitamins

Vitamin C losses into the dialysate are substantial and a minimal oral daily intake of 60 mg of vitamin C is recommended. Pyridoxine, (vitamin B_6) is low in plasma and red blood cells, and a pyridoxine supplement of 10 mg/day improves lymphocyte function and, possibly, immune function; the supplement is recommended. Despite the water solubility of thiamin, riboflavin, pantothenic acid, and biotin, these vitamins are frequently found in the normal range in dialysis patients. The loss of these vitamins into the dialysate might be offset by reduced renal metabolism or urine losses. Therefore, the nutritional requirements for these vitamins are not well defined, but water-soluble supplements are safe and should be prescribed. Vitamin A is increased in the serum of dialysis patients and its supplementation is not recommended. Vitamin K deficiency is infrequent, and vitamin D administration is reviewed in Chapter 4.

Trace Elements

Dietary requirements for trace elements have not been well defined in maintenance peritoneal dialysis patients. Because of the pivotal role of the kidney in trace element excretion, they might accumulate. Also, trace elements are bound to serum protein, and small quantities of trace elements contained in the dialysate may be absorbed against a concentration gradient.

The extent of zinc deficiency in dialysis patients is a subject of debate, and the need for a supplement is not established. Some reports indicate that dysgeusia and, in men, impotence is improved by giving zinc supplements. These findings have not been confirmed, but dialysis patients should receive the recommended dietary allowance of zinc (i.e., 15 mg/day). There are dangers associated with excess vitamin and mineral ingestion, especially vitamin C, vitamin A, and vitamin D, and caution in their use is required.

TREATMENT OF MALNOURISHED PATIENTS ON PERITONEAL DIALYSIS

The presence of malnutrition (10% to 15% severe; 30% mild to moderate) in CAPD patients is usually suspected because of abnormal anthropometric indices, SGA, hypoalbuminemia, decreased creatinine production, and so forth. Part of the evaluation of mechanisms is to assess the reduction in food intake.

The Dietary History

This is an essential element of the assessment of the malnourished patient; it revises treatment options, some of which may be simple and easy to implement. A dietary history should include personal and ethnic food preferences, but if preferences interfere with food intake, the physician or dietitian should work with the patient to add more of the preferred foods to the diet. With severe malnutrition, most or all dietary limitations may have to be removed to encourage a greater calorie, protein, and nutrient intake. The role of the dietitian cannot be overemphasized.

Oral Supplements

Oral dietary supplements including Ensure, Isocal, Nephro, Replete, and Sustacal, can provide additional calories and protein for dialysis patients. The choice of a preparation is dictated by local availability, patient preference, palatability, presence or absence of lactose intolerance, and, importantly, cost. Other factors that need to be taken into account when choosing an oral supplement are the amounts of sodium, potassium, and phosphorous per gram of protein. These amounts may have an important bearing on the choice of the supplement depending on the patient's clinical status and the need for restricting these elements.

Oral Essential Amino Acids and Ketoacids

In malnourished patients, the evidence that essential amino acids are of value is sadly lacking. Part of the reason may be the unpalatability of some preparations, but the use of small amounts of oral essential amino acids may improve protein utilization and reduce the degree of catabolism.

Maneuvers That Aid Patients

1. Malnourished patients with loss of appetite may be helped by draining the peritoneal fluid just before meals so that the abdomen is empty at meal times.
2. They may also tolerate frequent, small meals better than the usual three large meals.
3. Peritoneal dialysis patients in general have fewer dietary restrictions than those treated with hemodialysis because CAPD patients are continuously dialyzed.
4. The concept that peritoneal dialysis patients can have ad libitum fluid intake is incorrect because it necessitates fluid removal with 3.86% glucose in the dialysis fluid. The ensuing increase in glucose absorption can cause hyperglycemia, which directly suppresses appetite. Avoidance of an excess fluid intake is therefore desirable and in the long run helps maintain the nutritional status.

Nasoantral Feeding

If the preceding regimens are unsuccessful for patients with severe anorexia, therapies based on enteral or parenteral supplementation are used. Overnight supplementation by a nasoantral feeding tube can lead to a sufficient improvement in nutritional status and overall well-being, in addition to helping a patient resume an oral diet. Patients with severe gastric problems (e.g., gastroparesis in diabetes) may be unable to tolerate any form of oral supplementation. Here, insertion of a gastrostomy tube through a percutaneous route (percutaneous endoscopic gastrostomy) is a viable option and can lead to an adequate diet. This is managed at home but must be initiated in the hospital setting. Total parenteral nutrition is necessary for those with persistent malnutrition but inability to take the supplements. This is a short-term undertaking to get the patient into a reasonable state before commencing oral/enteral therapy.

Amino Acid-Based Dialysis Fluids

Short-term studies have shown that dialysate solutions containing amino acids may reverse the daily losses of amino acids during dialysis with glucose-based solutions. A new, 1% amino acid solution containing increased buffers (lactate 35 mmol/l) and mainly essential amino acids in proportions designed to correct the amino acid abnormalities in uremic patients resulted in some improvements in the plasma amino acid pattern and nutritional parameters. Acidosis and increased serum urea level persisted. These experiences show that:

1. The altered amino acid composition of this solution was beneficial.
2. Patients included should have signs of protein malnutrition and low DPI to benefit from intraperitoneal amino acids.
3. Even more buffer is needed.
4. It is important that the energy intake is sufficient to prevent amino acids being used as an energy source.

An improved 1.1% amino acid solution with lactate (40 mmol/l) was tested in a metabolic balance study of 19 malnourished CAPD patients (protein intake 0.8 g protein/kg/day and energy intake of 25 to 30 cal/kg/day). The patients were treated with one exchange of this amino acid solution and three glucose-based dialysates. Treatment with the amino acid solution resulted in a positive nitrogen balance, a significant net increase in protein anabolism, an improved fasting plasma amino acid pattern, and significant increases in serum total protein and transferrin. Although this carefully conducted metabolic study over the course of a few weeks showed positive results, larger trials with this solution have not been as promising. For example, 134 malnourished peritoneal dialysis patients were randomized to receive either one or two exchanges of this amino acid solution or the usual dialysis solutions for a 3-month period. Overall, there was no significant difference in nutritional parameters measured in the amino acid group compared with the control group; subset analysis showed some improvement in nutritional parameters in the severely malnourished patients. Evidence from several French studies of amino acid dialysates also indicated that severely malnourished diabetic patients did not show any improvement in nutritional state as measured by transferrin, lean body mass, and albumin levels, whereas nondiabetic patients showed a marginal improvement.

In conclusion, amino acid solutions should be considered for malnourished patients, especially if attempts to increase the dose of dialysis or dietary intake fail. Although the evidence so far is not very striking or convincing, this regimen could be used for severely malnourished patients. In patients who suffer from severe peritonitis, intraperitoneal amino acid use may well be of some advantage.

Hormonal Treatment of Malnutrition in Peritoneal Dialysis Patients

The dramatic evolution of molecular biology and the advent of new biotechnological tools have resulted in the possibility of producing recombinant human hormones. These include:

1. Erythropoietin
2. Growth hormone and IGF
3. Anabolic steroids

Correction of Anemia With Recombinant Human Erythropoietin

Achieving this goal can improve nutritional status to a moderate degree in hemodialysis patients, but the results are less clear in CAPD patients. A positive effect was shown retrospectively in a small group of CAPD patients treated with erythropoietin (increased body weight and albumin, improvement in appetite and well-being).

Growth Hormone and Insulin-Like Growth Factors

Growth hormone has been used almost exclusively to promote normal or catch-up growth in children with chronic renal failure. There is no doubt that it has a markedly beneficial effect.

Regarding the use of growth hormone in adults, most studies have been in maintenance hemodialysis patients, and suffer because they are short term and have inconclusive results.

Patients who show the most improved nitrogen balance, the largest fall in predialysis serum urea nitrogen, and an increase in serum IGF-1 also have the highest nitrogen intake as well as low acute catabolic stress. Malnourished, stressed hemodialysis patients could benefit from the administration of recombinant IGF-1 because growth hormone does not promote protein anabolism in severely stressed, nonuremic patients. A few short-term studies of the effects of growth hormone in CAPD patients showed a net anabolic effect, with decreased serum urea levels, increased IGF-1 levels, and increased body weight and midarm muscle circumference. The role of growth hormone in dialysis patients is therefore still very much in the realm of experimentation.

Treatment of Malnourished CAPD
Patients With Recombinant Human IGF-1

Insulin-like growth factor-1 belongs to a group of serum proteins that are produced in the liver and exert insulin-like metabolic effects. A low serum level of IGF-1 is a good marker of malnutrition in dialysis patients. The rationale for administering IGF-1 is that some patients become resistant to the anabolic effects of growth hormone because of malnutrition or uremia, a response that is partly associated with a low IGF-1 response to growth hormone and reduced IGF-1 bioactivity in uremic serum. Malnourished CAPD patients treated for 35 days with IGF-1 had a positive nitrogen balance and a slight fall in serum phosphorus and calcium, but no significant changes in serum albumin, potassium, amino acids, or anthropometric values. These data indicate that IGF-1 may improve protein balance in stable but malnourished CAPD patients. The increased protein balance may be largely in the form of somatic protein because serum phosphorus decreased but serum albumin did not rise significantly during this study.

Potential Limitations of the Use of Growth Factors

Little is known about the short- and long-term benefits or adverse effects of growth hormone or IGF-1 administration in adult patients with renal failure. In adults, the anabolic effects of these hormones may be limited to short periods of time and useful only for the treatment of acute illnesses or transient states of catabolism or malnutrition. Moreover, it has not been shown that these agents reduce morbidity or improve the quality of life in adults with renal insufficiency, or under what circumstances these hormones may cause undesirable sequelae. IGF-1 has been implicated as a factor stimulating cancer growth, and these hormones may increase the risk of cancer, which is already high in patients with renal failure.

OTHER FACTORS AFFECTING NUTRITION

Drug Toxicity and Drug Treatment

Drugs that can impair appetite or make meals less palatable should be reduced or eliminated. In severe cases, the patient may benefit from temporary cessation of oral phosphate binders because these can cause nausea. Metoclopramide can be given but the dose must be reduced in patients with kidney failure because of toxicity.

Gastroparesis

Gastroparesis can contribute to decreased food intake by delaying gastric emptying, thereby increasing the feeling of fullness. Gastroparesis is common in diabetics, but can also occur in nondiabetics, and is diagnosed by measuring the rate of gastric emptying using radiology (barium meal) or radiolabeled test meal with simultaneous gastric scanning. If there is delayed gastric emptying, several therapeutic options are available:

1. Metoclopramide can be given, but the dose must be limited to avoid toxicity.
2. Patients with diabetes have been successfully treated with erythromycin for gastroparesis.
3. Those not responsive may respond to agents such as cisapride.

Dialysis Dose, Anorexia, and Nutritional Intake

To maintain an adequate nutritional intake, it seems logical that the patient should be receiving adequate dialysis (solute clearance), and raising the dialysis dose should always be considered. There is debate about the level of dialysis dose necessary to achieve an adequate protein and calorie intake. The amelioration of anorexia with an increase in appetite is characteristic of patients commencing CAPD, but attempts to quantify the relationship between small solute clearance and protein intake have predominantly focused on cross-sectional correlations between fractional urea clearance (Kt/V) and DPI estimated as the normalized protein catabolic rate (nPCR). Although there may be a physiologic relationship between these two parameters, the evidence points to the relationship being a mathematical artifact, and no credence can be put on relying on increasing dialysis to raise protein intake. A summary of five studies is given in Table 13-7. Two studies showed an increased protein intake and three did not, but most did not estimate protein intake from dietary history, and no study showed an increase in serum albumin. An important factor is that the increase in dialysate volume required to increase clearance was counterbalanced by a spontaneous, gradual decrease in residual renal function, so that there was no change in small solute clearance. The dialysis dose increase needs to be substantial to have an impact on nutrition; this level of solute clearance may not be attainable with standard CAPD.

SUMMARY AND CONCLUSION

A large proportion of peritoneal dialysis patients have signs of protein and calorie malnutrition due to various factors, including disturbances in protein and energy metabolism, hormonal derangements, infections, and other superimposed factors that lead to poor food intake; in addition, there are anorexia and nausea. Signs of malnutrition are correlated with clinical outcome among CAPD patients, although a slight decrease in serum albumin levels does not always seem to reflect impaired nutritional status or to be associated with increased morbidity and mortality in CAPD patients.

The safe protein requirement in CAPD patients appears to be at least 1 g/kg/day, although some patients are in neutral balance when the protein intake is as low as 0.8 g/kg/day. Nitrogen balance is strongly dependent on the energy intake, but it is often lower than the recommended 35 kcal/kg/day. It is important to monitor protein intake and nutritional status in CAPD patients, but success in improving the diet when malnutrition is present is rare. Anorexia with low protein and energy intake may result from a variety of factors, of which underdialysis may be one. Evidence that increasing the dialysis dose improves nutritional status is not available.

Nevertheless, malnutrition is associated with high morbidity and mortality. Improvement must be sought in an attempt to better the quality of life and duration of survival in these patients.

SELECTED READINGS

Avram MM, Goldwasser P, Erroa M, et al. Predictors of survival in continuous ambulatory peritoneal dialysis patients: the importance of prealbumin and other nutritional and metabolic markers. *Am J Kidney Dis* 1994;23:91–98.

Bergstrom J. Why are dialysis patients malnourished? *Am J Kidney Dis* 1995;26:229–241.

Bergstrom J, Furst P, Alvestrand A, et al. Protein and energy intake, nitrogen balance and nitrogen losses in patients treated with continuous ambulatory peritoneal dialysis. *Kidney Int* 1993;44: 1048–1057.

Blake PG, Flowerdew G, Blake RM, et al. Serum albumin in patients on continuous ambulatory peritoneal dialysis: predictors and correlation with outcome. *J Am Soc Nephrol* 1993;3:1501–1507.

Blake PG, Oreopoulos DG. Answers to all your questions about peritoneal urea clearance and nutrition in CAPD patients. *Perit Dial Int* 1996;16:248–251.

CANUSA Peritoneal Dialysis Study Group. Adequacy of dialysis and nutrition in continuous peritoneal dialysis: association with clinical outcomes. *J Am Soc Nephrol* 1996;7:198–207.

Cianciaruso B, Brunor G, Kopple JD, et al. Cross-sectional comparison of malnutrition in continuous ambulatory peritoneal dialysis and haemodialysis patients. *Am J Kidney Dis* 1995;26:475–486.

Davies SJ, Russell L, Bryan J, et al. Co-morbidity, urea kinetics, and appetite in continuous ambulatory peritoneal dialysis: their interrelationship and prediction of survival. *Am J Kidney Dis* 1995;26: 353–361.

Enia G, Sicuso C, Alati G, et al. Subjective global assessment of nutrition in dialysis patients. *Nephrol Dial Transplant* 1993;8: 1094–1098.

Faller B, Aparicio M, Faict D. Clinical evaluation of an optimised 1.1% amino acid solution for peritoneal dialysis. *Nephrol Dial Transplant* 1995;10:1432–1437.

Fenton SA, Johnson N, Delamore T, et al. Nutritional assessment of CAPD patients. *Trans Am Soc Artif Intern Organs* 1987;33: 650–653.

Harty J, Conway L, Keegan M, et al. Energy metabolism during CAPD: a controlled study. *Adv Perit Dial* 1995;11:229–233.

Harty J, Gokal R. Nutritional status in peritoneal dialysis. *Journal of Renal Nutrition* 1995;5:2–10.

Harty JC, Boulton H, Curwell J, et al. The normalised protein catabolic rate is a flawed marker of nutrition in CAPD patients. *Kidney Int* 1994;45:103–109.

Harty JC, Boulton H, Uttley L, et al. Limitations of urea kinetic modelling as predictors of nutritional and dialysis adequacy in CAPD. *Am J Nephrol* 1993;13:454–463.

Heide B, Pierratos A, Khanna R, et al. Nutritional status of patients undergoing CAPD. *Peritoneal Dialysis Bulletin* 1983;5:138–141.

Heimburger O, Traneaus A, Bergstrom J, et al. The effect of increasing peritoneal dialysis on Kt/V, protein catabolic rate and serum albumin. *Perit Dial Int* 1992;12(Suppl 1):S19.

Ikizler TA, Greene JH, Wingard RL, et al. Spontaneous dietary protein intake during progression of chronic renal failure. *J Am Soc Nephrol* 1995;6:1386–1391.

Jones MR. Etiology of severe malnutrition: results of an international cross-sectional study in continuous ambulatory peritoneal dialysis patients. *Am J Kidney Dis* 1994;23:412–420.

Kopple JD, Bernard D, Messana J. Treatment of malnourished CAPD patients with an amino-acid based dialysate. *Kidney Int* 1995;47:1148–1157.

Kopple JD, Blumenkrantz MJ. Nutritional requirements for patients undergoing continuous ambulatory peritoneal dialysis. *Kidney Int* 1983;24(Suppl 16):S295–S302.

Lindsay RM, Spanner E. A hypothesis: the protein catabolic rate is dependent upon the type and treatment in dialyzed uraemic patients. *Am J Kidney Dis* 1989;13:382–389.

Malhotra D, Tzamaloukas AH, Murata GH, et al. Serum albumin in continuous peritoneal dialysis: its predictors and relationship to urea clearance. *Kidney Int* 1996;50:243–249.

Markman P. Nutritional status of patients on hemodialysis and CAPD. *Clin Nephrol* 1988;29:75–78.

McCusker FX, Teehan BP, Thorpe KE, et al. How much peritoneal dialysis for the maintenance of a good nutritional state? *Kidney Int* 1996;50(Suppl 56):S56–S61.

Nelson E, Hong C, Pesce A, et al. Anthropometric norms for dialysis populations. *Am J Kidney Dis* 1990;16:32–37.

Pollock CA, Ibels LS, Allen BJ, et al. Total body nitrogen as a prognostic marker in maintenance dialysis. *J Am Soc Nephrol* 1995;6:82–88.

Struijk DG, Krediet RT, Koomen GCM, et al. The effect of serum albumin at the start of CAPD on patient survival. *Perit Dial Int* 1994;14:121–126.

Tzamaloukas AH, Malhotra D, Murata GH, et al. Increasing the dose of CAPD on serum albumin. *Perit Dial Int* 1995;15(Suppl 4):S31.

Williams P, Jones J, Marriott J. Do increases in dialysis dose in CAPD lead to nutritional improvement? *Nephrol Dial Transplant* 1994;9:1841–1842.

Young GA, Kopple JD, Lindholm B, et al. Nutritional assessment of CAPD patients: an international study. *Am J Kidney Dis* 1991;27:462–471.

Nutritional Requirements of Renal Transplant Patients

J. Andrew Bertolatus
and Lawrence G. Hunsicker

Successful transplantation of a kidney into a patient with renal failure restores near-normal renal function and is expected to correct the nutritional abnormalities arising from renal insufficiency. In the minds of both patients and physicians, one of the major benefits of renal transplantation is an end to the dietary restrictions required for therapy during periods of progressive renal failure and dialysis. Typically, renal transplant recipients experience an improvement in general sense of well-being along with a marked improvement in appetite and increase in dry body weight. These patients nevertheless face many nutritional challenges because of the metabolic complications of preexisting medical conditions and as a consequence of transplant-related immunosuppression.

The implications of proper nutritional therapy of the transplant recipient are far-reaching. Immunosuppressive therapies used to maintain the renal allograft, especially glucocorticoids, cyclosporine, and tacrolimus, are associated with metabolic side effects, including protein hypercatabolism, obesity, hyperlipidemia, glucose intolerance, hypertension, hyperkalemia, and interference with the metabolism and action of vitamin D. These metabolic effects of immunosuppression tend to interact with the aspects of nutrition and metabolism most likely to have affected patients during the period of renal failure: protein depletion, hyperlipidemia, hypertension, calcium malabsorption, and hyperparathyroidism. Many of these factors contribute to accelerated atherosclerosis and consequent cardiovascular disease, the major cause of death among renal transplant recipients. Some have postulated that the fate of the graft itself may be affected by the amount of dietary protein by virtue of the glomerular hyperfiltration response, or by the degree of hyperlipidemia. For these reasons, careful attention to the nutritional and metabolic state of the renal transplant is warranted. Because metabolic problems tend to occur early after transplantation, a nutritional plan should be formulated at the time of transplantation and the patient should be introduced to this plan in the immediate posttransplantation period. The plan should consider the following elements: protein intake in the immediate posttransplantation period and during long-term therapy; maintenance of appropriate weight for height; dietary lipid composition; and calcium, phosphate, and vitamin D intake. Patients with preexisting diabetes need continued attention to carbohydrate metabolism, as will those in whom steroid-induced diabetes develops after transplantation. Finally, some patients may need iron supplementation, sodium or potassium restriction, or supplementation with water-soluble vitamins.

294

PROTEIN METABOLISM

Posttransplantation Period

One of the principal metabolic effects of glucocorticoid hormones is to increase hepatic gluconeogenesis associated with increased catabolism of amino acids and proteins. Thus, it is not surprising that the large doses of steroids used early in the posttransplantation period, together with the stresses of surgery, are associated with evidence of markedly increased protein catabolism. Protein hypercatabolism is further increased when rejection episodes are treated with high-dose intravenous methylprednisolone. As described elsewhere in this volume, patients with chronic renal insufficiency who present for transplantation may already have preexisting protein malnutrition, especially if they are diabetic. Although it is remarkable how benign the clinical course of such patients is after transplant surgery, excess protein catabolism combined with preexisting protein depletion may add substantially to problems such as poor wound healing and susceptibility to infection. These problems are likely to be exaggerated in patients in whom there is delayed onset of function of the transplanted kidney and in whom continued dialysis may be needed early in the posttransplantation course.

Fortunately, several investigators have shown convincingly that it is possible to prevent negative nitrogen balance during the immediate posttransplantation period simply by increasing dietary protein. Their studies have shown that steroid therapy increases the protein catabolic and urea appearance rates to a degree dependent on the total corticosteroid dose but independent of the dietary protein intake, such that patients receiving less than 1 g of dietary protein/kg/day invariably are in negative nitrogen balance. An isocaloric increase in dietary protein does not result in a significant increase in the protein catabolic rate. Rather, as illustrated in Fig. 14-1, increases in dietary protein restore nitrogen balance. There is a consensus among these investigators that neutral (or zero) net nitrogen balance occurs in patients treated with typical posttransplantation doses of steroid when daily protein intake is 1.3 to 1.5 g/kg. Given the protein depletion seen in many pretransplantation patients and the frequent need for pulse steroid therapy for rejection episodes, it would seem prudent to prescribe a protein intake at the upper end of this range. Higher levels are unlikely to be acceptable to patients accustomed to protein-restricted diets.

The diet must also contain adequate calories to ensure that the dietary protein is used for anabolism; in general, an intake of 30 to 35 kcal/kg/day is prescribed for the first several weeks after transplantation. This dietary approach may not complicate the clinical course of the patient with delayed graft function; the higher protein intake should not increase the protein catabolic rate or the urea appearance rate further, so there should be no increased need for dialysis. Finally, it is possible that a relatively high protein intake in the weeks after transplantation may minimize some of the steroid-induced side effects other than muscle wasting. Whittier and colleagues found that patients on a high-protein, low-carbohydrate diet had only a mild cushingoid appearance 4 weeks after trans-

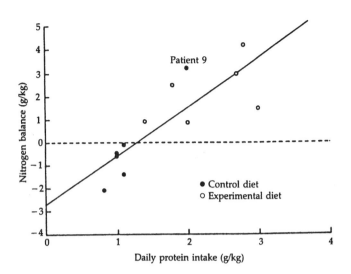

Fig. 14-1. Relationship of nitrogen balance to daily protein intake. Patients on the control diet were told to eat 1.0 g/kg protein daily, but patient 9 actually consumed 2.0 g/kg daily. Those on the experimental diet were told to eat 3.0 g/kg protein daily, but actual intake ranged from 1.4 to 3.0 g/kg daily. There is a direct relationship between protein intake and nitrogen balance (r = 0.83, P < 0.01), with zero nitrogen balance at an intake of approximately 1.3 g/kg daily. (From Whittier FC, Evans DH, Dutton S. Nutrition in renal transplantation. *Am J Kidney Dis* 1985;6:405–411.)

plantation, whereas patients on lower protein intakes had moderate to severe cushingoid changes.

Maintenance Prescription for Dietary Protein

Although a high-protein intake is clearly indicated early in the posttransplantation course (and probably during any subsequent therapy for acute rejection), the optimal dietary prescription is less well established for renal transplant patients being treated with maintenance immunosuppression. This uncertainty results from the conflicting goals of optimizing protein nutrition and, at the same time, optimizing long-term renal function.

The argument for maintaining a relatively generous dietary protein intake during long-term therapy after successful renal transplantation rests on the evidence that there is a continued increase in protein catabolism even in patients receiving glucocorticoids at relatively low maintenance dosages (equivalent to 0.15 to 0.20 mg prednisone/kg/day). That steroids continue to cause protein wasting in these patients is evidenced by the high frequency of steroid-induced side effects seen in long-term transplant recipients, including truncal obesity with wasting of the musculature of the extremities, fragile and atrophied skin, and delayed wound healing.

The extent of muscle wasting in these patients has been documented by several authors. Miller and colleagues studied 24 diabetic and 21 nondiabetic patients for approximately 2 years after successful renal transplantation. All had adequate renal function at the time of final study (creatinine < 2.5 mg/dl in 42 of the patients and < 3.6 mg/dl in the other 3). All had been eating a diet containing 1.0 g protein/kg and 25 to 35 kcal/kg/day. All were clinically stable while taking an average dose of 16.6 mg prednisone per day. Despite an increase in body weight to normal, overcorrection of cutaneous fat (the triceps skinfold thickness in 14% exceeded the 95th percentile of normal control values), and correction of any low values of serum albumin and transferrin, many of these patients continued to show evidence of reduced muscle mass. Half of the diabetic patients and one fourth of the nondiabetic patients had midarm muscle circumferences that were less than the fifth percentile of normal control subjects.

Similarly, Horber and associates studied nine clinically stable renal transplant patients at least 6 months after transplantation at a time when their average serum creatinine level was 1.46 mg/dl and their dose of prednisone was 9.6 mg/day. All had been fully rehabilitated and had returned to work or full activities, and none had any known musculoskeletal disease or neuropathy. Compared with matched normal subjects, these patients had 20% less midthigh muscle area and 36% more midthigh fat as measured quantitatively by computed tomography. The reduction in midthigh muscle area correlated with a reduction in the peak torque and total work output from these muscles. Biopsy specimens of the thigh muscles of these patients showed a reduction in cross-sectional area of all three types of muscle fiber and an increased muscle cell lipid content compared with control subjects. Thus, even patients with excellent renal transplant function and excellent rehabilitation exhibit evidence of significantly reduced muscle mass. Horber and coworkers showed that this muscle atrophy and weakness could be reversed by physical training, at least in those patients receiving < 0.20 mg prednisone/kg/day. Unfortunately, these authors did not report the amount of protein eaten by their patients, who appear to have been on unregulated diets. It remains uncertain, but likely, that dietary intakes above 1.0 g protein/kg/day together with exercise might minimize muscle wasting and possibly the other evidences of protein depletion.

The argument to restrict protein stems from the hypothesis that excess protein intake induces a hyperfiltration injury through mechanisms analogous to those suggested for other patients with reduced renal function. Indirect evidence to support this hypothesis is based on observations that transplant recipients who would be expected to have more hyperfiltration in the glomeruli of their allografts, such as large people receiving kidneys from small donors, have poorer graft survival. Feehally and coworkers carried out a more direct investigation of the hyperfiltration hypothesis in five renal transplant recipients exhibiting well established progressive renal insufficiency and with renal biopsy specimens showing the typical findings of chronic rejection. The dietary protein of these patients was reduced to 0.6 g/kg/day, and immunosuppressive therapy, including the dose of prednisone, was not changed. Four of the five patients had a distinct change in the slope of reciprocal serum creatinine (1/serum creatinine) values, with stabilization of their previously declining renal function (Fig. 14-2). The diet appears to have been well tolerated by the patients, whose weight remained stable after a small initial drop and whose midarm muscle circumference did not change. However, the follow-up was short, averaging 6 months, and three of the five patients progressed to renal failure during this time. These measures may not have been sufficiently sensitive to permit detection of early protein malnutrition. It should also be noted that stabilization of serum creatinine in Feehally and colleagues' patients might have resulted from a decrease in endogenous creatinine synthesis caused by progressive muscle wasting or from a decreased endogenous creatinine intake, rather than from preservation of renal function (see Chapter 10).

Two short-term studies assessed the feasibility and nutritional consequences of a 0.55- to 0.6-g/kg protein diet on transplant recipients on stable immunosuppressive regimens. Both used assessment of glomerular filtration rate (GFR) by inulin clearance and assessment of nitrogen balance, as well as determinations of lymphocyte counts and serum protein, albumin, transferrin, and prealbumin concentrations to assess adequacy of

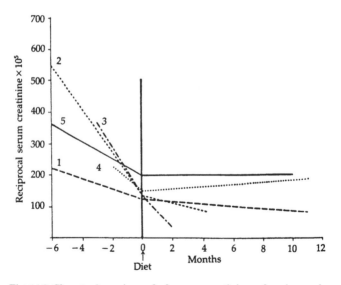

Fig. 14-2. Changes in reciprocal of serum creatinine values in renal transplant recipients with chronic graft rejection on introduction of dietary protein restriction to 0.6 g/kg/day. Four of five patients had a significant change in the slope of the reciprocal creatinine clearance. This may reflect either a slowing in the progression of renal failure or a reduction in creatinine excretion, possibly from reduction of dietary creatinine intake or loss of muscle mass. (From Feehally J, Harris KP, Bennett SE, et al. Is chronic renal transplant rejection a non-immunological phenomenon? *Lancet* 1986;2:486–488.)

nutrition. Windus and colleagues studied eight of their most compliant transplant recipients over a 4-week period out of the hospital while they were on a 0.6-g/kg protein diet. Their patients were noted to have negative nitrogen balances during baseline, with a statistically insignificant trend toward worsening during the study diet. Despite these observations, the authors noted no worsening of total lymphocyte count or serum protein levels suggestive of malnutrition. They found no correlation of nitrogen balance with protein intake, but did note a significant positive correlation with caloric intake. They demonstrated neutral nitrogen balance in all patients eating > 25 kcal/kg/day. These authors concluded that although neutral nitrogen balance could be achieved in this population with a protein intake of 0.6 g/kg/day, these most compliant patients had great difficulty maintaining sufficient caloric intake necessary to achieve balance, even over the short 4-week observation period.

Salahudeen and associates studied 14 transplant recipients with biopsy-documented chronic rejection over an 11-day period during which they received a 0.55-g/kg protein, 35-kcal/day diet in a clinical research center setting. They reported neutral nitrogen balance during the study period, but significant reductions in serum protein, albumin, and transferrin concentrations after this dietary manipulation. There was no significant change in blood pressure or GFR, but there was a significant reduction in proteinuria. These investigators later reported that the subjects on the low-protein diet also had reduced activity of the renin–angiotensin system, which could be important in reducing glomerular hyperfiltration and hypertrophy, thereby preserving renal function. They concluded that a low-protein diet may be beneficial, although these patients may require a higher minimum protein intake to maintain nutritional balance.

It is clear that additional studies of protein metabolism are needed in transplant patients before therapeutic decisions can be rendered from established and accepted fact rather than from hypothesis and opinion. In the interim, a defensible approach for most patients is to prescribe a diet containing about 1.0 g/kg/day of protein and to encourage regular exercise as a way to avoid muscle wasting. Patients with progressive graft failure may be considered for a more restricted protein intake (0.6 g/kg/day), but only if the caloric intake can be maintained above 25 kcal/kg/day and the prednisone dose does not exceed 0.2 mg/kg. Such patients should be monitored closely for any evidence of protein wasting.

OBESITY

Obesity is a major problem in the transplant recipient population. Several reports provide an overview of the problem. Approximately 15% to 20% of recipients meet some definition of obesity at the time of transplantation. By 1 year after transplantation, approximately 60% of recipients have gains in weight of 10% or more, and the percentage who are overweight more than doubles, to 43% in one study. Women, and African Americans of either gender, have higher weight gains. Although obesity may not be a risk factor for short-term posttransplantation complications, it is clearly a risk factor for chronic graft loss (Fig. 14-3). Potential mechanisms for the negative effect of obe-

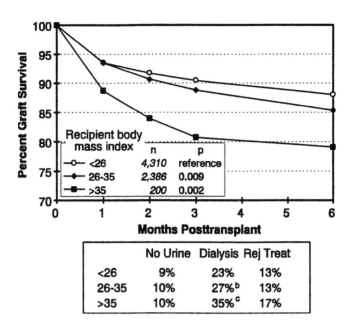

Fig. 14-3. Effect of recipient body mass index on graft survival. Recipients with body mass index (weight in kg/[height in cm]²) > 26 had significantly reduced graft survival, with the effect being particularly large for those with body mass index > 36. The larger people also had a greater need for dialysis in the posttransplantation period. (From Cho YW, Terasaki PI, Cecka JM. New variables reported to the UNOS Registry and their impact on cadaveric renal transplant outcomes: a preliminary study. In: Cecka JM, Terasaki PI, eds. *Clinical transplants 1995.* Los Angeles: UCLA Tissue Typing Laboratory; 1996:405–415.)

sity include a greater chance for mismatches in recipient and donor size, and hence for nephron underdosing and hyperfiltration; underdosing or perhaps impaired bioavailability of immunosuppressive agents; or the effect of hyperlipidemia in promoting chronic graft dysfunction. Importantly, in one study only those patients experiencing weight gain over the first year posttransplantation had significant increases in cholesterol and triglycerides. Recipients who did not gain weight did not show worsened serum lipid status, indicating that control of body weight through a combination of diet and exercise is critical in this patient population.

HYPERLIPIDEMIA

As the success rate of transplantation has improved, and the number of life-threatening infections has decreased, atherosclerotic cardiovascular disease has emerged as the most significant health risk and most common cause of death among transplant recipients. A multitude of factors contribute to posttransplantation atherosclerosis: a history of nephrotic syndrome with hyperlipidemia and hypertension induced by the underlying renal disease, the effects of altered lipid metabolism during the dialysis period, and the metabolic effects of immunosuppressive therapy with glucocorticoids and calcineurin inhibitors (cyclosporine or tacrolimus). The prevalence of hyperlipidemia after renal transplantation has been variably reported to be between 16% and 60%. Some of this variability may be related to different patient populations and different immunosuppressive protocols, but much of the variability remains unexplained. Unlike chronic renal failure and dialysis patients, who more frequently have isolated hypertriglyceridemia, transplant recipients are more likely to have hypercholesterolemia, either isolated or associated with hypertriglyceridemia. In fact, hypertriglyceridemia improves shortly after transplantation, only to be replaced by an increase in cholesterol. The rise in cholesterol is associated with a rise in low-density lipoprotein (LDL) cholesterol as well as a rise in high-density lipoprotein (HDL) cholesterol from very low levels toward normal. Ettinger and coworkers reported that whereas total HDL was increased, the HDL_2 subfraction, which is believed to be cardioprotective, remained low.

Two longitudinal studies involving large numbers of similarly treated patients best highlight the natural history of hyperlipidemia. Of 201 patients treated between 1976 and 1983, Kasiske and Umen observed hypertriglyceridemia in 36% before transplantation and 23% and 29% at 1 and 5 years, respectively, after transplantation. They found hypercholesterolemia in 8% of patients before transplantation and in 27% and 30% at 1 and 5 years after transplantation. These patients received an immunosuppressive regimen including splenectomy, azathioprine (2.5 mg/kg/day), and prednisone (15 mg/day to 15 mg on alternate days). The average serum cholesterol level increased nearly 25% from about 200 to over 250 mg/dl. Similar findings were reported by Vathsala and colleagues among 500 patients treated either with cyclosporine and prednisone or with azathioprine and prednisone. They found no significant differences in the severity of hypercholesterolemia between cyclosporine–prednisone- and azathioprine–prednisone-treated patient groups. Multivariate analyses in these and other studies demonstrated that each of the following was independently correlated with serum cholesterol: age, diabetes, pretransplantation lipid levels, cumulative prednisone dose, serum creatinine, the amount of urine protein excretion, and obesity.

Clearly, the most significant factors contributing to posttransplantation hypercholesterolemia are the immunosuppressive agents used, prednisone and cyclosporine. The mechanisms by which prednisone exerts its hypercholesterolemic effects are becoming clarified. Krausz and associates demonstrated in rats that there is a glucocorticoid-dependent rise in hepatic synthesis of cholesterol and of the components of very–low-density lipoprotein and HDL. These changes were related to the marked hyperinsulinemia caused by peripheral insulin resistance, whereas hepatic responsiveness to insulin was unaffected. In addition, the activity of adipose tissue lipoprotein lipase, an enzyme whose synthesis is stimulated by insulin, was decreased. Chan and colleagues studied the clearance of intravenously infused fat emulsions in 19 stable renal transplant recipients approximately 3 years after successful transplantation; their serum creatinine levels averaged 1.7 mg/dl. These investigators found that the fractional clearance of lipids in these patients was significantly and substantially reduced compared with that of normal control subjects. The increase in plasma lipids was directly correlated with the increase in plasma insulin levels, which in turn were inversely correlated with the fractional lipid clearance rates. They also found suggestive evidence for increased hepatic synthesis of lipoproteins. Taken together, these and other supporting studies indicate that the underlying cause of hyperlipidemia after glucocorticoid therapy is insulin resistance in peripheral tissues with impaired synthesis of lipoprotein lipase, together with persistent responsiveness of the liver to the elevated plasma insulin levels, leading to enhanced lipoprotein synthesis.

Although the hyperlipidemic effects of glucocorticoids have been well described and investigated, the hyperlipidemic effects of cyclosporine and the magnitude of these effects remain controversial. Ellis and coworkers noted increased LDL cholesterol and triglyceride levels in 21 psoriasis patients treated with cyclosporine monotherapy for 4 weeks, followed by return to baseline levels within 2 weeks. In 35 renal transplant recipients receiving cyclosporine and azathioprine after successful withdrawal from prednisone, Hricik and associates demonstrated that serum cholesterol improved modestly but remained significantly elevated above normal and pretransplantation levels. Several investigators have reported improvement in lipid abnormalities among transplant patients treated with cyclosporine and prednisone on conversion to an azathioprine–prednisone regimen. However, Vathsala and colleagues reported similar elevations of cholesterol and triglycerides among 566 patients treated either with cyclosporine and prednisone or azathioprine and prednisone, and found a negative correlation between cyclosporine dose and serum cholesterol levels. Little is known about the etiology of hypercholesterolemia associated with cyclosporine. It has been postulated that cyclosporine may interfere with the feedback mechanism that regulates LDL cholesterol synthesis by altering the binding kinetics of LDL and its receptor. Princen and colleagues reported that cyclosporine inhibits 26-hydroxylase and postulated that hypercholesterolemia could ensue by inhibition of the synthesis of bile acids from cholesterol. Finally, Derfler and coworkers noted decreased hepatic lipase and lipoprotein lipase activity in hyperlipidemic transplant recipients. This could decrease the conversion of very–low-density lipoprotein to intermediate-density lipoprotein and LDL.

The newer calcineurin inhibitor, tacrolimus (FK506), is now available as an alternative to cyclosporine. Most of the clinical experience with this drug has been in liver transplant recipients, who experience less weight gain and less marked elevations in serum cholesterol when on a tacrolimus-based regimen compared with cyclosporine-based immunosuppression. Preliminary results from a randomized trial comparing tacrolimus and cyclosporine in kidney recipients also suggest a lessened hyperlipidemic effect with use of the newer agent.

It is likely that dietary factors contribute to posttransplantation hyperlipidemia. Disler and colleagues found that before institution of intensive diet therapy, 21 renal transplant recipients with hyperlipidemia averaged 129% of ideal body weight; the major weight gain occurred during the first 6 months after transplantation. They noted, however, that compared with the average diet of the surrounding community, the hyperlipidemic transplant patients ate a diet lower in cholesterol content and with a higher polyunsaturated/saturated fat ratio. Moore and colleagues noted that before dietary intervention, 12 of 17 patients had a cholesterol intake greater than 250 mg/day. Few reports have examined the effectiveness of diet therapy in controlling posttransplantation hypercholesterolemia, and unfortunately none has investigated the long-term efficacy of dietary manipulations in this population. Disler and colleagues studied the effects of a 1-year weight reduction diet featuring no more than 300 mg of cholesterol daily, elimination of simple sugars, and the addition of 30 ml of sunflower seed oil to increase polyunsaturated fat intake. They reported a modest weight loss from 129% ideal body weight to 121%, and a significant fall in cholesterol from 356 to 294 mg/dl. Shen and associates studied the effects of a weight reduction diet composed of < 500 mg/dl cholesterol, < 35% calories from fat, < 50% from carbohydrate, a polyunsaturated/saturated fat ratio of > 1.0, and a limited alcohol consumption, on 12 posttransplantation patients over a 3-month period. They noted an average weight loss of 1.3 kg, and a modest reduction in cholesterol from 313 to 248 mg/dl. They noted, however, that dietary treatment was considered undesirable by 48% of their patient population and that of those who agreed to participate in dietary manipulation, none was totally compliant. Most recently, Moore and colleagues studied the effect of the American Heart Association (AHA) Step One diet over an 8-week period on 17 stable posttransplantation patients with hyperlipidemia. They reported that most members of their study population were able to adhere to the diet and lower their weight, leading to a modest reduction in serum cholesterol from 262 to 241 mg/dl. However, they noted no decrease in LDL cholesterol and suggested that long-term compliance with this diet would likely diminish with time, and that the altered lipid metabolism of transplantation may render dietary therapy alone ineffective. A Scandinavian study reached similar conclusions.

The long-term control of hyperlipidemia after renal transplantation depends on some dietary intervention, whether this is effective alone or requires the addition of pharmacotherapy. Because obesity is an important contributor to hyperlipidemia in transplant patients, and because the greatest weight gain in this population is within the first 6 months, it is important for transplant recipients to receive intensive calorie and cholesterol counseling before and immediately after transplantation. We believe that the AHA Step One diet is a reasonable initial approach for transplant patients. This diet, consisting of < 300 mg of cholesterol per day (with a goal of < 250 mg/day), 30% total calories as fat, 50% as carbohydrate, and 20% as protein, is an easily attainable diet and familiar to nutritionists. Unfortunately, a recent survey of renal transplant diet recommendations reported that fully 64% of renal dietitians were not restricting cholesterol after transplantation, and that polyunsaturated/saturated fat ratios were not being followed by 56%.

GLUCOSE METABOLISM

An increasing fraction of patients presenting for renal transplantation, currently about 25%, have renal failure resulting from diabetes mellitus, either type I or type II. The posttransplantation nutritional care of these patients is considerably complicated by diabetes, and the treatment of diabetes is complicated by the insulin resistance induced by steroid therapy. Nutritional deficits tend to be more severe in diabetic patients with chronic renal failure. Because the nutritional problems of diabetics with nephropathy are discussed in Chapter 8, treatment of these patients is not discussed further here. However, the nutritional as well as the other aspects of the medical care of these patients occupy a disproportionate share of the time physicians and dietitians spend caring for transplant recipients.

In addition to the patients who come to transplantation with diabetes, there are a large number of patients in whom clinical diabetes develops as a result of immunosuppressive therapy with glucocorticoids and calcineurin inhibitors (cyclosporine or tacrolimus). Perhaps not surprisingly, even transplant recipients with overtly normal glucose tolerance have evidence of insulin resistance when studied by the insulin clamp technique. The development of clinical diabetes appears to occur when relative insulin deficiency develops, such that insulin production is inadequate, relative to the degree of insulin resistance. There is some evidence that posttransplantation diabetes is more common with tacrolimus-based immunosuppression, although one randomized study in liver recipients suggested that this is not always the case. Others have argued that even if tacrolimus is more diabetogenic in the first few months after transplantation, the effects of tacrolimus on glucose metabolism are dose related, such that with proper dose adjustment the long-term rate of diabetes need not be higher than what is observed in cyclosporine-treated patients.

In one of the larger reported surveys, Friedman and colleagues found that clinical diabetes developed in 15.7% of previously nondiabetic recipients after transplantation; diabetes was defined as three consecutive, fasting blood glucose values greater than 150 mg/dl. More than half became diabetic within 3 weeks of starting steroid therapy. Other factors were clearly important, however, because the average steroid dose of the recipients who became diabetic was actually less than that of a matched group of recipients whose blood glucose values remained normal. The diabetic patients and nondiabetic control patients had similar body weights, a similar male/female ratio, similar serum creatinine values, and a similar incidence of diabetes in family members. The only significant difference between the two groups was that the diabetic group had a higher proportion of African Americans. In just over 50% of the patients in whom diabetes developed, no specific therapy was needed. The other half of the group required dietary therapy and either an oral hypoglycemic agent or insulin. With time and lowering of the dose of prednisone, steroid-induced diabetes tended to improve. Only 33% of patients still had clinical diabetes after 6 months, and only 28% after 1 year. Despite this apparently benign course, the 2-year survival rate of patients in whom posttransplantation diabetes developed was significantly lower than that of other patients (diabetics 67%; control patients 83%; $P < 0.05$), primarily because of more frequent and severe infections. Thus, posttransplantation diabetes remains a major metabolic problem.

METABOLISM OF CALCIUM, PHOSPHORUS, AND VITAMIN D

Metabolic bone disease, including osteonecrosis and osteopenia, remains a major source of morbidity and mortality after successful renal transplantation. The incidence of osteonecrosis after renal transplantation has been variably reported to be from 3.5% to 5.0% to almost 30%. Much of the variability depends on different methods for identifying cases, differences in the transplant populations, and varying immunosuppressive regimens. Julian and coworkers reported on the continuing problems of vertebral osteopenia in renal transplantation, related primarily to steroid therapy. The metabolism of calcium, phosphorus, and vitamin D in renal transplant recipients is determined by a complex interplay of factors resulting from the patients' previous period of renal insufficiency, from the immunosuppressive therapy, and from incomplete restoration of normal renal function by the transplant (Table 14-1). In addition, observations suggest that in some people there may be a genetic susceptibility to increased bone loss after transplantation, based on polymorphisms in the vitamin D receptor. Although all recipients (regardless of receptor genotype) lost bone density to the same degree in the first 3 months after transplantation, those with the favorable genotype showed significantly better recovery of bone density at the end of the first posttransplantation year. Perhaps, in the future, pretransplantation testing for receptor genotype will identify those people with the highest risk for bone loss, and therefore the greatest need for monitoring and intervention.

Table 14-1. Factors affecting mineral metabolism in renal transplant recipients

Residua of previous renal insufficiency
  Hyperplastic, poorly suppressible parathyroid glands with hyperparathyroidism
  Preexisting parathyroid bone disease or osteomalacia with depletion of bone mineral
Effects of glucocorticoid immunosuppressive therapy
  Inhibition of osteoblast division, maturation, and function
  Inhibition of calcitriol-dependent absorption of calcium and phosphorus by the gut
  Increased urinary excretion of calcium and phosphorus
Effects of incomplete restoration of normal renal function
  Persistent hyperparathyroidism related to reduced glomerular filtration rate
  Parathyroid hormone-independent renal leak of phosphate
Other factors
  Vitamin D receptor genotype

Preexisting Hyperparathyroidism and Osteopenia

Factors leading to metabolic bone disease in the preuremic and dialysis patient have been reviewed in Chapter 4. Many patients have marked hyperparathyroidism, aluminum overload, or both; significant osteopenia is often present. The restoration of near-normal renal mass after transplantation immediately leads to correction or overcorrection of phosphate excretion, and to a restoration of vitamin D metabolism to produce its active form, calcitriol. These changes, as well as steroid-induced bone resorption, lead to an increase in serum calcium to normal or elevated levels. Although the expected effect of these changes on parathyroid gland function should be its complete suppression, this does not usually occur. Gonzalez and associates reported that immunoreactive parathyroid hormone levels remained elevated in 22 of 47 prospectively studied transplant patients with stable renal function, and necessitated parathyroidectomy in 8 more. Similarly, Cotorruelo and coworkers reported that 11 of 22 patients with pretransplantation hyperparathyroidism maintained elevated hormone levels at 1 year. The persistent inappropriate secretion of parathyroid hormone is widely believed to be secondary to some degree of functional autonomy of the gland, either because of the large size of the gland from years of chronic stimulation, or, rarely, because of the development of a parathyroid adenoma. Others argued that steroid use also participates in a maladaptive oversecretion of parathyroid hormone. The consequences of posttransplantation hyperparathyroidism are hypercalcemia, hypophosphatemia, and hyperphosphaturia, with persistent bone resorption and consequent osteopenia. It has been shown that

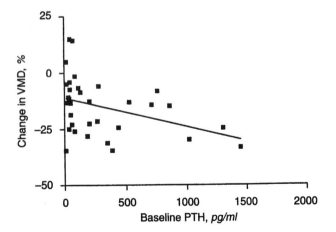

Fig. 14-4. Effect of pretransplantation parathyroid hormone (PTH) level on loss of vertebral mineral density (VMD) in first 3 months after transplantation. Patients with higher levels of PTH pretransplantation had significantly greater reduction in VMD ($r = -0.40$, $P < 0.05$). (From Torres A, Machado M, Concepcion MT, et al. Influence of vitamin D receptor genotype on bone mass changes after renal transplantation. *Kidney Int* 1996;50:1726–1733.)

the rate of reduction in bone density during the first 3 months after transplantation is highly correlated with pretransplantation parathyroid hormone levels (Fig. 14-4).

GLUCOCORTICOID EFFECTS

Preexisting bone disease notwithstanding, it is likely that the single most important determinant of posttransplantation osteopenia and osteonecrosis is steroid use. The effects of glucocorticoids on bone metabolism are numerous, and although not completely understood, are believed to be mediated by the nuclear mechanisms that depend on the glucocorticoid receptor. Glucocorticoids exert direct inhibitory effects on osteoblast function, inhibiting a variety of cellular functions including cell growth, multiplication, and differentiation and synthesis of type I collagen and noncollagenous proteins. Although bone resorption (by osteoclasts) and formation (by osteoblasts) are normally sequentially linked, the alterations in osteoblast function favor net resorption of bone. Using osteocalcin as a marker of osteoblast numbers, several investigators demonstrated a reduction in bone formation that occurs rapidly after initiation of steroid treatment and is maintained even with small doses of steroid. Julian and colleagues showed that stable transplant recipients on low doses of glucocorticoids exhibit a halving of the rate of vertebral bone formation, leading to progressive vertebral bone loss even as their parathyroid hormone and vitamin D metabolism is returning to normal. This effect of glucocorticoid can be partially reversed with calcitriol therapy.

Glucocorticoids have also been shown to impair end-organ responsiveness to vitamin D. Impaired active calcium absorption in the gut, a vitamin D-dependent process, has been observed in steroid-treated patients and is partially dose dependent. Because diffusional calcium absorption is unaltered, this effect can be minimized by increased dietary calcium, and partially reversed by pharmacologic doses of calcitriol. Although some have reported decreased conversion of 25-hydroxyvitamin D to the active calcitriol in the renal tubules, others have contradicted this finding, and calcitriol levels have been reported to be low, normal, or high in glucocorticoid-treated patients. Glucocorticoids also increase urinary excretion of both calcium and phosphate, which some ascribe to steroid-induced secondary hyperparathyroidism, whereas others postulate a direct suppression of renal tubular calcium resorption. Whether glucocorticoids have any direct effect on the parathyroid hormone level remains controversial. Thus, the net effects of long-term glucocorticoid therapy favor osteopenia through impaired calcium absorption in the gut, impaired calcium and phosphate resorption by the renal tubule, and impaired bone formation by osteoblasts.

Persistently Reduced Renal Function

Finally, although the renal transplant may restore a substantial degree of renal function, transplantation rarely returns renal function completely to normal. Hyperparathyroidism tends to resolve incompletely even for years after successful transplantation, so reduced tubular resorption of phosphate resulting in hypophosphatemia is not uncommon. It has been speculated that persistent hyperparathyroidism may result in part from a moderate reduction in GFR, even in successful transplants, through the same mechanisms that produce hyperparathyroidism in early renal insufficiency. Because the renal tubular phosphate "leak" correlates poorly with parathyroid hormone levels and is not corrected with phosphate restriction, it may also result in part from tubular injury or steroid effects on the tubule, independent of the level of parathyroid hormone.

The result of all these factors is to produce, in the immediate posttransplantation period, modest hypercalcemia and hypophosphatemia in about 50% of subjects, with increased urinary losses of both calcium and phosphorus and a further reduction in bone mineral. With regression of the hyperparathyroidism and lowering of the glucocorticoid dose, hypercalcemia tends to regress and serum calcium returns to normal in two thirds of patients within 3 years. The remaining patients have few symptoms related to hypercalcemia, and parathyroidectomy is rarely necessary. Without treatment, hypophosphatemia persists in many patients with good transplant function. Despite restoration of near-normal renal function, skeletal mineralization often worsens, leading to osteoporosis in many and to osteonecrosis in a significant fraction. The factors that are clearly associated with osteonecrosis include duration of uremia and dialysis, the degree of hyperparathyroidism before transplantation, and the total steroid dose.

To minimize the long-term metabolic bone complications after transplantation, careful attention must be paid to calcium and phosphate metabolism. In the presence of hypercalcemia, hypophosphatemia is usually managed by administration of supplemental oral phosphorus (sodium phosphates, approximately 150 mg three times daily). The diet should contain an adequate calcium and phosphorus content and be relatively free of phosphate binders, including magnesium oxide-based antacids because these compounds also bind phosphates. Administration of calcitriol can ameliorate the renal phosphate leak and hyperparathyroidism, the depressed intestinal absorption of calcium, and perhaps increase the rate of bone formation. One large, randomized, double-blinded study showed that use of calcitriol (0.5 to 1 µg/day) could significantly reduce bone loss from the lumbar spine in medical patients during 1 year of corticosteroid therapy given for a variety of indications, not including organ transplantation. The benefit was not observed in patients receiving calcium supplements alone. However, calcitriol must be used judiciously because it can cause hypercalcemia and hypercalciuria and lead to stone formation in the transplanted kidney.

OTHER NUTRIENTS

Sodium

The pathogenesis of hypertension in transplant recipients is multifactorial, resulting from cyclosporine therapy, glucocorticoid therapy with activation of the renin–angiotensin system, acute and chronic rejection, renal artery stenosis, and other factors. Although a thorough discussion of this topic is beyond the scope of this chapter, the issue is raised because cyclosporine-induced hypertension has been clearly shown to be sodium dependent and ameliorated by sodium restriction. Consequently, salt restriction should be part of the diet prescription for these patients. Conversely, there is little evidence that sodium restriction is helpful in patients who are not receiving cyclosporine. In fact, azathioprine-treated recipients who eat high-sodium diets do not have a disproportionate incidence of hypertension, nor is there any correlation of blood pressure with sodium intake in those patients. Sodium restriction in such patients is not sufficiently justified; it simply adds to the complexity of the dietary prescription, making compliance more difficult. Although tacrolimus may be associated with a lower incidence of post-transplantation hypertension than cyclosporine, this issue remains controversial. Both agents increase renal salt reabsorption to the same degree.

Potassium

Cyclosporine- and tacrolimus-based immunosuppressive regimens may also be associated with hyperkalemia, even when the GFR is relatively high. The predominant mechanism of hyperkalemia appears to be a tubular defect in potassium secretion with tubular insensitivity to mineralocorticoids. Other contributing factors may include suppression of the renin–aldosterone axis and altered distribution of potassium between the intracellular and extracellular compartments. This is most often seen in the early posttransplantation period when doses of cyclosporine or tacrolimus are highest, but hyperkalemia may be sustained in some patients. An occasional patient may require restriction of dietary potassium intake. Because many good sources of calories and virtually all high-protein foods have a high potassium content, dietary potassium restriction conflicts directly with the prescription of a high-protein, high-calorie diet and may cause significant malnutrition. β-Blockers and angiotensin-converting enzyme inhibitors appear to act synergistically with cyclosporine or tacrolimus to reduce aldosterone levels, and must be avoided in hyperkalemic patients. Measures used to increase potassium excretion in other instances of type IV renal tubular acidosis, such as administration of sodium bicarbonate, diuretic therapy, or use of ion exchange resins (e.g., sodium polystyrene sulfonate), may permit some liberalization of dietary potassium.

Iron

Iron stores vary widely in patients with renal failure who present for transplantation and may be reduced in hemodialysis patients as a result of blood loss during dialysis. Although iron absorption is normal in renal transplant recipients, the rapid expansion of the red blood cell mass after restoration of normal renal function may outstrip the iron absorption from foods, and some patients require supplemental ferrous sulfate. Other patients may have excessive iron stores as a result of frequent transfusions and should not receive iron supplements. The extensive use of recombinant erythropoietin in dialysis patients over the past several years has lessened both the incidence of iron overload and the degree of posttransplantation expansion of red blood cell mass seen previously. Therefore, iron studies should be performed before oral supplements are prescribed.

Vitamins

It is traditional to prescribe a supplement of water-soluble vitamins for transplant recipients; however, unlike dialysis patients (see Chapters 5 and 12), who can lose these vitamins during dialysis, there is little rationale for their use in transplant recipients. Vitamin A levels are elevated in patients with chronic renal failure and in recipients of renal transplants. The vitamin A circulates tightly bound to retinol-binding protein, the levels of which are also elevated, so that there may be no toxicity, but vitamin A supplements should not be given.

In the future, recommendations for vitamin supplementation in transplant recipients may be influenced by the growing evidence that these patients, like predialysis patients with chronic renal failure and those on dialysis, have elevated plasma levels of homocysteine, which appears to be a significant risk factor for atherosclerotic complications. The prevalence and degree of hyperhomocysteinemia in the transplant population appear to be similar to what is observed in other end-stage renal disease populations. The problem seems to be greater in those receiving cyclosporine than in patients on azathioprine. The elevated homocysteine levels observed in transplant patients are associated with a greater apparent risk of cardiovascular complications. Evidence suggests that supplementation with folic acid, but not with vitamins B_6 or B_{12}, can lower homocysteine levels in this population, but it is not yet known whether the reduction is associated with any decrease in risk of cardiovascular morbidity or mortality.

CONCLUSION

Recommended diets for the immediate posttransplantation period and for long-term therapy are summarized in Table 14-2. A recurrent theme in the preceding discussion of nutritional and metabolic abnormalities in transplant recipients is the adverse effects of glucocorticoid immunosuppressive therapy. Given all the problems that these steroids cause, it is not surprising that several studies have been undertaken to see whether they can be eliminated or the dose reduced. In smaller studies, patients removed from steroid therapy 6 months or more after transplantation seem to do very well, but a large, multicenter Canadian study suggests that there may be excess late graft losses when steroids are stopped completely. Few centers are now stopping steroid therapy completely, but there is a trend toward lower doses and use of alternate-day administration. Newer immunosuppressive agents such as mycophenolate mofetil and sirolimus (rapamycin) may facilitate steroid avoidance or withdrawal, although this remains to be demonstrated in clinical experience.

**Table 14-2. Recommended nutrition
for renal transplant recipients**

**First month after transplantation and during therapy
for acute rejection**

Protein	1.3–1.5 g/kg/d
Calories	30–35 kcal/kg/d

After first month

Protein	1.0 g/kg/d
Calories	Sufficient to achieve and maintain optimal weight for height

At all times

Carbohydrates	50% of calories
Fats	Not > 30% of calories
Cholesterol	Not > 300 mg/d
Polyunsaturated/ saturated fats ratio	> 1
Calcium	1200 mg/d
Phosphorus	1200 mg/d
Calcitriol	1 µg/d (unless patient is hypercalcemic or hypercalciuric)
Ferrous sulfate	300 mg/d if iron stores are reduced
Sodium	No added salt diet (3–4 g/d sodium chloride) if patient is on cyclosporine; usually no salt restriction needed otherwise

SELECTED READINGS

Arnadottir M, Hultberg B, Vladov V, et al. Hyperhomocysteinemia in cyclosporine-treated renal transplant recipients. *Transplantation* 1996;61:509–512.

Bantle JP, Nath KA, Sutherland DE, et al. Effects of cyclosporine on the renin–angiotensin–aldosterone system and potassium excretion in renal transplant recipients. *Arch Intern Med* 1985;145:505–508.

Bradford DS, Szalapaki EW, Sutherland DE, et al. Osteonecrosis in the transplant recipient. *Surg Gynecol Obstet* 1984;159:328–334.

Brenner BM, Cohen RA, Milford EL. In renal transplantation, one size may not fit all. *J Am Soc Nephrol* 1992;3:162–169.

Brenner BM, Meyer TW, Hostetter TH. Dietary protein intake and the progressive nature of kidney disease: the role of hemodynamically mediated glomerular injury in the pathogenesis of progressive glomerular sclerosis in aging, renal ablation and intrinsic renal disease. *N Engl J Med* 1982;307:652–659.

Canzanello VJ, Textor SC, Taler SJ, et al. Renal sodium handling with cyclosporine A and FK506 after orthotopic liver transplantation. *J Am Soc Nephrol* 1995;5:1910–1917.

Chan MK, Persaud VW, Varghese Z, et al. Fat clearances and hyper-lipidaemia in renal allograft recipients: the role of insulin resistance. *Clin Chim Acta* 1981;114:61–67.

Cho YW, Terasaki PI, Cecka JM. New variables reported to the UNOS Registry and their impact on cadaveric renal transplant outcomes: a preliminary study. In: Cecka JM, Terasaki PI, eds. *Clinical transplants 1995.* Los Angeles: UCLA Tissue Typing Laboratory; 1996:405–415.

Cogan MG, Sargent JA, Yarbrough SG, et al. Prevention of pred-nisone-induced negative nitrogen balance: effect of dietary modification on urea generation rate in patients on hemodialysis receiving high-dose glucocorticoids. *Ann Intern Med* 1981;95:158–161.

Cotorruelo JG, De Francisco AL, Canga E, et al. Sequential changes in divalent ion metabolism after renal transplantation. *Transplant Proc* 1990;22:1414–1415.

Curtis JJ, Luke RG, Jones P, et al. Hypertension in cyclosporine-treated renal transplant recipients is sodium dependent. *Am J Med* 1989;85:134–138.

De Groen PC. Cyclosporine, low density lipoprotein, and cholesterol. *Mayo Clin Proc* 1988;63:1012–1021.

Dennis VW, Robinson K. Homocysteinemia and vascular disease in end-stage renal disease. *Kidney Int* 1996;50(Suppl 57):S11–S17.

Derfler K, Hande M, Heinz G, et al. Decreased postheparin lipolytic activity in renal transplant recipients with cyclosporine A. *Kidney Int* 1991;40:720–727.

Diethelm AG, Edwards RP, Whelchel JD. The natural history and surgical treatment of hypercalcemia before and after renal transplantation. *Surg Gynecol Obstet* 1982;154:481–490.

Disler PR, Goldberg RB, Kuhn L, et al. The role of diet in the pathogenesis and control of hyperlipidemia after renal transplantation. *Clin Nephrol* 1981;16:29–34.

Edwards MS, Doster S. Renal transplant diet recommendations: results of a survey of renal dietitians in the United States. *J Am Diet Assoc* 1990;90:843–846.

Ekstrand AV, Eriksson JG, Gronhagen-Riska C, et al. Insulin resistance and insulin deficiency in the pathogenesis of posttransplantation diabetes in man. *Transplantation* 1992;53:563–569.

Ellis CN, Gorsulowsky DC, Hamilton TA, et al. Cyclosporine improves psoriasis in a double blind study. *JAMA* 1981;256:3110–3116.

Ettinger WH, Bender WL, Goldberg AP, et al. Lipoprotein lipid abnormalities in healthy renal transplant recipients: persistence of low HDL_2 cholesterol. *Nephron* 1987;47:17–21.

Feehally J, Harris KP, Bennett SE, et al. Is chronic renal transplant rejection a non-immunological phenomenon? *Lancet* 1986;2:486–488.

Friedman EA, Shyh TP, Beyer MN, et al. Posttransplant diabetes in kidney transplant recipients. *Am J Nephrol* 1986;5:196–202.

Gonzalez MT, Gonzalez C, Grino JM, et al. Long-term evolution of renal osteodystrophy after kidney transplantation: comparative study between intact PTH levels and bone biopsy. *Transplant Proc* 1990;22:1407–1411.

Gray JR, Kasiske BL. Patient and allograft survival in the late post-transplant period. *Semin Nephrol* 1992;12:343–352.

Hahn TJ, Halstead LR, Teitelbaum SL, et al. Altered mineral metabolism in glucocorticoid-induced osteopenia: effect of 25-hydroxyvitamin D administration. *J Clin Invest* 1979;64:655–665.

Hayes JM, Streem SB, Graneto D, et al. Renal transplant calculi: a reevaluation of risks and management. *Transplantation* 1982;47: 949–952.

Hodgson SF. Corticoid-induced osteoporosis. *Endocrinol Metab Clin North Am* 1990;19:95–111.

Horber FF, Hoppeler H, Herren D, et al. Altered skeletal muscle ultrastructure in renal transplant patients on prednisone. *Kidney Int* 1986;30:411–416.

Horber FF, Scheidegger JR, Gruing BE, et al. Evidence that prednisone-induced myopathy is reversed by physical training. *J Clin Endocrinol Metab* 1985;61:83–88.

Hoy WE, Sargent JA, Hall D, et al. Protein catabolism during the postoperative course after renal transplantation. *Am J Kidney Dis* 1985;5:186–190.

Hricik DE, Mayes JT, Schulak JA. Independent effects of cyclosporine and prednisone on posttransplant hypercholesterolemia. *Am J Kidney Dis* 1991;17:353–358.

Hricik DE, Whalen CC, Lautman J, et al. Withdrawal of steroids after renal transplantation: clinical predictors of outcome. *Transplantation* 1992;53:41–45.

Johnson CP, Gallagher-Lepak S, Zhu Y-R, et al. Factors influencing weight gain after renal transplantation. *Transplantation* 1993;56: 822–827.

Jowell PS, Epstien S, Fallon MD, et al. 1,25-Dihydroxyvitamin D3 modulates glucocorticoid-induced alteration in serum bone Gla protein and bone histomorphometry. *Endocrinology* 1987;120: 531–536.

Julian BA, Laskow DA, Dubousky J, et al. Rapid loss of vertebral mineral density after renal transplantation. *N Engl J Med* 1991; 325:544–550.

Kalbfleisch JH, Hebert LA, Lemann J, et al. Habitual excessive dietary salt intake and blood pressure levels in renal transplant recipients. *Am J Med* 1982;73:205–210.

Kamel K, Ethier JH, Quaggin S, et al. Studies to determine the basis for hyperkalemia in recipients of a renal transplant who are treated with cyclosporine. *J Am Soc Nephrol* 1991;2:1279–1284.

Kasiske BL, O Donnell MP, Cleary MP, et al. Treatment of hyperlipidemia reduces glomerular injury in obese Zucker rats. *Kidney Int* 1988;33:667–672.

Kasiske BL, Umen AJ. Persistent hyperlipidemia in renal transplant patients. *Medicine* 1987;66:309–316.

Kelleher J, Humphrey CS, Homer D, et al. Vitamin A and its transport protein in patients with chronic renal failure receiving maintenance hemodialysis and after renal transplantation. *Clin Sci* 1983;65:619–626.

Kopple JD. Abnormal amino acid and protein metabolism in uremia. *Kidney Int* 1978;14:340–348.

Krausz Y, Bar-On H, Shafrir E. Origin and pattern of glucocorticoid-induced hyperlipidemia in rats: dose-dependent bimodal changes in serum lipids and lipoproteins in relation to hepatic lipogenesis and tissue lipoprotein lipase activity. *Biochim Biophys Acta* 1981;663:69–82.

Laskow DA, Curtis JJ. Posttransplant hypertension. *Am J Hypertens* 1990;3:721–725.

Merion RM, Twork AM, Rosenberg L, et al. Obesity and renal transplantation. *Surg Gynecol Obstet* 1991;172:367–376.

Metselaar HJ, Van Steenbarge EJ, Bijen AB, et al. Incidence of osteo-necrosis after renal transplantation. *Acta Orthop Scand* 1985;56: 413–415.

Miller DG, Levine SE, D'Elia JA, et al. Nutritional status of diabetic and nondiabetic patients after renal transplantation. *Am J Clin Nutr* 1986;44:66–69.

Miller J, Pirsch JD, Vincenti F, et al, and the FK 506 Kidney Transplant Study Group. FK 506 in kidney transplantation: results of the U.S.A. randomized comparative phase III study. *Transplant Proc* 1997;29:304–305.

Milman N, Larsen L. Iron absorption after renal transplantation. *Acta Med Scand* 1976;200:25–30.

Moore RA, Callahan MF, Cody M, et al. The effect of the American Heart Association Step One diet on hyperlipidemia following renal transplantation. *Transplantation* 1990;49:60–62.

Mor E, Facklam D, Hasse J, et al. Weight gain and lipid profile changes in liver transplant recipients: long-term results of the American FK506 Multicenter Study. *Transplant Proc* 1995;27: 1126.

Nehme D, Rondeau E, Pollard F, et al. Aseptic necrosis of bone following renal transplantation: relationship with hyperparathyroidism. *Nephrol Dial Transplant* 1989;4:123–128.

Nuti R, Vattimo A, Turchetti V, et al. 25-Hydroxycholecalciferol as an agonist of adverse corticosteroid effects on phosphate and calcium metabolism in man. *J Endocrinol Invest* 1984;7:445–448.

Parfrey PS, Fage D, Parfrey NA, et al. The decreased incidence of aseptic necrosis in renal transplant recipients: a case control study. *Transplantation* 1986;41:182–187.

Pei Y, Richardson R, Greenwood C, et al. Extrarenal effect of cyclosporine A on potassium homeostasis in renal transplant recipients. *Am J Kidney Dis* 1993;22:314–319.

Pirsh JD, Miller J, Deiernoi MH, et al. A comparison of tacrolimus (FK506) and cyclosporine for immunosuppression after cadaveric renal transplantation. *Transplantation* 1997;63:977–983.

Pirsch JD, Armbrust MJ, Knechtle SJ, et al. Obesity as a risk factor following renal transplantation. *Transplantation* 1995;59: 631–647.

Princen HM, Meijer P, Wolthers BG, et al. Cyclosporine A blocks bile acid synthesis in cultured hepatocytes by specific inhibition of chenodeoxycholic acid synthesis. *Biochem J* 1991;275:501–505.

Prummel MF, Weirsinga WM, Lips P, et al. The course of biochemical parameters of bone turnover during treatment with corticosteroids. *J Clin Endocrinol Metab* 1991;72:382–386.

Raine AE, Carter R, Mann JL, et al. Adverse effect of cyclosporine on plasma cholesterol in renal transplant recipients. *Nephrol Dial Transplant* 1988;3:458–463.

Rosenberg ME, Salahudeen AK, Hostetter TH. Dietary protein and the renin–angiotensin system in chronic renal allograft rejection. *Kidney Int* 1995;48(Suppl 52):S102–S106.

Salahudeen AK, Hostetter TH, Raatz SK, et al. Effects of dietary protein in patients with chronic renal transplant rejection. *Kidney Int* 1992;41:183–190.

Sambrook P, Birmingham J, Kelly P, et al. Prevention of corticosteroid osteoporosis. A comparison of calcium, calcitriol, and calcitonin. *N Engl J Med* 1993;328:1747–1752.

Shapiro R. Tacrolimus (FK-506) in kidney transplantation. *Transplant Proc* 1997;29:45–47.

Shen SY, Lukens CW, Alongi SU, et al. Patient profile and effect of dietary therapy on post-transplant hyperlipidemia. *Kidney Int* 1983;24(Suppl):S147–152.

Short CD, Durrington PN. Hyperlipidemia and renal disease. *Baillieres Clin Endocrinol Metab* 1992;4:777–806.

Sinclair NR, and the Canadian Multicentre Transplant Study Group. Low-dose steroid therapy in cyclosporine-treated renal transplant recipients with well-functioning grafts. *Can Med Assoc J* 1992;147:645–657.

Slatopolsky E, Martin K. Glucocorticoids and renal transplant osteonecrosis. *Adv Exp Med Biol* 1984;171:353–359.

Steinmuller TM, Graf K-J, Schleicher J, et al. The effect of FK506 versus cyclosporine on glucose and lipid metabolism: a randomized trial. *Transplantation* 1994;58:669–674.

Suzuki Y, Ichikawa Y, Saito E, et al. Importance of increased urinary calcium excretion in the development of secondary hyperparathyroidism of patients under glucocorticoid therapy. *Metabolism* 1983; 32:151–156.

Terasaki PI, Koyama H, Cecka JM, et al. The hyperfiltration hypothesis in human renal transplantation. *Transplantation* 1994;57: 1450–1454.

Tonstad S, Holdaas H, Gorbitz C, et al. Is dietary intervention effective in post-transplant hyperlipidemia? *Nephrol Dial Transplant* 1995;10:82–85.

Torres A, Machado M, Concepcion MT, et al. Influence of vitamin D receptor genotype on bone mass changes after renal transplantation. *Kidney Int* 1996;50:1726–1733.

Ulmann A, Chkoff N, Lacour B. Disorders of calcium and phosphorus metabolism after successful kidney transplantation. *Advances in Nephrology* 1983;12:331–340.

The U.S. Multicenter FK506 Liver Study Group. A comparison of tacrolimus (FK506) and cyclosporine for immunosuppression in liver transplantation. *N Engl J Med* 1994;331:1110–1115.

Vathsala A, Wienberg RB, Schoenberg L, et al. Lipid abnormalities in cyclosporine–prednisone-treated renal transplant recipients. *Transplantation* 1989;48:37–43.

Whittier FC, Evans DH, Dutton S. Nutrition in renal transplantation. *Am J Kidney Dis* 1985;6:405–411.

Windus DW, Lacson S, Delmez JA. The short-term effects of a low-protein diet in stable renal transplant recipients. *Am J Kidney Dis* 1986;17:693–699.

Approaches to Successful Nutritional Intervention in Renal Disease

Sandra Newbill Powers

Nutritional intervention varies throughout the course of chronic renal disease. When end-stage renal insufficiency occurs, nutritional intervention must accommodate the mode of dialysis or the regimen required by a renal transplant. The dietary modifications that are used throughout the course of treating renal failure are often complex because of the need to alter the intake of multiple nutrients simultaneously. When comorbid conditions exist, such as hypertension, diabetes, and hyperlipidemia, additional dietary interventions are necessary, adding further complexity. In the presence of acute renal failure, diet or dialysis are required, usually for a brief period of time, until the kidney regains function. The nutritional intervention for chronic renal failure is more complicated. A complex diet, combined with sickness, frequent hospitalizations, and poor appetite, puts the patient with chronic kidney disease at serious risk for malnutrition (Table 15-1).

The challenge to create an effective and enjoyable nutritional intervention regimen should be approached as an art as well as a science. Dietitians can have a significant impact on the health of the patient with kidney disease by conveying the message that food is important to keep and improve health and alter abnormal physiologic conditions to bring about more normal conditions. Success is achieved by simplifying a complex dietary regimen and by effectively using individualized approaches to education and monitoring, a process that can be enhanced through the use of microcomputers. Success builds self-confidence and motivation, and patients who succeed in adhering to multiple dietary restrictions and who believe that the intervention will help are most likely to achieve their goals.

The clinical setting and tools available for successful nutritional intervention have improved, in part, because of the extensive published results from the Modification of Diet in Renal

Table 15-1. Challenges to successful intervention

The type of intervention varies throughout the course of chronic renal disease.

The intervention is complex because multiple nutrients must be altered.

Comorbid conditions require additional intervention.

Intercurrent illness and hospitalizations complicate the nutritional intervention.

Poor appetite and side effects of medications complicate the nutritional intervention.

Disease (MDRD) Study and the publication of the National Renal Diet from The American Dietetic Association. The MDRD Study was a long-term, multicenter study based on well designed nutritional intervention programs for patients randomly assigned to usual-protein, low-protein, or very–low-protein diets. The nutritional intervention program used a variety of approaches that resulted in a level of dietary compliance greater than expected. Detailed information about the MDRD dietary interventions, and patient characteristics and patterns associated with adherence, are found in the Selected Readings listed at the end of this chapter. The National Renal Diet was created by The American Dietetic Association's Renal Dietetic Practice Group and the National Kidney Foundation's Council on Renal Nutrition in an effort to provide a uniform and consistent tool for use by patients and professionals nationwide.

GOALS

The goals for nutritional intervention in renal disease are to 1) maintain or improve nutritional status and prevent malnutrition and wasting; 2) implement an appropriate diet and nutrition prescription based on nutritional status, food and nutritional intake, and clinical and physical condition; and 3) facilitate compliance with the nutritional intervention through education, evaluation, and monitoring.

Maintain or Improve Current Nutritional Status and Prevent Malnutrition and Wasting

Before planning the type of diet and nutritional intervention, the first step should be to evaluate nutritional status and nutrient intake. The methods used in these assessments also are used to monitor the patient's progress throughout the course of renal insufficiency. Assessment and evaluation create the foundation for an educational process and for establishing a stable and effective working relationship with the patient. This collaboration is important for achieving adherence to the recommended intervention.

Clinical and Biochemical Data

A baseline assessment should include a review of the patient's clinical history to determine the type of kidney disease, the level of kidney function or the type of renal replacement therapy, if the patient has received a transplant, and whether there are other medical conditions such as hypertension, diabetes, or hyperlipidemia. Laboratory data should include the serum albumin because the level will influence the diet, primarily the protein and calorie recommendations. Serum albumin is an index of visceral protein status; the level is reduced when protein stores are depleted. Serum albumin also is influenced by changes in body fluids; fluid retention can reduce the serum albumin, making it a poor marker of nutritional status for certain patients. Moreover, protein stores can become depleted before the serum albumin falls significantly because of its long half-life (16 to 21 days). Finally, infection can reduce albumin synthesis and its serum levels.

Serum transferrin, which binds and transports iron, is a more sensitive indicator of visceral protein status than serum albumin because it has a shorter half-life. However, serum transferrin can be falsely elevated in iron deficiency, so assessing protein status by this value alone should be done cautiously when serum iron is low.

Anthropometry

Measurements of weight, height, and frame size to estimate a standard or relative body weight, the ideal body weight, or body mass index are easy to obtain and provide a baseline for monitoring. If scoliosis is present, a knee height measurement can be used to estimate height more precisely. For dialysis patients, measurements should be made at the end of dialysis sessions to evaluate the "dry" weight. Frame size can be determined using either wrist measurements or elbow breadth. Procedures for measuring the wrist and elbow breadth as well as reference tables are found in several of the Selected Readings at the end of this chapter, including *Suggested Guidelines for Nutrition Care of Renal Patients* published by The American Dietetic Association, and for dialysis patients, "Anthropometric Norms for the Dialysis Population," by Nelson and colleagues. Additional measurements to assess muscle mass and body fat include arm muscle circumference and triceps, biceps, and subscapular skinfolds. These measurements establish a baseline physical assessment to compare with values in the normal range and serve as a reference point for monitoring.

When anthropometry is used, the quality of the measurements is important. The dietitian or health care provider who performs the measurements should be trained and use methods of quality control to ensure reliable and valid results. When standard procedures are followed, the measurements are reproducible.

Dietary and Nutrient Intake Assessment

Assessing dietary habits, food preferences, nutrient intake, and the intake of supplements is especially important for the patient at risk for nutritional problems. Common reasons for malnutrition in patients with chronic renal insufficiency are limited protein intake and inadequate calories.

By using 24-hour diet recalls and food records, the patient's usual calorie and nutrient intake can be compared with prescribed amounts to determine if dietary changes are needed. This process of obtaining information about food intake is also an opportunity for the patient to become more familiar with what he or she eats, especially in relation to portion sizes and specific nutrient content. The collaboration of the dietitian and the patient while examining the types and amounts of foods eaten is a good start to successful intervention.

Select an Appropriate Diet and Nutrition Prescription

The diet and nutritional prescription should be individualized to make it easy for the patient to follow. The prescription is based on the nutritional requirements and the patient's food preferences as well as the medical and clinical condition. The nutritional requirements for stages of renal disease (including renal replacement therapies), renal transplantation, malnutrition, and catabolic stress are found in Chapters 11, 12, 13, and 14. This chapter focuses on general factors to consider when planning a diet and nutrition prescription.

An appropriate diet improves the overall medical condition of the patient with renal disease. The kidneys perform many functions, including those that influence nutrient requirements by creating an internal balance so that intake equals output. The kidneys remove excess fluid and waste products, including urea, sodium, and potassium. Calcium and phosphorus balances also are regulated by the kidneys, through activation of vitamin D. The kidneys regulate blood pressure by varying sodium and water balance and through the production of renin. The production of red blood cells is stimulated by the hormone erythropoietin. When the kidneys function poorly, all or some of these functions are compromised. By altering specific nutrients, the clinician can reduce edema, accumulation of waste products, and acidosis, and improve the hypertension, anemia, and bone disease that occur with advancing renal failure. Designing a diet to serve these multiple purposes can be complex and overwhelming, but the diet can be very effective in correcting abnormal values and improving the clinical status.

The following sections list the factors to consider in selecting an appropriate diet prescription.

Weight and the Calculation of Protein and Calorie Needs

Prescriptions for protein and calorie recommendations frequently are based on a body weight in kilograms. The decision whether to use actual weight or an ideal, adjusted, usual, standard, or relative body weight depends on several factors (Table 15-2). Actual body weight is appropriate for most circumstances, as long as actual body weight is near to the ideal or standard body weight, when no significant weight change has occurred, and when the patient is not malnourished. The usual weight is appropriate for patients who have been slightly overweight or underweight for most of their lives. If a patient is obese, the actual body weight or the ideal body weight may be inappropriate because the protein and caloric needs will be excessive. A formula in the *Suggested Guidelines for Nutrition Care of Renal Patients* (The American Dietetic Association) for adjusting the body weight for obese patients is based on 25% of the weight as excessive body fat:

$$[(\text{Actual weight} - \text{ideal weight}) \times 0.25] + \text{ideal body weight (IBW)}$$

A variety of methods are used to establish "ideal" body weight. Tables or calculations usually specify a frame size that is visually estimated or determined from either the wrist circumference or elbow breadth. The ideal body weight tables from the Metropolitan Life Insurance Company are based on average weights for a given sex, age, height, and frame size derived from a population that should have the greatest longevity. The Hamwi method (see Table 15-2) is one of the easiest ways to estimate ideal body weight. It uses sex and height and adjusts for frame size. Standard body weight makes no correction for frame size and is based on average values from large populations of healthy people of similar sex, height, and age. The standard body weight or ideal body weight can be expressed as a percentage of relative body weight (RBW):

$$\% \text{RBW} - \frac{\text{Actual body weight}}{\text{Standard reference weight}} \times 100$$

Table 15-2. Considerations for selecting a weight for calculating protein and calorie recommendations

Use actual body weight (dry weight for dialysis patients) when:
    Weight is within reasonable range of ideal or standard body weight.
    Recent weight change has not occurred.
    Patient is not malnourished.

Use usual body weight when patients have been slightly overweight or underweight almost all of their lives.

Use adjusted body weight when patients are obese:
    [(Actual weight – ideal weight) × 0.25] + ideal body weight (IBW)

Ideal body weight can be selected from the Metropolitan Life Insurance Company Tables according to frame size. These weights are based on average weights from a population associated with the greatest longevity (ages 25–59 years for a given sex, age, and height).

Ideal body weight can be estimated using the Hamwi method based on sex, height, and frame size:
    Male: 106 pounds for the first 5 feet. Add 6 pounds for each inch over 5 feet.
    Female: 100 pounds for the first 5 feet. Add 5 pounds for each inch over 5 feet.
    For small frame, subtract 10%.
    For large frame, add 10%.

Tables of standard body weight are adjusted for sex, height, and age but not for frame size.

Relative body weight (RBW) is expressed as a percentage to assess actual body weight compared with a reference weight:

$$\text{RBW} = \frac{\text{Actual body weight}}{\text{Standard body weight or ideal body weight}} \times 100$$

Another method used to assess body weight is the body mass index (BMI):

$$\text{BMI} = \frac{\text{Actual weight (kg)}}{\text{Height m}^2}$$

Protein

Dietary protein is often restricted in patients with a chronic renal insufficiency and then increased when patients begin long-term dialysis treatment or transplantation. To determine if the protein intake should be lowered or raised, the usual protein intake should be estimated. The estimated protein intake (EPI) can be determined by dietary intake assessment or by laboratory methods based on the urinary nitrogen appearance (UNA) rate and then multiplying by 6.25 g protein/g nitrogen:

$$\text{EPI} = 6.25 \times [\text{UUn g/day} + (0.031 \times \text{body weight}) + \text{Uprotein g/day}]$$

when Uprotein is greater than 5 grams per 24 hours and UUN is urinary urea nitrogen.

In dialysis patients, protein intake is estimated from urea kinetic modeling, a mathematical method for calculating the protein catabolic rate. The protein catabolic rate should be equal to dietary protein intake in people who are stable, in nitrogen balance, and have adequate dialysis treatment. The formula takes into account total body water, dialyzer clearance, blood flow, dialysate flow, time of treatment, and residual renal function. A combination of dietary history and a laboratory assessment of urea kinetics will provide a more complete estimate of actual protein intake.

The validity of the assessment depends on the accuracy of the food intake data, including the amount of food eaten, the food description, and the completeness of the information. The accuracy of the urea kinetic calculations depends on the completeness of the 24-hour urine collection. In addition to estimating protein intake, a 24-hour urine collection can be used to calculate creatinine clearance and estimate sodium and potassium intake. Some patients or health care professionals may view a 24-hour urine collection as inconvenient, but if the patient knows that the results are used to evaluate and monitor renal function and the effectiveness of dietary changes, the patient usually is more willing to collect urine accurately. The patient should be given instruction to help ensure that the collection will be complete.

CHRONIC RENAL INSUFFICIENCY. The amount of protein prescribed for a patient with chronic renal insufficiency depends on several factors, including the degree of renal failure, the type of renal disease, and nutritional status. The recommended protein allowance for normal, healthy people is 0.75 g/kg/day (recommended dietary allowance), although the typical American eats more protein, usually between 1.0 to 1.5 g/kg/day. The time to initiate a protein restriction and the amount of the protein to recommend are not universally agreed on. In general, in moderate to advanced renal failure and before the onset of dialysis, a lower protein intake, around 0.6 g/kg/day, is recommended to retard the progression of advanced renal disease and reduce the uremic symptoms related to renal insufficiency. A reduced protein intake decreases the accumulation of nitrogenous waste products that cause uremic symptoms, such as nausea, vomiting, loss of appetite, and energy. Patients who are compliant with dietary protein restriction should be monitored regularly to assess their nutrient intake and nutritional status. Fearful of increasing the nutritional risk, some nephrologists are hesitant to prescribe a dietary protein restriction, especially in the presence of reduced appetite that frequently occurs near end-stage renal disease. Attention to the amount of dietary calories is necessary to ensure a neutral or positive nitrogen balance. When protein is restricted, most (about two thirds) of the protein should come from high-quality (high–biologic-value) protein sources found in animal products. High-quality protein contains a greater proportion of essential amino acids; these are used more efficiently by the body than the nonessential amino acids that are proportionally higher in low-quality proteins sources such as breads, grains, cereals, fruits, and vegetables.

ACUTE RENAL INSUFFICIENCY. With acute renal failure, protein intake is usually reduced to about 0.5 g/kg/day for a short time, until dialysis is initiated or until the kidney regains function. If dialysis is initiated, protein intake is increased to 1.0 to 1.5 g/kg/day. A comprehensive review of the nutritional management of acute renal failure is presented in Chapter 10 of this book.

DIALYSIS. Protein requirements are increased for dialysis patients because amino acids and peptides are lost during the dialysis procedure, and the process of dialysis appears to be catabolic. The protein intake recommended for hemodialysis patients is 1.1 g/kg ideal body weight/day, with the prescribed amount depending on nutritional status, degree of physical stress, and activity level. In peritoneal dialysis, protein intake should even be higher, at a level of 1.2 to 1.5 g/kg/day, because of the additional loss of protein during the procedure.

TRANSPLANTATION. After transplantation, the protein requirement depends, in part, on the amount of steroid therapy the patient is receiving. The steroids cause catabolism, which increases the protein requirements up to 1.5 g/kg/day with maximum doses. When the steroid dose is minimized or discontinued, protein intake can be returned to a normal level.

Phosphorus

As chronic renal insufficiency progresses, the serum phosphorus level increases and phosphate metabolism is altered. When this happens, a reduced phosphorus intake is recommended. Foods commonly identified as carriers of phosphorus are dairy products and foods that contain protein. By knowing the usual phosphorus intake as well as the major carriers of phosphorus in the patient's diet, recommendations can be made to avoid or reduce phosphorus intake. Medications such as calcium carbonate and calcium acetate can be used if dietary restriction is not effective. These medications bind phosphorus in the gut and should be taken with meals. Although they are effective in increasing the elimination of phosphorus, a common side effect of these phosphate binders is constipation.

Sodium

The intake of sodium is usually individualized and monitored regularly to avoid hypertension and volume overload. The amount recommended is usually around 2000 mg/day. Sodium intake can be estimated from the sodium excretion of a 24-hour urine collection or, with some difficulty, from a diet recall. Knowing the exact amount of salt added to prepared food or at the table can be difficult at best unless the added salt is measured. Asking about the use of salt substitutes is important because some brands have a significant amount of potassium.

Potassium

The amount of potassium in the diet usually depends on maintaining the serum potassium within normal limits. Patients with chronic renal insufficiency or receiving maintenance dialysis should be monitored on a regular basis to avoid hyperkalemia or hypokalemia. Hyperkalemia can result not only from excessive potassium intake, but from catabolism, acidosis, medications such as angiotensin-converting enzyme inhibitors, or potassium-sparing diuretics. Hypokalemia may be a problem for patients who take diuretics.

Potassium intake can be estimated by the 24-hour urinary excretion of potassium and by assessment of food intake.

Calcium

Calcium supplements are often prescribed for patients with chronic renal insufficiency, because the kidney no longer produces sufficient vitamin D 1,25-dihydroxycholecalciferol, which regulates the absorption of calcium. In addition, as renal disease progresses, calcium intake is often reduced because the intake of phosphorus and protein is reduced, therefore calcium supplements are needed. Unfortunately, dairy products, a primary source of calcium, are also rich sources of phosphorus and protein. If calcium supplements are prescribed, they should be taken between meals unless they are used as a phosphate binder. The most active form of vitamin D, 1,25-dihydroxycholecalciferol, is often prescribed to enhance the absorption of calcium and to decrease parathyroid hormone levels. Assessment of calcium intake is probably best achieved by diet recall or a food record analysis.

Iron

Iron supplements are often prescribed with a low-protein diet because such diets are low in heme-iron, the most highly bioavailable form of iron that is found in most animal products. When serum iron and hematocrit levels are low, iron supplements are recommended. Patients receiving erythropoietin therapy usually require iron supplementation.

Fat

The amount and type of fat are prescribed on an individual basis and depend on factors such as serum lipid levels, protein intake, and body weight. In renal failure, high serum lipid levels are associated with an increased rate of cardiovascular disease, but if the diet must have multiple modifications, the fat content should be changed only in cases when serum levels are significantly high. When protein is reduced, cholesterol intake is usually reduced; alternatively, when protein intake rises, cholesterol intake usually rises. Increasing the amount of polyunsaturated fats and reducing the saturated fat intake is effective in some cases for lowering cholesterol. Increasing the fiber content of the diet may be helpful in reducing the serum lipids if the additional fiber does not adversely effect the phosphorus content of the diet. Reducing concentrated sweets can be effective in reducing serum triglyceride levels. To assess serum lipids, a sample obtained after a 12-hour fast provides the most accurate result.

Calories

In chronic renal failure, calories should be adjusted to promote or maintain a desirable body weight. As the renal failure progresses, nonprotein calories can be added to the diet to maintain caloric intake and for a protein-sparing effect. If additional fat and simple carbohydrates are contraindicated, low-protein wheat-starch products are available (Table 15-3). The caloric prescription should always be individualized and depends on factors such as current body weight, age, sex, activity, nutritional state, and degree of stress. The range recommended is usually between 25 to 50 kcal/kg/day (Table 15-4). Calories should be higher as stress and activity increase. Patients treated by peritoneal dialysis absorb glucose from the dialysate; therefore, a lower calorie range

Table 15-3. Sources of low-protein and wheatstarch products

Dietary Specialties, Inc.
  PO Box 227
  Rochester, New York 14601
  716/263-2787 or 1/800/544-0099

Ener-G Foods, Inc.
  5960 1st Avenue South
  PO Box 84487
  Seattle, Washington 98124

Med-Diet Laboratories, Inc.
  3050 Randhview Lane
  Plymouth, Minnesota 55447
  1/800/MED-DIET

R & D Laboratories, Inc.
  4204 Glencoe Avenue
  Marina Del Ray, California 90292
  1/800/338-9066

Table 15-4. Guidelines for recommending calorie intake based on ideal body weight

Early chronic renal failure (~35 kcal/kg/d)
Obese patients may require less; more active
  or underweight patients may require more.

Adult hemodialysis

Maintenance of weight	30–35 kcal/kg/d
Weight reduction	20–30 kcal/kg/d
Weight gain	35 to 50 kcal/kg/d

Adult peritoneal dialysis—intermittent

Maintenance of weight	35 kcal/kg/d
Repletion/weight gain	35–50 kcal/kg/d
Weight reduction	20–25 kcal/kg/d
Stable diabetes	35 kcal/kg/d

Adult peritoneal dialysis—continuous ambulatory or automated

Maintenance of weight	25–35 kcal/kg/d
Repletion/weight gain	35–50 kcal/kg/d
Weight reduction	20–25 kcal/kg/d
Stable diabetes	35 kcal/kg/d

From American Dietetic Association. *A clinical guide to nutrition care in end-stage renal disease*. 2nd ed. Chicago: The American Dietetic Association; 1994.

is usually recommended. Energy needs in acute renal failure are usually high because of physical stress, and the recommendation is usually between 35 to 50 kcal/kg/day.

Vitamin Supplementation

If dietary protein and phosphorus are restricted during chronic renal insufficiency, the intake of certain vitamins may be inadequate. During dialysis, vitamins are lost into the dialysate. Water-soluble vitamins are usually recommended, and supplements, such as Nephro-Vite RX (R & D Laboratories; Marina Del Rey, CA), that contain vitamins B and C are designed especially for the patient with renal failure. The fat-soluble vitamins A, E, and K are usually not prescribed unless there is a deficiency. The oral form of vitamin D can be used when calcium levels are low, and the intravenous form is often used for dialysis patients.

Nutritional Supplementation

Oral nutritional supplements are prescribed when dietary intake is insufficient to meet nutritional needs. These liquid supplements are an effective and well tolerated means to increase protein or energy intake. A variety of brand names, formulations, and flavors are available to patients through grocery stores and pharmacies.

**Facilitate Compliance With Prescribed
Nutritional Intervention Through
Education, Evaluation, and Monitoring**

The fewer the diet and nutritional changes, the greater the chances of successful intervention. A simple, individualized diet plan that satisfies the patient is a critical component for long-term compliance. The approach to education and monitoring depends on several factors, including the patient's educational level, the complexity of the changes, the time available to the dietitian and patient for education and follow-up, and the motivation of the patient.

The educational process begins with an initial assessment and continues with individualized instructions for following the prescription. Patients who are taught about their disease, instructed how to change habits and life style to manage and improve their health, and given feedback about their efforts. These are the patients who are empowered to succeed. Knowledge and the awareness to make informed choices are part of the empowerment model approach to health care and patient education. This approach has been successfully used in diabetes care, and can increase the success of the desired intervention.

The dietitian can use several approaches to simplify and individualize the nutritional intervention program. The approach should incorporate foods the patient likes to demonstrate how the diet can be enjoyed despite the restrictions. Creating a setting whereby the patient can succeed at achieving the desired prescription fosters continued compliance and successful intervention (Table 15-5).

Dietary Intake Data

The 24-hour recall and food record help the patient and dietitian learn about portion sizes and the nutrient or calorie content of the foods usually eaten. The use of food scales, measur-

Table 15-5. Steps that increase success in modifying the diet

Simplify a complex regimen.

Minimize and prioritize dietary alterations.

Individualize the approach to the intervention.

Know the patient's food habits and preferences.

Build a stable working relationship with the patient and his or her family.

Start early in the course of renal insufficiency.

Build self-confidence and motivation for patients.

Educate and provide feedback to the patient.

ing cups and spoons, rulers, and food models demonstrates the importance of portion size and improves the accuracy of the recall. The diet recall gives the patient an example of information needed when recording a food record. The 24-hour recall plus a food record can be the first step in dietary education as well as a way of obtaining accurate information for food and nutrient intake assessment.

In the MDRD Study, 24-hour recalls and food records were successfully used prior to the dietary intervention for assessment and education. Before implementing the diet prescription, patients recorded their food intake and then personally determined the amount of protein in each portion of food eaten. In addition, patients calculated their daily protein intake by adding the protein eaten during the day as well as averaging the protein intake over several days. Patients were given a calculator along with instructions for calculating the protein content of any portion size. A digital scale, a ruler, and measuring cups and spoons were provided to increase the accuracy of portion sizes. Over time, patients became skilled at estimating portion sizes without weighing or measuring foods. Reference material included a "Protein Wise Counter," developed specifically for the MDRD Study by the Nutrition Coordinating Center at the University of Pittsburgh. This protein counter listed the protein, calorie, sodium, and phosphorus content of over 1400 foods. A similar counter was developed by the same group for convenience and fast foods, called "Shopping Wise." This self-learning approach was effective in teaching patients the protein content of the foods they usually eat, as well as how to determine their usual daily protein intake.

There are some limitations and shortcomings to using dietary intake data. For example, the days that are captured may not be representative of usual intake, and the reported data may not be accurate. The dietitian can improve the accuracy of the food record by clarifying the method of preparation and by using measuring cups, spoons, ruler, and food models to improve the accuracy of the portion size. If food records are a burden, a patient may not eat as much to avoid recording every food item. Alternatively, patients may adhere more closely to the dietary restrictions on food record days. Finally, patients may modify their intake during the food record days by omitting food or including foods to please the dietitian.

Diet histories and food frequencies are good for determining the types and amounts of food eaten over a long period of time, but are not as useful for assessing nutrient intake. The process may be time consuming but also can provide valuable information about food habits, especially with a skilled interviewer.

Self-Monitoring and Keeping Track

This approach, used successfully in the MDRD Study, was a vehicle not only for the patient to learn the protein content of foods eaten, but to facilitate compliance with the protein prescription. By recording intake, portion size, and protein content, this self-monitoring approach to achieving compliance allowed the patient to monitor protein intake throughout the day in an effort to stay within range of the protein goal.

Menus

Menus are one of the best educational tools a dietitian can use to translate a renal diet prescription into the appropriate foods to eat, especially when the menus contain foods the patient likes and when multiple nutrients are being controlled. Before the use of computers, individual patient menus were planned primarily by exchange lists, first developed in the 1950s for patients with diabetes. Even with exchange lists, menu planning can be considered a laborious task, especially with renal diets. Individualizing the menu planned with exchanges is limited by the number of food choices within each list, forcing a patient to use only foods in the exchange lists. By taking advantage of computers, dietitians can plan individualized menus and demonstrate how to combine food choices and adjust the amounts to achieve the desired diet. Computer software such as the Professional Diet Analyzer, by The CBORD Group, Inc. (Ithaca, New York) has a menu planning component that is user-friendly and can be used by the dietitian or patient. Computerized spreadsheets can be designed for planning and calculating menus, a process very similar to planning menus on paper, but faster and more accurate because of automatic calculations.

One of the most effective ways to plan menus is to take a patient's 24-hour recall and modify the food choices and amounts as little as possible to achieve the desired prescription. Tables 15-6 through 15-13 are examples of two different patients' baseline 24-hour recalls and demonstrate how food choices and amounts were modified to achieve a low-protein prescription for moderate renal insufficiency and higher-protein prescriptions for hemodialysis or peritoneal dialysis. The menus were planned using the Professional Diet Analyzer from The CBORD Group, Inc., with a nutrient database developed and maintained by the Department of Epidemiology and Biostatistics at Case Western Reserve University (Cleveland, OH).

When planning menus with either a computerized spreadsheet or with a computer program, each menu can be saved under a different file name so that changes in foods or amounts can easily create multiple new menus. Changes in the nutrient content are reflected immediately by the totals on the screen.

When foods and amounts from the 24-hour recall are entered into the computer while the patient is recalling food intake, the results are immediate for both the dietitian and patient. Once

Table 15-6. 24-hour diet recall calculated using CBORD Professional Diet Analyzer for Patient Example 1 (weight, 70 kg)

Food name Usual Week-day Food Intake	Amount	PRO (g)	Kcal	Phos (mg)	APRO (g)	Sod (mg)	Pot (mg)
Breakfast							
Coffee, regular or decaffeinated	8 ozv	0.2	5	2.368	0.0	5	128
Sugar, white	1 tbsp	0.0	46	0.0000	0.0	0	1
Orange juice	8 ozv	1.6	112	39.84	0.0	2	474
English muffin	1 avg	4.5	134	63.64	0.0	364	318
Jam/jelly, all flavors	0.5 tbsp	0.1	27	0.9000	0.0	1	9
Lunch							
Lettuce, iceberg, raw	2 cup	1.1	14	22.00	0.0	10	174
Carrots, raw	1 med	0.7	31	31.68	0.0	25	233
Celery, raw	2 stalk	0.5	13	20.80	0.0	70	227
Broccoli, raw	.25 cup	0.7	6	14.52	0.0	6	72
Cauliflower, raw	.25 cup	0.5	6	11.50	0.0	4	89
Cheddar cheese	1 ozw	7.0	114	145.40	7.0	176	28
Ham, cured	1 ozw	6.1	69	60.66	6.1	337	81
Italian or French dressing	2 tbsp	0.2	136	1.460	0.0	230	4

Ritz cracker	8 each	1.7	124	59.00	0.0	243	19
Margarine, soft	0.5 tbsp	0.1	50	1.401	0.1	75	3
Apples w/skin, raw	1 large	0.3	109	12.88	0.0	0	212
Tea, instant beverage w/sugar and lemon	12 ozv	0.5	132	3.885	0.0	36	74
Dinner							
Chicken breast, half	3 ozw	23.1	129	184.6	23.1	42	201
White rice	1 cup	3.4	182	80.52	0.0	6	86
Beans, lima	0.5 cup	4.8	80	59.50	0.0	200	192
Summer squash	0.5 cup	0.8	18	35.10	0.0	1	173
Margarine, soft	0.5 tbsp	0.1	50	1.401	0.1	75	3
Vanilla ice cream, regular	1 cup	4.8	270	134.3	4.8	116	256
Snacks							
Cheese crackers	10 each	0.8	43	19.71		149	8
Pear, raw w/skin	1 med	0.6	98	18.26	0.0	0	208
Fruit-flavored soda, carbonated beverage	12 ozv	0.0	179	11.16	0.0	53	38
Total		64.0	2175	1036	41.1	2224	3308
Percentage of goal							

PRO, protein; Kcal, Kilocalories; Phos, phosphorus; APRO, animal protein; Sod, sodium; Pot, potassium; ozv, ounces by volume; ozw, ounces by weight; tbsp, tablespoon.

The CBORD Group, Inc., The Professional Diet Analyzer, version 1.0.7, Ithaca, NY.

Table 15-7. Menu for Patient Example 1, modified for reduced protein in moderate renal insufficiency and based on 24-hour recall (weight, 70 kg; the prescription is 0.6 g protein/kg body weight and 30 kcal/kg body weight)

Food name Renal Insufficiency—0.6 g PRO/kg/day	Amount	PRO (g) 42.0	Kcal 2100	Phos (mg)	APRO (g) 18.0	Sod (mg)	Pot (mg)
Breakfast							
Coffee, regular or decaffeinated	8 ozv	0.2	5	2.368	0.0	5	128
Sugar, white	1 tbsp	0.0	46	0.0000	0.0	0	1
Apple juice or cider	8 ozv	0.1	117	17.36	0.0	7	295
English muffin	1 avg	4.5	134	63.64	0.0	364	318
Jam/jelly, all flavors	2 tbsp	0.2	109	3.600	0.0	5	35
Lunch							
Lettuce, iceberg, raw	2 cup	1.1	14	22.00	0.0	10	174
Carrots, raw	1 med	0.7	31	31.68	0.0	25	233
Celery, raw	2 stalk	0.5	13	20.80	0.0	70	227
Broccoli, raw	0.25 cup	0.7	6	14.52	0.0	6	72
Cauliflower, raw	0.25 cup	0.5	6	11.50	0.0	4	89
Italian or French dressing	4 tbsp	0.4	272	2.920	0.0	460	8
Ritz cracker	8 each	1.7	124	59.00	0.0	243	19

Food	Serving	PRO	Kcal	Phos	APRO	Sod	Pot
Margarine, soft	1 tbsp	0.1	99	2.801	0.1	149	5
Apples w/skin, raw	1 large	0.3	109	12.88	0.0	0	212
Tea, instant beverage w/sugar and lemon	12 ozv	0.5	132	3.885	0.0	36	74
Dinner							
Chicken breast, half	3 ozw	23.1	129	184.6	23.1	42	201
White rice	1 cup	3.4	182	80.52	0.0	6	86
Beans, green	1 cup	1.8	36	32.40	0.0	18	152
Summer squash	0.5 cup	0.8	18	35.10	0.0	1	173
Margarine, soft	1 tbsp	0.1	99	2.801	0.1	149	5
Fruit ice or sorbet	0.5 cup	0.4	118	0.0000	0.0	0	3
Snacks							
Cheese crackers	10 each	0.8	43	19.71		149	8
Pear, raw w/skin	1 med	0.6	98	18.26	0.0	0	208
Fruit flavored soda, carbonated beverage	12 ozv	0.0	179	11.16	0.0	53	38
Total		42.5	2118	653.5	23.3	1801	2763
Percentage of goal		101%	101%		129%		

PRO, protein; Kcal, kilocalories; Phos, phosphorus; APRO, animal protein; Sod, sodium; Pot, potassium; ozv, ounces by volume; tbsp, tablespoon; ozw, ounces by weight; tbsp, tablespoon.

The CBORD Group, Inc., The Professional Diet Analyzer, version 1.0.7, Ithaca, NY.

Table 15-8. Menu for Patient Example 1, modified for hemodialysis and based on 24-hour recall (weight, 70 kg; the prescription is 1.0 g protein/kg body weight and 35 kcal/kg body weight)

Food name Hemodialysis—1.0 g PRO/kg/day	Amount	PRO (g)	Kcal 70.0	Phos (mg) 2450	APRO (g)	Sod (mg)	Pot (mg)
Breakfast							
Coffee, regular or decaffeinated	8 ozv	0.1	3	1.184	0.0	3	64
Sugar, white	0.5 tbsp	0.0	23	0.0000	0.0	0	0
Cranberry juice cocktail	4 ozv	0.0	72	2.528	0.0	3	23
English muffin	1 avg	4.5	134	63.64	0.0	364	318
Jam/jelly, all flavors	2 tbsp	0.2	109	3.600	0.0	5	35
Lunch							
Lettuce, iceberg, raw	2 cup	1.1	14	22.00	0.0	10	174
Carrots, raw	1 med	0.7	31	31.68	0.0	25	233
Celery, raw	2 stalk	0.5	13	20.80	0.0	70	227
Broccoli, raw	0.25 cup	0.7	6	14.52	0.0	6	72
Cauliflower, raw	0.25 cup	0.5	6	11.50	0.0	4	89
Turkey, light meat	1 ozw	8.5	45	62.14	8.5	18	87
Ham, cured	0.5 ozw	3.0	34	30.33	3.0	168	40
Italian or French dressing	4 tbsp	0.4	272	2.920	0.0	460	8

		PRO	Kcal	Phos	APRO	Sod	Pot
Ritz cracker	8 each	1.7	124	59.00	0.0	243	19
Margarine, soft	1 tbsp	0.1	99	2.801	0.1	149	5
Candy corn	2 ozw	0.0	206	3.402	0.0	120	2
Apple juice or cider	4 ozv	0.1	59	8.680	0.0	4	148
Dinner							
Chicken breast, half	5 ozw	38.5	215	307.6	38.5	70	335
White rice	1 cup	3.4	182	80.52	0.0	6	86
Beans, green	1 cup	1.8	36	32.40	0.0	18	152
Summer squash	0.5 cup	0.8	18	35.10	0.0	1	173
Margarine, soft	2 tbsp	0.2	198	5.602	0.2	298	10
Pound cake	1 slice	1.9	121	30.59	1.2	53	23
Snacks							
Cheese crackers	10 each	0.8	43	19.71		149	8
Jelly beans, candy	2 ozw	0.0	208	2.268	0.0	6	0
Pear, raw w/skin	1 med	0.6	98	18.26	0.0	0	208
Fig bar cookie	2 avg	1.1	100	16.80	0.3	71	55
Total		71.2	2468	889.6	51.8	2322	2595
Percentage of goal		102%	101%				

PRO, protein; Kcal, kilocalories; Phos, phosphorus; APRO, animal protein; Sod, sodium; Pot, potassium; ozw, ounces by weight; tbsp, tablespoon; ozv, ounces by volume; ozw, ounces by weight; tbsp, tablespoon.
The CBORD Group, Inc, The Professional Diet Analyzer, version 1.0.7, Ithaca, NY.

Table 15-9. Menu for Patient Example 1, modified for peritoneal dialysis and based on 24-hour recall (weight, 70 kg; the prescription is 1.2 g protein/kg body weight and 30 kcal/kg body weight)

Food name Peritoneal Dialysis—1.2 g PRO/kg/day	Amount	PRO (g) 84.0	Kcal 2100	Phos (mg)	APRO (g)	Sod (mg)	Pot (mg)
Breakfast							
Coffee, regular or decaffeinated	4 ozv	0.1	3	1.184	0.0	3	64
Sugar, white	0.5 tbsp	0.0	23	0.0000	0.0	0	0
Cranberry juice cocktail	4 ozv	0.0	72	2.528	0.0	3	23
English muffin	1 avg	4.5	134	63.64	0.0	364	318
Jam/jelly, all flavors	2 tbsp	0.2	109	3.600	0.0	5	35
Lunch							
Lettuce, iceberg, raw	2 cup	1.1	14	22.00	0.0	10	174
Carrots, raw	1 med	0.7	31	31.68	0.0	25	233
Celery, raw	2 Stalk	0.5	13	20.80	0.0	70	227
Broccoli, raw	0.25 cup	0.7	6	14.52	0.0	6	72
Cauliflower, raw	0.25 cup	0.5	6	11.50	0.0	4	89
Turkey, light meat	2 ozw	17.0	90	124.3	17.0	36	174
Ham, cured	0.5 ozw	3.0	34	30.33	3.0	168	40

		PRO	Kcal	Phos	APRO	Sod	Pot
Egg, whole cooked	1 large	6.1	79	90.05	6.1	69	65
Italian or French dressing	4 tbsp	0.4	272	2.920	0.0	460	8
Ritz cracker	8 each	1.7	124	59.00	0.0	243	19
Margarine, soft	1 tbsp	0.1	99	2.801	0.1	149	5
Candy corn	2 ozw	0.0	206	3.402	0.0	120	2
Dinner							
Chicken breast	5 ozw	38.5	215	307.6	38.5	70	335
White rice	1 cup	3.4	182	80.52	0.0	6	86
Beans, green	1 cup	1.8	36	32.40	0.0	18	152
Summer squash	0.5 cup	0.8	18	35.10	0.0	1	173
Margarine, soft	1 tbsp	0.1	99	2.801	0.1	149	5
Pound cake	1 slice	1.9	121	30.59	1.2	53	23
Snacks							
Cheese crackers	10 each	0.8	43	19.71		149	8
Pear, raw w/skin	1 med	0.6	98	18.26	0.0	0	208
Total		84.6	2127	1011	66.0	2179	2539
Percentage of goal		101%	101%				

PRO, protein; Kcal, kilocalories; Phos, phosphorus; APRO, animal protein; Sod, sodium; Pot, potassium; ozv, ounces by volume; ozw, ounces by weight; tbsp, tablespoon.

The CBORD Group, Inc., The Professional Diet Analyzer, version 1.0.7, Ithaca, NY.

Table 15-10. 24-hour recall calculated using CBORD Professional Diet Analyzer for Patient Example 2 (weight, 55 kg)

Food name Usual week-day food Intake	Amount	PRO (g)	Kcal	Phos (mg)	APRO (g)	Sod (mg)	Pot (mg)
Breakfast							
Coffee, regular or decaffeinated	16 ozv	0.4	10	4.736	0.0	10	256
Cranberry/apricot/grape juice drink	4 ozv	0.2	78	6.120	0.0	2	75
Corn flakes, cereal	1 cup	1.6	88	9.564	0.0	243	22
Sugar, white	2 tbsp	0.0	92	0.0000	0.0	0	1
Nondairy creamer, liquid	4 ozv	1.2	162	77.04	0.0	96	228
Lunch							
Hamburger bun or roll	1 avg	3.2	120	34.00	tr	202	38
Chicken breast, half	2 ozw	15.4	86	123.0	15.4	28	134
Lettuce, iceberg, raw	2 leaf	0.4	5	8.000	0.0	4	63
Tomato, raw	2 slice	0.4	8	9.430	0.0	3	85
Mayonnaise	2 tbsp	0.4	198	7.728	0.0	156	10

Food	Measure	PRO	Kcal	Phos	APRO	Sod	Pot
Apples w/skin, raw	1 large	0.3	109	12.88	0.0	0	212
Caramel candy	1 ozw	1.2	114	34.57	tr	64	54
Fruit-flavored soda, carbonated beverage	12 ozw	0.0	179	11.16	0.0	53	38
Dinner							
White rice	0.5 cup	1.7	91	40.26	0.0	3	43
Asparagus, green	0.5 cup	2.8	26	52.26	0.0	4	208
Summer squash	0.5 cup	0.8	18	35.10	0.0	1	173
Soft roll	1 avg	2.2	83	23.61	0.1	141	27
Margarine, regular	1 tbsp	0.1	99	3.160	0.1	130	6
Tea, instant beverage w/sugar and lemon	8 ozv	0.3	88	2.590	0.0	24	49
Chocolate chip cookie	1 avg	0.4	34	8.323	0.1	29	10
Orange sherbet	0.5 cup	1.1	135	37.15	1.1	44	99
Snacks							
Jelly beans, candy	1 ozw	0.0	104	1.134	0.0	3	0
Total		34.1	1926	541.9	16.8	1240	1830
Percentage of goal							

PRO, protein; Kcal, kilocalories; Phos, phosphorus; APRO, animal protein; Sod, sodium; Pot, potassium; ozv, ounces by volume; ozw, ounces by weight; tbsp, tablespoon; tr, trace.
The CBORD Group, Inc., The Professional Diet Analyzer, version 1.0.7, Ithaca, NY.

Table 15-11. Menu for Patient Example 2, modified for reduced protein in moderate renal insufficiency and based on 24-hour recall (weight, 55 kg; the prescription is 0.6 g protein/kg body weight and 35 kcal/kg body weight)

Food name Renal Insufficiency—0.6 g PRO/kg/day	Amount	PRO (g) 33.0	Kcal 1925	Phos (mg)	APRO (g)	Sod (mg)	Pot (mg)
Breakfast							
Coffee, regular or decaffeinated	16 ozv	0.4	10	4.736	0.0	10	256
Cranberry/apricot/grape juice drink	4 ozv	0.2	78	6.120	0.0	2	75
Corn flakes, cereal	1 cup	1.6	88	9.564	0.0	243	22
Sugar, white	2 tbsp	0.0	92	0.0000	0.0	0	1
Nondairy creamer, liquid	4 ozv	1.2	162	77.04	0.0	96	228
Lunch							
Hamburger bun or roll	1 avg	3.2	120	34.00	tr	202	38
Chicken breast, half	2 ozw	15.4	86	123.0	15.4	28	134
Lettuce, iceberg, raw	2 leaf	0.4	5	8.000	0.0	4	63
Tomato, raw	2 slices	0.4	8	9.430	0.0	3	85
Mayonnaise	2 tbsp	0.4	198	7.728	0.0	156	10
Apples w/skin, raw	1 large	0.3	109	12.88	0.0	0	212

	Amount	PRO	Kcal	Phos	APRO	Sod	Pot
Caramel candy	1 ozw	1.2	114	34.57	tr	64	54
Fruit-flavored soda, carbonated beverage	12 ozv	0.0	179	11.16	0.0	53	38
Dinner							
White rice	0.5 cup	1.7	91	40.26	0.0	3	43
Asparagus, green	0.5 cup	2.8	26	52.26	0.0	4	208
Summer squash	0.5 cup	0.8	18	35.10	0.0	1	173
Soft roll	1 avg	2.2	83	23.61	0.1	141	27
Margarine, regular	1 tbsp	0.1	99	3.160	0.1	130	6
Tea, instant beverage w/sugar and lemon	8 ozv	0.3	88	2.590	0.0	24	49
Chocolate chip cookie	1 avg	0.4	34	8.323	0.1	29	10
Orange sherbet	0.5 cup	1.1	135	37.15	1.1	44	99
Snacks							
Jelly beans, candy	1 ozw	0.0	104	1.134	0.0	3	0
Total		34.1	1926	541.9	16.8	1240	1830
Percentage of goal		103%	100%				

PRO, protein; Kcal, kilocalories; Phos, phosphorus; APRO, animal protein; Sod, sodium; Pot, potassium; ozv, ounces by volume; ozw, ounces by weight; tbsp, tablespoon; tr, trace.
The CBORD Group, Inc., The Professional Diet Analyzer, version 1.0.7, Ithaca, NY.

Table 15-12. Menu for Patient Example 2, modified for hemodialysis and based on 24-hour recall (weight, 55 kg; the prescription is 1.0 g protein/kg body weight and 35 kcal/kg body weight)

Food name Hemodialysis—1.0 g PRO/kg/day	Amount	PRO (g) 55.0	Kcal 1925	Phos (mg)	APRO (g)	Sod (mg)	Pot (mg)
Breakfast							
Coffee, regular or decaffeinated	4 ozv	0.1	3	1.184	0.0	3	64
Plain or fruit muffin	1 avg	3.2	119	60.89	1.3	177	50
Margarine, soft	1 tbsp	0.1	99	2.801	0.1	149	5
Jam/jelly, all flavors	1 tbsp	0.1	55	1.800	0.0	3	18
Lunch							
Hamburger bun or roll	1 avg	3.2	120	34.00	tr	202	38
Chicken breast, half	3 ozw	23.1	129	184.6	23.1	42	201
Lettuce, iceberg, raw	2 leaf	0.4	5	8.000	0.0	4	63
Mayonnaise	2 tbsp	0.4	198	7.728	0.0	156	10

	Amount	PRO	Kcal	Phos	APRO	Sod	Pot
Apples w/skin, raw	1 large	0.3	109	12.88	0.0	0	212
Butterscotch candy	1 ozw	0.0	113	1.701	0.0	19	1
Dinner							
Beef pot roast	2 ozw	18.8	132	152.0	18.8	38	164
Corn cooked on cob	1 med	2.6	84	79.30	0.0	14	192
Beans, green	1 cup	1.8	36	32.40	0.0	18	152
Margarine, soft	1 tbsp	0.1	99	2.801	0.1	149	5
Chocolate chip cookie	2 avg	0.8	69	16.65	0.1	59	19
Applesauce	1 cup	0.5	194	17.85	0.0	7	155
Snacks							
Jelly beans, candy	2 ozw	0.0	208	2.268	0.0	6	0
Candy corn	2 ozw	0.0	206	3.402	0.0	120	2
Total		55.5	1977	622.2	43.5	1165	1351
Percentage of goal		101%	103%				

PRO, protein; Kcal, kilocalories; Phos, phosphorus; APRO, animal protein; Sod, sodium; Pot, potassium; ozv, ounces by volume; ozw, ounces by weight; tbsp, tablespoon; tr, trace.
The CBORD Group, Inc., The Professional Diet Analyzer, version 1.0.7, Ithaca, NY.

Table 15-13. Menu for Patient Example 2, modified for peritoneal dialysis and based on 24-hour recall (weight, 55 kg; the prescription is 1.2 g protein/kg body weight and 30 kcal/kg body weight)

Food name Peritoneal Dialysis—1.2 g PRO/kg/day	Amount	PRO (g) 55.0	Kcal 1650	Phos (mg)	APRO (g)	Sod (mg)	Pot (mg)
Breakfast							
Coffee, regular or decaffeinated	4 ozv	0.1	3	1.184	0.0	3	64
Plain or fruit muffin	1 avg	3.2	119	60.89	1.3	177	50
Margarine, soft	1 tbsp	0.1	99	2.801	0.1	149	5
Jam/jelly, all flavors	1 tbsp	0.1	55	1.800	0.0	3	18
Lunch							
Hamburger bun or roll	1 avg	3.2	120	34.00	tr	202	38
Chicken breast, half	3 ozw	23.1	129	184.6	23.1	42	201
Lettuce, iceberg, raw	2 leaf	0.4	5	8.000	0.0	4	63
Mayonnaise	1 tbsp	0.2	99	3.864	0.0	78	5
Apples w/skin, raw	1 large	0.3	109	12.88	0.0	0	212

		PRO	Kcal	Phos	APRO	Sod	Pot
Dinner							
Beef pot roast	3 ozw	28.2	198	227.9	28.2	57	246
Corn cooked on cob	1 med	2.6	84	79.30	0.0	14	192
Beans, green	0.5 cup	0.9	18	16.20	0.0	9	76
Soft roll	1 avg	2.2	83	23.61	0.1	141	27
Margarine, soft	2 tsp	0.1	66	1.867	0.1	99	3
Chocolate chip cookie	2 avg	0.8	69	16.65	0.1	59	19
Applesauce	1 cup	0.5	194	17.85	0.0	7	155
Snacks							
Jelly beans, candy	2 ozw	0.0	208	2.268	0.0	6	0
Total		66.0	1657	695.7	53.0	1050	1374
Percentage of goal		120%	100%				

PRO, protein; Kcal, kilocalories; Phos, phosphorus; APRO, animal protein; Sod, sodium; Pot, potassium; ozv, ounces by volume; ozw, ounces by weight; tbsp, tablespoon; tr, trace.
The CBORD Group, Inc., The Professional Diet Analyzer, version 1.0.7, Ithaca, NY.

the recall has been entered and calculated, it can be modified to meet the recommended prescription. Menus planned with the aid of a computer are fun, easy, and quick, and demonstrate to the patient what changes must be made in the usual diet to comply with the new diet prescription.

Another way to individualize menus is through a "what-if" type analysis, a process easy to do with a computer. For example, if a patient who is prescribed a protein-controlled diet has requested a fast-food burger with French fries for lunch, what choices would be appropriate for the rest of the day? A computer program such as the Professional Diet Analyzer can be used quickly to plan food choices and determine what would be appropriate without exceeding the protein prescription (Table 15-14).

Other features of the Professional Diet Analyzer include choosing the number and type of nutrient columns to be printed or viewed on the screen, entering additional food items, sorting foods in ascending or descending order for a specific nutrient, meal planning using an exchange list, creating food databases for specific patients, calculating and adding recipes, changing the font size of the printed menu, and calculating food diaries and food frequencies. An outstanding feature is the flexibility to select the source of the food and nutrient database. The MDRD Study used two databases, one created by the Department of Epidemiology and Biostatistics at Case Western Reserve University for the pilot study, and one compiled by the University of Pittsburgh Nutrition Coordinating Center, Graduate School of Public Health, for the full-scale clinical trial.

Computerized spreadsheets designed for menu planning do not have the advantage of a food database, but are relatively inexpensive. When computer programs such as the Professional Diet Analyzer and Nutritionist IV are not available, the computerized spreadsheet can be an effective alternative to planning the menus by hand. In addition, spreadsheets can quickly create menu patterns (Table 15-15) using exchange lists (Table 15-16) by entering formulas into the template for automatic calculations. Information about how to design and use spreadsheet applications for menu planning can be found in *Nutrition Counseling Skills*, edited by L. G. Snetselaar.

Exchange Lists

Exchange lists are one of the oldest methods used for teaching the renal diet. Foods are grouped according to similar nutritional value, and food choices within the same group can be exchanged or swapped with other foods within the same group. Based on the patient's usual food habits, the dietitian determines how many food choices from each exchange list can be used to meet the daily prescription. Menus can then be planned using the appropriate food choices throughout the day. Menus planned by exchange lists may not be as accurate as those planned when using the actual nutrient content of the food items, but the accuracy can be improved when portion sizes are measured or weighed rather than estimated.

The National Renal Diet, published by The American Dietetic Association, is a comprehensive educational tool based on exchange lists for patients with pre–end-stage renal disease and

Table 15-14. Menu using a "what-if" analysis for selecting a fast-food meal in a protein-controlled diet

Food name	Amount	PRO (g) 55.0	Kcal 1900	Phos (mg)	APRO (g)	Sod (mg)	Pot (mg)
Breakfast							
Bagel	20 g	2.2	59	13.40	0.0	72	15
Jam/jelly, all flavors	2 tbsp	0.2	109	3.600	0.0	5	35
Grape juice, canned or bottled	4 ozv	0.7	77	13.91	0.0	4	167
Lunch							
McDonald's quarter pounder	1 order	24.6	427		18.2	720	
McDonald's medium French fries	1 svg	4.4	320			150	
Cola carbonated beverage	12 ozv	0.0	152	44.20	0.0	15	3
Dinner							
Pork chop, loin	2 ozw	18.2	130	138.3	18.2	44	238
Corn cooked on cob	1 med	2.6	84	79.30	0.0	14	192
Beans, green	0.5 cup	0.9	18	16.20	0.0	9	76
Applesauce	1 cup	0.5	194	17.85	0.0	7	155
Margarine, soft	2 tsp	0.1	66	1.867	0.1	99	3
Tea, instant beverage w/sugar and lemon	8 ozv	0.3	88	2.590	0.0	24	49
Cookies, assorted packaged	2 avg	0.9	84	28.36	0.2	64	12
Snacks							
Candy corn	1 ozw	0.0	103	1.701	0.0	60	1
Total		55.6	1910	361.3	18.5	1288	947
Percentage of goal		101%	101%				

PRO, protein; Kcal, kilocalories; Phos, phosphorus; APRO, animal protein; Sod, sodium; Pot, potassium; ozv, ounces by volume; ozw, ounces by weight; tbsp, tablespoon; svg, serving.
The CBORD Group, Inc., The Professional Diet Analyzer, version 1.0.7, Ithaca, NY.

Table 15-15. Example of meal patterns using a spreadsheet template with amplified exchange lists **

Prescription: 55 g protein, 2000 calories

Food Group	Number Exchanges	Protein (g)	Sodium (mg)	Potassium (mEq)	Kilocalories
Meal Pattern 1					
Meat	5	35	125	12.5	325
Milk	1	4	80	5	120
Fruit	4	2	20	16	240
Vegetable	5	5	75	20	125
Starch	4	8	600	4	320
Fats	6	0	120	6	600
Other Foods*	3				300
Totals†		54	1020	63.5	2030
Meal Pattern 2					
Meat	7	49	175	17.5	455
Milk	0	0	0	0	0
Fruit	1	0.5	5	4	60
Vegetable	2	2	30	8	50
Starch	2	4	300	2	160
Fats	6	0	120	6	600
Other foods*	4				400
Totals†		55.5	630	37.5	1725

*100 calories estimated per serving for this example; the amount of sodium and potassium varies with this group.
†The total for sodium is a guide for the dietitian and is an estimate because the sodium values vary for different foods within each exchange group.
**Published by The Community Dialysis Center, P.O. Box 12220, East Cleveland, OH 44112.

Table 15-16. Example of simplified exchange list*

Food Group (1 serving)	Protein (g)	Sodium (mg)	Potassium (mEq)	Kilocalories
Meat	7	25	2.5	65
Milk	4	80	5	120
Fruit	0.5	5	4	60
Vegetable	1	15	4	25
Starch	2	150	1	80
Fats	0	20	1	100
Other foods	0	0	0	100

*Published by The Community Dialysis Center, P.O. Box 12220, East Cleveland, OH 44112

those on dialysis. The exchange lists are modified for patients with diabetes and have food choices that are high in sodium, potassium, and phosphorus content. In addition to exchange lists, the booklets include tips for dining out, selecting fast foods, planning holiday meals, and ethnic diet choices. Table 15-17 shows the average calculations for the diabetic and nondiabetic renal diets. Tables 15-18 through 15-23 are case examples from the *National Renal Diet: Professional Guide* for diet prescriptions, meal plans, and menus for patients with and without diabetes for renal insufficiency, hemodialysis, and peritoneal dialysis.

Handouts

When only one nutrient is modified, one-page handouts for foods that are allowed or not allowed can be very effective. Patients can look quickly over the list to determine which foods commonly eaten should be avoided and what foods to substitute.

Food Labels

Dietitians and patients can take advantage of the information on the labels of foods to learn more about their nutrient content as well as the amount of a specific nutrient in relation to portion size. Portion sizes are noted by measures as well as grams or ounces.

Reference Material

Food composition books including references for fast foods and convenience foods, cookbooks, and recipes can be used effectively to increase the knowledge and stimulate ideas. *Bowes and Church's Food Values of Portions Commonly Used* is found in most book stores and can supplement the information provided by the dietitian.

Graphs

Graphs can be very effective for education and monitoring. They draw attention to numeric data and show trends much better than a series of numbers. Figure 15-1 is an example of a line graph used to demonstrate the change in serum iron levels in relation to a patient's compliance with iron supplements. Bar

Table 15-17. Average calculation figures for nondiabetic and diabetic renal diets

Food Choices*	kcal	PRO (g)	CHO (g)	Fat (g)	Na (mg)	K (mg)	P (mg)
Nondiabetic							
Milk	120	4.0	12	6	80	185	110
Nondairy milk substitute	140	0.5	12	10	40	80	30
Meat	65	7.0	—	4	25	100	65
Starch	90	2.0	18	1	80	35	35
Vegetable							
Low potassium	25	1.0	5	Trace	15	70	20
Medium potassium	25	1.0	5	Trace	15	150	20
High potassium	25	1.0	5	Trace	15	270	20
Fruit							
Low potassium	70	0.5	17	—	Trace	70	15
Medium potassium	70	0.5	17	—	Trace	150	15
High potassium	70	0.5	17	—	Trace	270	15
Fat	45	—	—	5	55	10	5
High-calorie	100	Trace	25	—	15	20	5
Beverage	Varies	Varies	Varies	Varies	Varies	Varies	Varies
Salt	—	—	—	—	250	—	—

Diabetic

Milk	100	4.0	8	5	80	185	110
Nondairy milk substitute	140	0.5	12	10	40	80	30
Meat	65	7.0	—	4	25	100	65
Starch	80	2.0	15	1	80	35	35
Vegetable							
Low potassium	25	1.0	5	Trace	15	70	20
Medium potassium	25	1.0	5	Trace	15	150	20
High potassium	25	1.0	5	Trace	15	270	20
Fruit							
Low potassium	60	0.5	17	—	Trace	70	15
Medium potassium	60	0.5	17	—	Trace	150	15
High potassium	60	0.5	17	—	Trace	270	15
Fat	45	—	—	5	55	10	5
High-calorie	60	Trace	15	—	15	20	5
Beverage	Varies	Varies	Varies	Varies	Varies	Varies	Varies
Salt	—	—	—	—	250	—	—

*Serving sizes for each food choice are shown in the client booklets.

Table 15-18. Sample calculation of diet plan for patient with renal insufficiency secondary to hypertension

Food Choices*	kcal	PRO (g)	CHO (g)	Fat (g)	Na (mg)	K (mg)	P (mg)
Nondiabetic							
Milk	120	4.0	12	6	80	185	110
Nondairy milk substitute	140	0.5	12	10	40	80	30
Meat	65	7.0	—	4	25	100	65
Starch	90	2.0	18	1	80	35	35
Vegetable							
Low potassium	25	1.0	5	Trace	15	70	20
Medium potassium	25	1.0	5	Trace	15	150	20
High potassium	25	1.0	5	Trace	15	270	20
Fruit							
Low potassium	70	0.5	17	—	Trace	70	15
Medium potassium	70	0.5	17	—	Trace	150	15
High potassium	70	0.5	17	—	Trace	270	15
Fat	45	—	—	5	55	10	5
High-calorie	100	Trace	25	—	15	20	5
Beverage	Varies	Varies	Varies	Varies	Varies	Varies	Varies
Salt	—	—	—	—	250	—	—

Diabetic

Milk	100	4.0	8	5	80	185	110
Nondairy milk substitute	140	0.5	12	10	40	80	30
Meat	65	7.0	—	4	25	100	65
Starch	80	2.0	15	1	80	35	35
Vegetable							
Low potassium	25	1.0	5	Trace	15	70	20
Medium potassium	25	1.0	5	Trace	15	150	20
High potassium	25	1.0	5	Trace	15	270	20
Fruit							
Low potassium	60	0.5	17	—	Trace	70	15
Medium potassium	60	0.5	17	—	Trace	150	15
High potassium	60	0.5	17	—	Trace	270	15
Fat	45	—	—	5	55	10	5
High-calorie	60	Trace	15	—	15	20	5
Beverage	Varies	Varies	Varies	Varies	Varies	Varies	Varies
Salt	—	—	—	—	250	—	—

*Serving sizes for each food choice are shown in the client booklets.

continued

Table 15-18. *Continued.*

The patient is a 50-year-old woman with renal insufficiency secondary to hypertension. She is 60 in tall, weighs 142 lb (64.5 kg) with trace edema, and has a medium frame. Her ideal weight adjusted for obesity is 113.4 lb (51.6 kg). Her laboratory values are: blood urea nitrogen, 35 mg/dl; creatinine, 2.1 mg/dl; albumin, 3.9 g/dl; potassium, 3.7 mEq/l; sodium, 136 mEq/l; calcium, 9.5 mg/dl; phosphorus, 4.2 mg/dl. Her 24-hour urine output is 1900 ml. Currently, her blood pressure is under fair control.

Nutrient	Level	Rationale
Calories	1800	35 kcal/kg IBW
Protein	31 g	0.6 g/kg IBW
Sodium	2000 mg	Urine output normal, trace edema, blood pressure under fair control
Potassium	No restriction	Urine output adequate, serum potassium within normal range
Phosphorus	410–620 mg	8–12 mg/kg IBW

Sample diet calculation

Food Choices	No. of Choices	kcal	Pro (g)	Na (mg)	P (mg)
Goals		1800	31	2000	≤620
Nondairy milk substitute	1	140	0.05	40	30
Meat	3	195	21.0	75	195
Starch	4	360	8.0	320	140
Vegetable	1	25	1.0	15	20
Fruit	3	210	1.5	Trace	45
Fat	8	360	—	440	40
High-calorie	5	500	—	75	25
Salt	4	—	—	1000	—
Totals		1790	32	1965	495

Sample menu

Breakfast	Choices
¾ cup cornflakes	1 Starch + 1 Salt
½ cup nondairy creamer	1 Nondairy milk substitute
½ banana	1 Fruit
1 slice toast	1 Starch
1 tsp margarine	1 Fat
1 tbsp jam	½ High-calorie
1 tbsp sugar	½ High-calorie

Lunch	Choices
Sandwich	
1 oz deli-style ham	1 Meat + 1 Salt
2 slices low-protein bread, toasted	2 High-calorie
1 tbsp mayonnaise	3 Fat
½ oz dill pickle	1 Salt
⅛ small cantaloupe	1 Fruit
1 cup lemonade	1 High-calorie

Dinner	Choices
2 oz broiled steak	2 Meat
2½ tsp steak sauce	1 Salt
1 small baked potato	1 Starch
½ cup glazed carrots	1 Vegetable
1 small French roll	1 Starch
4 tsp margarine	4 Fat
1 fresh pear	1 Fruit
Iced tea with lemon and 2 tbsp sugar	1 High-calorie

IBW, ideal body weight; CHO, carbohydrate; Pro, protein.

Table 15-19. Sample calculation of diet plan for patient with renal insufficiency secondary to diabetes

The patient is a 50-year-old woman with renal insufficiency secondary to diabetes mellitus. She is 60 in tall, weighs 142 lb (64.5 kg), and has a medium frame. Her ideal weight adjusted for obesity is 113.4 lb (51.6 kg). Her laboratory values are: blood urea nitrogen, 35 mg/dl; creatinine, 2.1 mg/dl; albumin, 3.9 g/dl; potassium, 4.3 mEq/l; sodium, 140 mEq/l; calcium, 9.4 mg/dl; phosphorus, 3.6 mg/dl. Her 24-hour urine output is 2100 ml. The 24-hour urinary protein measurement reveals an excretion of 1.5 g. She has a history of edema and congestive heart failure.

Nutrient	Level	Rationale
Calories	1800	35 kcal/kg IBW
Protein	41 g	0.8 g/kg IBW
Sodium	2000 mg	Urine output normal, history of edema and congestive heart failure, blood pressure controlled
Potassium	No restriction	Urine output adequate, serum potassium within normal limits
Phosphorus	410–620 mg	8–12 mg/kg IBW

Sample diet calculation

Food Choices	No. of Choices	kcal	CHO (g)	Pro (g)	Fat (mg)	Na (mg)	P (mg)
Goals		1800		41		2000	≤620
Nondairy milk substitute	1	140	12	0.05	10	40	30
Meat	4	260	—	28.0	16	100	260
Starch	4	320	60	8.0	4	320	140
Vegetable	3	75	15	3.0	—	45	60
Fruit	4	240	60	2.0	—	—	60
Fat	8	360	—	—	40	440	40
High-calorie	6	360	90	—	—	90	30

					750	
Salt	—	—	—	—	1785	—
Totals	1755	237	41.5	70		620

3

Sample menu

Breakfast	Choices
3/4 cup cornflakes	1 Starch + 1 Salt
1/2 cup nondairy creamer	1 Nondairy milk substitute
1/2 banana	1 Fruit
1 slice toast	1 Starch
1 egg, soft-cooked	1 Meat
2 tsp margarine	2 Fat
Coffee with sugar substitute	

Lunch	Choices
Sandwich	
1 oz roast beef	1 Meat
1 tsp mayonnaise	1 Fat
2 slices low-protein bread, toasted	4 High-calorie
1/8 small cantaloupe	1 Fruit
1 cup lettuce with 1 medium tomato	2 Vegetable
1 tbsp Italian salad dressing	1 Fat
Diet ginger ale	

Dinner	Choices
2 oz broiled steak	2 Meat
2 tbsp barbecue sauce	1 Salt
2/3 cup low-protein pasta	2 High-calorie
1/2 cup carrots	1 Vegetable
4 tsp margarine	4 Fat
1 fresh pear	1 Fruit
Coffee with sugar substitute	

Snacks	Choices
3/4 oz pretzels	1 Starch + 1 Salt
Diet lemon-lime soda	
3 graham cracker squares	1 Starch
1 medium apple	1 Fruit
Iced tea with lemon	

IBW, ideal body weight; CHO, carbohydrate; Pro, protein.

Table 15-20. Sample calculation of diet plan for patient on hemodialysis

The patient is a 55-year-old man who works full time in an office and has a sedentary lifestyle. He is 5 ft, 10 in tall, has a medium frame, and weighs 76 kg. His ideal and usual weight is 68 kg. For the past 6 to 9 months, he has been anorectic and has experienced intermittent nausea and vomiting. His appetite is improving but is not at its previous level. He is on hemodialysis for 4 hours, three times a week. His predialysis laboratory values include: blood urea nitrogen, 63 mg/dl; sodium, 135 mEq/l; potassium, 4.0 mEq/l; phosphorus, 6.2 mg/dl; calcium, 9.0 mg/dl; albumin, 3.3 g/dl. His urine output ranges between 800 and 1000 ml.

Nutrient	Level	Rationale
Calories	3000	40 kcal/kg IBW; anorexia, nausea, and vomiting
Protein	91 g	1.2 g/kg IBW
Sodium	2000 mg	Limited to decrease thirst, control fluid weight gains
Potassium	3000 mg (75 mEq)	~40 mg/kg IBW
Phosphorus	1300 mg	≤17 mg/kg IBW
Fluid	1500–1750 ml	750 ml + urine output or 1000 ml if anuric

Sample diet calculation

Food Choices	No. of Choices	kcal	Pro (g)	Na (mg)	K (mg)	P (mg)
Goals		3000	91	2000	3000	1300
Milk	1	120	4.0	80	185	110
Nondairy milk substitute	1	140	0.5	40	80	30
Meat	9	585	63.0	225	900	585
Starch	10	900	20.0	800	350	350
Vegetable	2	50	2.0	30	—	40
Low potassium	(1)	—	—	—	150	—
Medium potassium	(1)	—	—	—	270	—
High potassium						
Fruit	3	210	1.5	—	—	45
Low potassium	(1)	—	—	—	150	—
Medium potassium	(2)	—	—	—	540	—
High potassium						
Fat	10	450	—	550	100	50
High-calorie	5	500	—	75	100	25
Salt	1	—	—	250	—	—
Totals		2955	91.0	2050	2825	1235

continued

Table 15-20. *Continued.*

Sample menu Breakfast	Choices	Lunch	Choices
2 slices French toast (1 egg + 1/4 cup nondairy creamer)	2 Starch 1 Meat, 1/2 Nondairy milk substitute	Sandwich 2 oz sliced turkey	2 Meat
1 tbsp margarine	3 Fat	1 tbsp mayonnaise	3 Fat
2 tbsp syrup	1 High-calorie	Lettuce	
1/4 honeydew melon	2 high-potassium Fruit	2 slices light rye bread	2 Starch
1 cup cranberry juice cocktail	1 High-calorie	1 small raw carrot	1 medium-potassium Vegetable
		4 sugar cookies	1 Starch
		1 cup lemonade	1 High-calorie

Dinner	Choices	Snacks	Choices
6 oz broiled steak	6 Meat	1 pouch chewy fruit snacks	1 High-calorie
1 cup herbed rice	2 Starch	1 cup lemon-lime soda	1 High-calorie
4 tsp margarine	4 Fat	Cinnamon raisin bagel	2 Starch
1/2 cup Brussels sprouts	1 high-potassium Vegetable	3 tbsp cream cheese	1 Milk
1 slice angel food cake	1 Starch	1/8 tsp salt used during day	1 Salt
1/2 cup strawberries	1 medium-potassium Fruit		
1/4 cup nondairy frozen dessert topping	1/2 Nondairy milk substitute		

IBW, ideal body weight; Pro, protein.

Table 15-21. Sample calculation of diet plan for patient on hemodialysis with diabetes

The patient is a 32-year-old woman with insulin-dependent diabetes mellitus and a history of nephrotic syndrome. She is married and has an 8-year-old child. She does not work outside the home and has felt so tired this past year that she has had difficulty keeping up with housework. She is 5 ft, 5 in tall, has a small frame (IBW, 51 kg), and weighs 48 kg. She is on hemodialysis for 3 hours, three times a week. Her predialysis laboratory values include: blood urea nitrogen, 43 mg/dl; sodium, 133 mEq/l; potassium, 3.9 mEq/l; glucose, 350 mg/dl; phosphorus, 5.8 mg/dl; calcium, 9.2 mg/dl; albumin, 2.7 g/dl. Her appetite is only fair, and she occasionally vomits after eating. She has almost no urine output.

Nutrient	Level	Rationale
Calories	1800	35 kcal/kg IBW
Protein	66 g	1.3 g/kg IBW because low serum albumin level indicates protein depletion
Sodium	2000 mg	No urine output; some increased thirst that may be secondary to high blood sugar level
Potassium	2000 mg (51 mEq)	~40 mg/kg IBW
Phosphorus	870 mg	≤17 mg/kg IBW
Fluid	100 ml	No urine output

continued

Table 15-21. *Continued.*

Sample diet calculation

Food Choices	No. of Choices	kcal	CHO (g)	Pro (g)	Fat (g)	Na (mg)	K (mg)	P (mg)
Goals		1800		66		2000	2000	870
Milk	0	—	—	—	—	—	—	—
Nondairy milk substitute	1	140	12	0.5	10	40	80	30
Meat	7	455	—	49.0	28	175	700	455
Starch	7	560	105	14.0	7	560	245	245
Vegetable								
Low potassium	—	—	—	—	—	—	—	—
Medium potassium	(1)	25	5	1.0	—	15	150	20
High potassium	—	—	—	—	—	—	—	—
Fruit								
Low potassium	5	300	75	2.5	—	—	140	75
Medium potassium	(2)	—	—	—	—	—	300	—
High potassium	(2)	—	—	—	—	—	270	—
Fat	7	315	—	—	35	385	70	35
Salt	3	—	—	—	—	750	—	—
Totals		1795	197	67	80	1925	1955	860

Sample menu

Breakfast	Choices
3/4 cup cornflakes	1 Starch + 1 Salt
1/2 cup nondairy creamer	1 Nondairy milk substitute
1/2 cup blueberries	1 low-potassium Fruit
1/2 bagel	1 Starch
1 tsp margarine	1 Fat

Lunch	Choices
Sandwich	
2 oz unsalted tuna	2 Meat
1 tbsp mayonnaise	3 Fat
Lettuce	
2 slices white bread	2 Starch
1 cup low-calorie cranberry juice cocktail	1 low-potassium Fruit

Dinner	Choices
4 oz broiled chicken	4 Meat
2 tbsp barbecue sauce	1 Salt
1/2 cup herbed rice	1 Starch
2 tsp margarine	2 Fat
1/2 cup broccoli	1 medium-potassium Vegetable
1 slice angel food cake (1/20 cake)	1 Starch
1/2 cup strawberries	1 medium-potassium Fruit

Snacks	Choices
2 tbsp raisins	1 medium-potassium Fruit
Small orange	1 high-potassium Fruit
1/4 cup cottage cheese	1 Meat
3 oblong pieces Melba toast	1 Starch
1 tsp margarine	1 Fat
1/8 tsp salt used in cooking	1 Salt

Table 15-22. Sample calculation of diet plan for patient on continuous ambulatory peritoneal dialysis (CAPD)

The patient is a 55-year-old man who works full time as a salesman. He is 5 ft, 8 in tall, has a medium frame, and weighs 70 kg. His laboratory values are: blood urea nitrogen, 60 mg/dl; creatinine, 10.4 mg/dl; sodium, 140 mEq/l; potassium, 4.5 mEq/l; calcium, 9.5 mg/dl; phosphorus, 5.0 mg/dl; albumin, 3.8 g/dl. His CAPD regimen is two exchanges of 1.5% dextrose, one exchange of 2.5% dextrose, and one exchange of 4.25% dextrose. Exchanges are 2 l each. The dialysate supplies approximately 400 kcal/d.

Nutrient	Level	Rationale
Calories	2100	30 kcal/kg IBW including contribution of dextrose from dialysate
Protein	84 g	1.2 g/kg IBW
Sodium	2000–3000 mg	To maintain normal blood pressure and fluid balance
Potassium	No restriction	Serum potassium levels are within normal limits
Phosphorus	1190 mg	≤17 mg/kg IBW

Sample diet calculation

Food Choices	No. of Choices	kcal	Pro (g)	Na (mg)	P (mg)
Goals		2100	84	2000–3000	1190
Milk	1	120	4	80	110
Meat	9	585	63	225	585
Starch	7	630	14	560	245
Vegetable	2	50	2	30	40
Fruit	2	140	1	Trace	30
Fat	4	180	0	220	20
Salt	6	—	—	150	—
Totals		1705	84	2615	1030
Dialysate kcal		400			
Total kcal		2105			

Sample menu

Breakfast	Choices
1/8 cantaloupe	1 Fruit
3/4 cup cornflakes	1 Starch + 1 Salt
1 slice raisin toast	1 Starch
1 tsp margarine	1 Fat
1/2 cup milk	1 Milk
Coffee	

Lunch	Choices
Sandwich	
3 oz sliced deli turkey	3 Meat + 3 Salt
2 slices white bread	2 Starch
1 tbsp low-calorie mayonnaise	1 Fat
Sliced tomato	1 Vegetable
Iced tea with lemon	

Dinner	Choices
6 oz dilled baked fish	6 Meat
1/2 cup mashed potato	1 Starch
1/2 cup carrots	1 Vegetable
1 small dinner roll	1 Starch
1 tsp margarine	1 Fat
Ginger ale, sugar-free	

Snacks	Choices
1 slice toast	1 Starch
1 tsp margarine	1 Fat
1/2 cup pineapple	1 Fruit
1/2 tsp salt used in cooking	2 Salt

IBW, ideal body weight; Pro, protein.

Table 15-23. Sample calculation of diet plan for patient on continuous ambulatory peritoneal dialysis (CAPD) with diabetes

The patient is a 50-year-old woman with glucose intolerance. She is 5 ft tall and weighs 55 kg. Her ideal weight is 52 kg. Her laboratory values are: blood urea nitrogen, 55 mg/dl; creatinine, 8.5 mg/dl; sodium, 4.4 mEq/l; potassium, 140 mEq/l; calcium, 9.2 mg/dl; phosphorus, 4.7 mg/dl; albumin, 3.6 g/dl. Her CAPD regimen of 4 l of 1.5% dextrose and 4 l of 2.5% dextrose provides approximately 265 kcal/d.

Nutrient	Level	Rationale
Calories	1550	30 kcal/kg IBW including contribution of dextrose from dialysate
Protein	62 g	1.2 g/kg IBW
Sodium	2000 mg	To maintain normal blood pressure and fluid balance
Potassium	Unrestricted	Serum potassium in normal range
Phosphorus	885 mg	≤17 mg/kg IBW

Sample diet calculation

Food Choices	No. of Choices	kcal	CHO (g)	Pro (g)	Fat (g)	Na (mg)	P (mg)
Goals		1550		62		2000	885
Nondairy milk substitute	1	140	12	0.5	10	40	30
Meat	7	455	—	49.0	28	175	455
Starch	6	480	90	12.0	6	480	210
Vegetable	2	50	10	2.0	—	30	40
Fruit	2	120	30	1.0	—	—	30
Fat	1	45	—	—	5	55	5
Salt	4	—	—	—	—	1000	—

Totals	1290	142	64.5	49	1780	770
Dialysate calories	265					
Total calories	1555					

Sample menu

Breakfast	Choices
¾ cup cornflakes	1 Starch + 1 Salt
½ banana	1 Fruit
1 slice raisin toast	1 Starch
1 tsp margarine	1 Fat
½ cup nondairy creamer	1 Nondairy milk substitute
Coffee	

Lunch	Choices
Sandwich	2 Meat + 2 Salt
2 oz ham	2 Starch
2 slices bread	1 Vegetable
Lettuce, sliced tomato	
Ginger ale, sugar-free	

Dinner	Choices
4 oz dilled baked fish	4 Meat
½ cup mashed potato	1 Starch
½ cup carrots	1 Vegetable
Iced tea with lemon	
⅛ tsp salt used in cooking	1 Salt

Snacks	Choices
1 medium apple	1 Fruit
½ sandwich	
1 slice bread	1 Starch
1 oz sliced chicken	1 Meat
Fat-free mayonnaise	
Orange soda, sugar-free	

IBW, ideal body weight; CHO, carbohydrate; Pro, protein.

graphs are easy to understand and can be used creatively for comparing, for example, the protein content of popular fast foods (see Fig. 15-1). Graphs can help the patient focus on the interventions that need priority attention as well as those that have been successful.

Supportive Relationship

From the start, establishing a stable, supportive, effective, and enjoyable relationship with the patient is important. Clinic visits that are regular, timely, and conducted in a private and pleasant setting enhance the quality of the nutrition intervention.

Computerized Approach

Computers are now common in health care settings as well as in the homes of patients. With new, easy-to-use software available, dietitians can use computers for menu planning and computer-assisted nutritional counseling. Computer-assisted counseling should include spreadsheets to plan menus, to enter and calculate 24-hour recalls, to generate graphs to show changes over time and to demonstrate comparisons, and to create menus using exchange lists. Nutrition-related software such as the Professional Diet Analyzer by CBORD and Nutritionist IV are user-friendly and can be used with the patient. Being creative with computer applications facilitates compliance and promotes time efficiency for both the patient and dietitian.

A Renal Nutrition Expert

A dietitian with expertise in renal nutrition, including knowledge about food and nutrients, food combinations, nutritional assessment, renal disease and treatment, and methods for effective education and evaluation, is essential for a successful intervention. By utilizing research results in the clini-

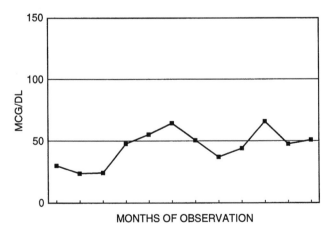

Fig. 15-1. Serum iron—40-year-old man.

cal setting and using the computer to enhance creativity and time efficiency, individualized nutritional intervention programs can be designed to facilitate compliance.

BARRIERS TO SUCCESSFUL NUTRITION INTERVENTION

When dietary compliance is poor, look for barriers that might interfere. Once recognized, the barriers can be discussed with the patient and steps taken to reduce the impact of the barriers. Common barriers in the renal disease population include:

1. *Poor appetite and anorexia.* These are common causes of decreased food intake. Helping the patient focus on foods that taste good improves food intake. Oral nutritional supplements can be used to boost calories and protein and do not require food preparation.
2. *Food costs.* The cost of high-quality protein foods, such as beef, fresh pork, and poultry, can be excessive for some dialysis patients or after renal transplantation. Plan lower-cost menus and discuss ways to lower the cost of the grocery bill without compromising nutrient intake.
3. *Inadequate understanding of the diet.* A lack of understanding of the purpose of the dietary modifications and inadequate instructions to achieve the modifications are common barriers. Make it clear what foods to eat and which foods to avoid. Simplify and individualize menus and meal plans.
4. *Lack of motivation to follow the diet.* No matter how simple the diet, without appropriate motivation, dietary compliance will be difficult. Provide simple guidelines and suggestions that focus on what each patient likes to eat. Make as few changes as possible. Increase the frequency of follow-up and contact with the dietitian.
5. *Lack of family and social support.* Family and other forms of social support are important to the educational process. Involving friends and family in counseling sessions often has a positive influence on compliance.
6. *Hospitalizations and extended illnesses.* Hospitalizations and extended periods of illness can cause nutritional depletion even in well-nourished people with renal disease and cause a nutritional setback in those who are already at nutritional risk. Follow up by phone, letter, or an office visit shortly after the period of illness to reinforce the importance of adequate nutrition. Recommend simple and easy-to-prepare foods to boost calories and protein.

SELECTED READINGS

The American Dietetic Association. *A clinical guide to nutrition care in end-stage renal disease.* 2nd ed. Chicago: The American Dietetic Association; 1997.

The American Dietetic Association. *National renal diets.* Chicago: The American Dietetic Association; 1993.

Blagg CR. Importance of nutrition in dialysis patients. *Am J Kidney Dis* 1991;17:458–461.

Blumenkrantz MJ, Kopple JD, Gutman RA, et al. Methods for assessing nutritional status of patients with chronic renal failure. *Am J Clin Nutr* 1980;33:1567–1585.

Cianciaruso B, Capuano A, D'Amaro E, et al. Dietary compliance to low protein and phosphate diet in patients with chronic renal failure. *Kidney Int* 1989;27(Suppl):173–176.

Coyne T, Olson M, Bradham K, et al, for Modification of Diet in Renal Disease Study Group. Dietary satisfaction correlated with adherence in the modification of diet in renal disease study. *J Am Diet Assoc* 1995;95:1301–1306.

Feste C. *The physician within.* 2nd ed. Minneapolis, MN: Chronimed Publishing; 1993.

Gillis BP, Caggiula AW, Chiavacci AT, et al, for the Modification of Diet in Renal Disease Group. Nutrition intervention program of the modification of diet in renal disease study: a self-managed approach. *J Am Diet Assoc* 1995;95:1288–1294.

Hamwi G. Changing dietary concepts. In: Danowski TS, ed. Diabetes mellitus: diagnosis and treatment. New York: American Diabetes Association.

Insull W. Dietitians as intervention specialists: a continuing challenge for the 1990s. *J Am Diet Assoc* 1992;92:551.

Klahr S, Levey AS, Beck GJ, et al. The effects of dietary protein restriction and blood pressure control on the progression of chronic renal disease. *N Engl J Med* 1994;330:877–884.

Levey AS, Adler S, Caggiula AW, et al, for the Modification of Diet in Renal Disease Study Group. Effects of dietary protein restriction on the progression of advanced renal disease in the Modification of Diet in Renal Disease (MDRD) Study. *Am J Kidney Dis* 1996;27: 652–663.

Lowrie EG, Lew NL. Death risk in hemodialysis patients: the predictive value of commonly measured variables and evaluation of death rate differences between facilities. *Am J Kidney Dis* 1990; 15:458–482.

Maroni BJ, Steinman TI, Mitch WE. A method for estimating nitrogen intake of patients with chronic renal failure. *Kidney Int* 1985; 27:58–65.

Maschio G, Oldrizzi L, Tessitori N, et al. Effects of dietary protein and phosphorus restriction on the progression of early renal failure. *Kidney Int* 1992;22:371–376.

Modification of Diet in Renal Disease Nutrition Coordinating Center. *Protein wise kit.* Pittsburgh, PA: University of Pittsburgh; 1990.

Modification of Diet in Renal Disease Study Group, prepared by Levey AS, Adler S, Caggiula AW, et al. Effects of dietary protein restriction on the progression of moderate renal disease in the Modification of Diet in Renal Disease Study. *J Am Soc Nephrol* 1996;7:2616–2626.

Milas NC, Nowalk MP, Akpele L, et al, for the Modification of Diet in Renal Disease Study. Factors associated with adherence to the dietary protein intervention in the modification of diet in renal disease study. *J Am Diet Assoc* 1995;95:1295–1300.

Miller RW, St. Jour ST, Hershey MS. Compliance with renal diets: a review and analysis. *Dial Transplant* 1980;9:968.

Mitch WE, May RC, Maroni BJ, et al. Protein and amino acid metabolism in uremia: influence of metabolic acidosis. *Kidney Int* 1989; 27(Suppl):205–207.

National Research Council. *Recommended dietary allowances.* 10th ed. Washington, D.C.: National Academy Press; 1989.

Nelson EE, Hong CD, Pesce AL, et al. Anthropometric norms for the dialysis population. *Am J Kidney Dis* 1990;16:32–37.

Pennington JAT. *Bowes and Church's food values of portions commonly used*. 16th ed. Philadelphia: JB Lippincott; 1994.

Powers SN. Computerized spreadsheets to plan and assess menus for therapeutic diets. *Clin Nutr* 1987;6:192–197.

Powers SN., Stumbo PJ, Computer assisted nutrition counseling. In: Snetselaar LG, ed. *Nutrition counseling skills: assessment, treatment, and evaluation*. Rockville, MD: Aspen Publications; 1989: 123–149.

Schoenfield PY, Henry RR, Laird NM, et al. Assessment of nutritional status of the National Cooperative Dialysis Study population. *Kidney Int* 1983;23:S80–S88.

Thompson JK, Dwyer JT. Computer applications in out-patient nutrition services: fostering the computer connection. *Clin Nutr* 1987;6:185–191.

Underwood BA. Evaluating the nutritional status of individuals: a critique of approaches. *Nutr Rev* 1986;44:213.

United States Department of Agriculture. *Composition of foods*. Handbook 8. Washington, D.C.: Government Printing Office; 1976–1989.

United States Department of Agriculture. *Nutritive value of American foods in common units*. Handbook 456. Washington, D.C.: Government Printing Office; 1975.

Wilkens KG, Schiro KB, eds. *Suggested guidelines for nutrition care of renal patients*. 2nd ed. Chicago: American Dietetic Association; 1992.

Wolfson M. Use of nutritional supplements in dialysis patients. *Semin Dial* 1992;5:85.

Yamamoto ME, Averback FM, Caggiula AW, et al. The production of quality dietary data: a collaborative effort of the modification of diet in renal disease study. *Journal of Renal Nutrition* 1992;2: 117–125.

Subject Index